Advances in Diffusion-weighted Imaging

Editor

KEI YAMADA

MAGNETIC RESONANCE IMAGING CLINICS OF NORTH AMERICA

www.mri.theclinics.com

Consulting Editors
SURESH K. MUKHERJI
LYNNE S. STEINBACH

May 2021 • Volume 29 • Number 2

ELSEVIER

1600 John F. Kennedy Boulevard • Suite 1800 • Philadelphia, Pennsylvania, 19103-2899

http://www.mri.theclinics.com

MRI CLINICS OF NORTH AMERICA Volume 29, Number 2
May 2021 ISSN 1064-9689, ISBN 13: 978-0-323-75996-0

Editor: John Vassallo (j.vassallo@elsevier.com)
Developmental Editor: Arlene Campos

Magnetic Resonance Imaging Clinics of North America (ISSN 1064-9689) is published quarterly by Elsevier Inc., 360 Park Avenue South, New York, NY 10010-1710. Months of issue are February, May, August, and November. Business and Editorial Offices: 1600 John F. Kennedy Blvd., Ste. 1800, Philadelphia, PA 19103-2899. Customer Service Office: 3251 Riverport Lane, Maryland Heights, MO 63043. Periodicals postage paid at New York, NY and additional mailing offices. Subscription prices are $404.00 per year (domestic individuals), $1037.00 per year (domestic institutions), $100.00 per year (domestic students/residents), $450.00 per year (Canadian individuals), $1063.00 per year (Canadian institutions), $567.00 per year (international individuals), $1063.00 per year (international institutions), $100.00 per year (Canadian students/residents), and $275.00 per year (international students/residents). International air speed delivery is included in all *Clinics* subscription prices. All prices are subject to change without notice. **POSTMASTER:** Send address changes to *Magnetic Resonance Imaging Clinics*, Elsevier Health Sciences Division, Subscription Customer Service, 3251 Riverport Lane, Maryland Heights, MO 63043. Customer Service (orders, claims, online, change of address): Elsevier Health Sciences Division, Subscription **Customer Service, 3251 Riverport Lane, Maryland Heights, MO 63043. Tel:1-800-654-2452 (U.S. and Canada); 314-447-8871 (outside U.S. and Canada). Fax: 314-447-8029. E-mail: journalscustomerservice-usa@elsevier.com (for print support); journalsonlinesupport-usa@elsevier.com (for online support).**

Reprints. For copies of 100 or more of articles in this publication, please contact the Commercial Reprints Department, Elsevier Inc., 360 Park Avenue South, New York, NY 10010-1710. Tel.: 212-633-3874; Fax: 212-633-3820; E-mail: reprints@elsevier.com.

Magnetic Resonance Imaging Clinics of North America is covered in the *RSNA Index of Imaging Literature, MEDLINE/PubMed (Index Medicus),* and *EMBASE/Excerpta Medica*.

Contributors

CONSULTING EDITORS

SURESH K. MUKHERJI, MD, MBA, FACR
Clinical Professor, Marian University, Director of Head and Neck Radiology, ProScan Imaging, Regional Medical Director, Envision Physician Services, Carmel, Indiana, USA

LYNNE S. STEINBACH, MD, FACR
Emeritus Professor of Radiology on Full Recall, Department of Radiology and Biomedical Imaging, University of California, San Francisco, San Francisco, California, USA

EDITOR

KEI YAMADA, MD, PhD
Professor and Chairman, Department of Radiology, Kyoto Prefectural University of Medicine, Kyoto, Japan

AUTHORS

FELIX BOUCHER, MD
Fellow, Neuroradiology Division, Radiology, Michigan Medicine, Ann Arbor, USA

CHENG-YU CHEN, MD
Department of Medical Imaging, Translational Imaging Research Center, Taipei Medical University Hospital, Department of Radiology, School of Medicine, College of Medicine, Taipei Medical University, Taipei, Taiwan

SHO-JEN CHENG, MD
Department of Medical Imaging, Taipei Medical University Hospital, Taipei, Taiwan

HSIAO-WEN CHUNG, PhD
Graduate Institute of Biomedical Electronics and Bioinformatics, National Taiwan University, Department of Electrical Engineering, National Taiwan University, Taipei, Taiwan

CHRISTIAN FEDERAU, MD, MSc
University and ETH Zürich, Institute for Biomedical Engineering, Zürich, Switzerland; Ai Medical AG, Zollikon, Switzerland

KHADER M. HASAN, PhD
Professor of Diagnostic and Interventional Imaging, Department of Diagnostic and Interventional Radiology, The University of Texas Health Science Center at Houston, McGovern Medical School, Houston, Texas, USA

MASAAKI HORI, MD, PhD
Professor and Chairperson, Department of Radiology, Toho University Omori Medical Center, Tokyo, Japan

KOUHEI KAMIYA, MD, PhD
Lecturer, Department of Radiology, Toho University Omori Medical Center, Tokyo, Japan

YUN-TING LEE, MS
Translational Imaging Research Center, Taipei Medical University Hospital, Taipei, Taiwan

YI-TIEN LI, PhD
Translational Imaging Research Center, Taipei Medical University Hospital, Taipei, Taiwan

ERIC LIAO, MD
Assistant Professor, Neuroradiology Division, Radiology, Michigan Medicine, Ann Arbor, USA

STEVEN P. MEYERS, MD, PhD, FACR
Professor of Radiology/Imaging Sciences, Neurosurgery and Otolaryngology, University of Rochester Medical Center, University Medical Imaging, Rochester, New York, USA

KATSUTOSHI MURATA, MSc
MR Research & Collaboration, Collaboration Manager, Siemens Healthcare Japan KK, Tokyo, Japan

SHIGEO MURAYMA, MD, PhD
Brain Bank for Aging Research, Tokyo Metropolitan Geriatric Hospital and Institute of Gerontology, Itabashi-ku, Tokyo, Japan; Brain Bank for Neurodevelopmental, Neurological and Psychiatric Disorders, United Graduate School of Child Development, Osaka University, Osaka-fu, Japan

JEFFREY J. NEIL, MD, PhD
Departments of Neurology, Pediatrics, and Radiology, Washington University School of Medicine, St Louis, Missouri, USA

YUKO SAITO, MD, PhD
Brain Bank for Aging Research, Tokyo Metropolitan Geriatric Hospital and Institute of Gerontology, Itabashi-ku, Tokyo, Japan

KOJI SAKAI, PhD
Clinical AI Research Laboratory, Department of Radiology, Kyoto Prefectural University of Medicine, Kyoto, Japan

CHRISTOPHER D. SMYSER, MD, MSCI
Departments of Neurology, Pediatrics, and Radiology, Washington University School of Medicine, St Louis, Missouri, USA

GIANVINCENZO SPARACIA, MD
Neuroradiologist, Department of Diagnostic and Therapeutic Services, IRCCS-ISMETT, Palermo, Italy

ASHOK SRINIVASAN, MD
Professor and Division Director, Neuroradiology Division, Radiology, Michigan Medicine, Ann Arbor, USA

TOSHIAKI TAOKA, MD, PhD
Professor, Department of Innovative Biomedical Visualization (iBMV), Department of Radiology, Nagoya University Graduate School of Medicine, Nagoya, Aichi, Japan

AYA MIDORI TOKUMARU, MD, PhD
Department of Diagnostic Radiology, Tokyo Metropolitan Geriatric Hospital and Institute of Gerontology, Itabashi-ku, Tokyo, Japan

PING-HUEI TSAI, PhD
Department of Medical Imaging and Radiological Sciences, Chung-Shan Medical University, Taichung, Taiwan

KEI YAMADA, MD, PhD
Professor and Chairman, Department of Radiology, Kyoto Prefectural University of Medicine, Kyoto, Japan

Contents

MAGNETIC RESONANCE IMAGING CLINICS OF NORTH AMERICA

FORTHCOMING ISSUES

August 2021
MR Imaging of Chronic Liver Diseases and Liver Cancer
Khaled M. Elsayes and Claude B. Sirlin, *Editors*

November 2021
Pediatric Neuroimaging: State-of-the-Art
Mai-Lan Ho, *Editor*

February 2022
MR Imaging of Head and Neck Cancer
Ahmed Abdel Khalek Abdel Razek, *Editor*

RECENT ISSUES

February 2021
7 Tesla MRI
Meng Law, *Editor*

November 2020
MR Safety
Robert E. Watson, *Editor*

August 2020
Advanced MR Techniques for Imaging the Abdomen and Pelvis
Sudhakar K. Venkatesh, *Editor*

PROGRAM OBJECTIVE

The goal of *Magnetic Resonance Imaging Clinics of North America* is to keep practicing physicians up to date with current clinical practice by providing timely articles reviewing the state of the art in patient care.

TARGET AUDIENCE

All practicing physicians and healthcare professionals who provide patient care utilizing findings from Magnetic Resonance Imaging.

LEARNING OBJECTIVES

Upon completion of this activity, participants will be able to:

1. Review research/clinical topics related to diffusion imaging.
2. Discuss varying perspectives on CNS/head and neck pathologies.
3. Recognize new developments in the field of neuroimaging.

ACCREDITATION

The Elsevier Office of Continuing Medical Education (EOCME) is accredited by the Accreditation Council for Continuing Medical Education (ACCME) to provide continuing medical education for physicians.

The EOCME designates this journal-based CME activity enduring material for a maximum of 10 *AMA PRA Category 1 Credit(s)*™. Physicians should claim only the credit commensurate with the extent of their participation in the activity.

All other healthcare professionals requesting continuing education credit for this enduring material will be issued a certificate of participation.

DISCLOSURE OF CONFLICTS OF INTEREST

The EOCME assesses conflict of interest with its instructors, faculty, planners, and other individuals who are in a position to control the content of CME activities. All relevant conflicts of interest that are identified are thoroughly vetted by EOCME for fair balance, scientific objectivity, and patient care recommendations. EOCME is committed to providing its learners with CME activities that promote improvements or quality in healthcare and not a specific proprietary business or a commercial interest.

The planning committee, staff, authors and editors listed below have identified no financial relationships or relationships to products or devices they or their spouse/life partner have with commercial interest related to the content of this CME activity:

Felix Boucher, MD; Regina Chavous-Gibson, MSN, RN; Cheng-Yu Chen, MD; Sho-Jen Cheng, MD; Hsiao-Wen Chung, PhD; Christian Federau, MD, MSc; Khader M. Hasan, PhD; Masaaki Hori, MD, PhD; Kouhei Kamiya, MD, PhD; Yun-Ting Lee, MS; Yi-Tien Li, PhD; Eric Liao, MD; Steven P. Meyers, MD, PhD, FACR; Shigeo Murayma, MD, PhD; Jeffrey J. Neil, MD, PhD; Yuko Saito, MD, PhD; Koji Sakai, PhD; Christopher D. Smyser, MD, MSCI; Gianvincenzo Sparacia, MD; Ashok Srinivasan, MD; Pradeep Kuttysankaran; Toshiaki Taoka, MD, PhD; Aya Midori Tokumaru, MD, PhD; Ping-Huei Tsai, PhD; John Vassallo; Kei Yamada, MD, PhD

The planning committee, staff, authors and editors listed below have identified financial relationships or relationships to products or devices they or their spouse/life partner have with commercial interest related to the content of this CME activity:

Katsutoshi Murata, MSc: employed by Siemens Healthcare Japan KK

UNAPPROVED/OFF-LABEL USE DISCLOSURE

The EOCME requires CME faculty to disclose to the participants:

1. When products or procedures being discussed are off-label, unlabelled, experimental, and/or investigational (not US Food and Drug Administration [FDA] approved); and
2. Any limitations on the information presented, such as data that are preliminary or that represent ongoing research, interim analyses, and/or unsupported opinions. Faculty may discuss information about pharmaceutical agents that is outside of FDA-approved labelling. This information is intended solely for CME and is not intended to promote off-label use of these medications. If you have any questions, contact the medical affairs department of the manufacturer for the most recent prescribing information.

TO ENROLL

To enroll in the *Magnetic Resonance Imaging Clinics of North America* Continuing Medical Education program, call customer service at 1-800-654-2452 or sign up online at http://www.theclinics.com/home/cme. The CME program is available to subscribers for an additional annual fee of USD 281.00.

METHOD OF PARTICIPATION

In order to claim credit, participants must complete the following:

1. Complete enrolment as indicated above.
2. Read the activity.

3. Complete the CME Test and Evaluation. Participants must achieve a score of 70% on the test. All CME Tests and Evaluations must be completed online.

CME INQUIRIES/SPECIAL NEEDS

For all CME inquiries or special needs, please contact elsevierCME@elsevier.com.

Foreword

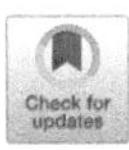

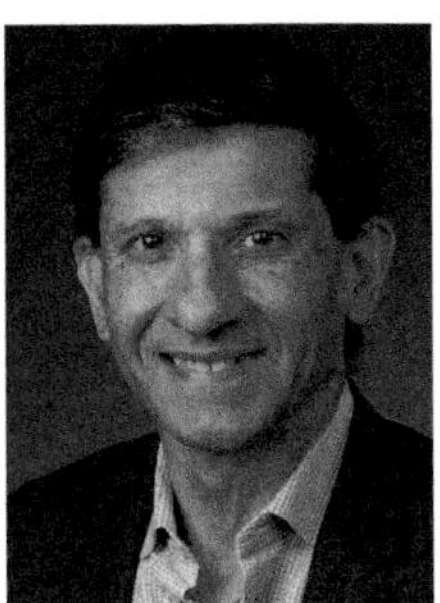

Suresh K. Mukherji, MD, MBA, FACR
Consulting Editor

This issue of *Magnetic Resonance Imaging Clinics of North America* is focused on diffusion-weighted imaging (DWI). There are articles devoted to the basics of DWI and various clinical applications, which include DWI assessment of the spinal cord, intracranial pathologic conditions, and numerous other disease sites. There is also a specific article devoted to imaging of infants.

I would also like to personally thank all the chapter authors for their superb contributions. All the contributors are recognized experts and leaders in the field. This excellent issue would not be possible without their efforts, and all of us at *Magnetic Resonance Imaging Clinics of North America* greatly appreciate their efforts.

I want to especially thank Dr Kei Yamada for accepting our invitation to guest edit this wonderful issue. DWI is a very important technique, whose "time has come," and I thank Dr Yamada for sharing his knowledge, insights, and experience with our global readership. Thank you, Kei!

Suresh K. Mukherji, MD, MBA, FACR
Clinical Professor, Marian University
Director of Head & Neck Radiology
ProScan Imaging
Regional Medical Director
Envision Physician Services
Carmel, Indiana, USA

E-mail address:
sureshmukherji@hotmail.com

Magn Reson Imaging Clin N Am 29 (2021) xi
https://doi.org/10.1016/j.mric.2021.03.002

Preface

Advances in Diffusion-Weighted Imaging

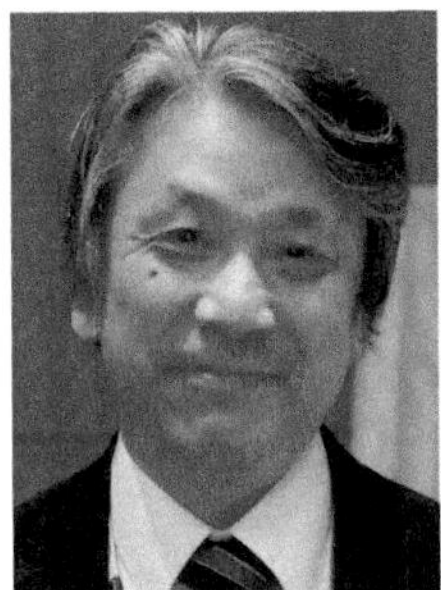

Kei Yamada, MD, PhD
Editor

My career as a radiologist started in the early 1990s when only the very basic MR imaging techniques were available. They included the spin-echo sequence, without any adjectives such as fast-, 3D-, or turbo. MR examinations were lengthy and pastoral back then. I was, however, busy enough catching up with the very basic MR physics and therefore had no complaints about this simplicity. A few years of neuroradiology training passed by, and I then quickly became aware of the rise of a new tool, that is, echo-planar imaging (EPI). This ultrafast imaging technique became available on clinical scanners in the late 1990s, which coincides with the time when I started participating in MR research.

Clinical application of EPI has led to 3 new methods for evaluating the central nervous system (CNS): functional MR imaging, perfusion-weighted imaging, and diffusion-weighted imaging (DWI). Of all these, DWI is currently one of the most widely used techniques, owing to its short acquisition time and robustness in elucidating pathologic conditions. It is now part of our daily practice and indeed an indispensable part of study protocols. Further evolution of this technique has led to visualization of anisotropic diffusion in the white matter using diffusion-tensor imaging. It has also evolved to enable perfusion estimation using intravoxel incoherent motion.

For this month's issue of *Magnetic Resonance Imaging Clinics of North America*, I had the privilege of gathering together some of the new developments in this field as a guest editor. I was blessed with the opportunity to become acquainted with a few of the outstanding, world-renowned researchers from the global village (the world is much smaller now even amid the pandemic). These leaders in this field kindly agreed to write about the cutting-edge research/ clinical topics related to diffusion imaging. This issue not only covers the research aspects of the technique but also elaborates on the CNS/head and neck pathologic conditions from multiple perspectives. I would like to extend my deepest gratitude to all these contributors for their diligent efforts. I hope that reading this issue of *Magnetic Resonance Imaging Clinics of North America*is enjoyable and educational.

Kei Yamada, MD, PhD
Department of Radiology
Kyoto Prefectural University of Medicine
465 Kajii-cho
Kamigyo-ku
Kyoto 6028566, Japan

E-mail address:
kyamada@koto.kpu-m.ac.jp

Magn Reson Imaging Clin N Am 29 (2021) xiii
https://doi.org/10.1016/j.mric.2021.03.001

Technical Basics of Diffusion-Weighted Imaging

Masaaki Hori, MD, PhD[a,*], Kouhei Kamiya, MD, PhD[a], Katsutoshi Murata, MSc[b]

KEYWORDS

• Diffusion • Time-dependent • Diffusion time

KEY POINTS

- Diffusion-weighted images provide a unique contrast that shows the ability to assess tissue structure and condition on a micrometer scale.
- Although the Einstein–Smoluchowski equation shows the relation between the mean square displacement and diffusion coefficient, it is not appropriate for simulating the actual diffusion-weighted MR signal.
- One of the emerging fields of diffusion MR imaging is to probe the tissue microstructure by altering the diffusion time t, the time interval over which spin displacements are sampled.

For diffusion-weighted images, MR imaging is performed to measure the displacement of water molecules on various scales and provide a way to display this information as quantitative maps and images. Unlike other MR imaging methods, diffusion-weighted images can be used to assess the structure and condition of tissues on a micrometer scale. The principle of this method was proposed in 1965,[1] but it was not applied to clinical practice until the 1980s.[2,3]

The physical principles underlying diffusion-weighted imaging (DWI) can be understood mathematically through the following equations.

The first equations of note are Fick's laws, which govern mass transport under some general assumptions. Fick's first law is written as follows:

$$N(x,t) = -D\frac{\partial c}{\partial x},$$

where x is the linear displacement, t is time, N is the net number of particles passing a given x coordinate at time t, D is the diffusion coefficient (an experimental constant dependent on the solvent, solute, pressure, and temperature), and c is the local volumetric concentration of particles at position x and time t. This formula simply indicates that the diffusion flux is proportional to the concentration gradient.

From this equation, the following equation, called Fick's second law, can be derived:

$$\frac{\partial c}{\partial t} = D\frac{\partial^2 c}{\partial x^2}$$

This equation governs how the local concentration of diffusing particles changes with time.

Various methods for estimating the diffusion coefficient D exist, but one of the particular interests is the Stokes–Einstein equation, which is valid for flows with low Reynolds numbers, a condition that is typical in biological systems. The equation reads

$$D = \frac{kT}{6\pi\eta r},$$

where k is the Boltzmann constant, T is the absolute temperature, η is the viscosity, and r is the radius of the particles.

[a] Department of Radiology, Toho University Omori Medical Center, 6-11-1 Omorinishi, Ota-ku, Tokyo 143-8541, Japan; [b] MR Research & Collaboration, Siemens Healthcare Japan KK, Gate City Osaki West Tower, 11-1 Osaki 1-Chome, Shinagawa-ku, Tokyo 141-8644, Japan

* Corresponding author.
E-mail address: masahori@med.toho-u.ac.jp

Magn Reson Imaging Clin N Am 29 (2021) 129–136
https://doi.org/10.1016/j.mric.2021.01.001
1064-9689/21/

The authors do not provide a detailed explanation of these expressions in this article, as detailed explanations have already been given in previously published texts. Note also that these equations are necessary for the theoretic understanding of diffusion MR imaging but not for pragmatic applications of imaging in clinical practice. The structure of various tissues and cells usually results in restricted diffusion, and the ideal conditions assumed by theory may not be attainable.

Consider the following example. Although the Einstein-Smoluchowski equation can be used, together with the theory of Brownian motion, to derive a relation between the mean square displacement of diffusing particles and the diffusion coefficient, use of the diffusion coefficient obtained by substituting the mean square displacement into Fick's laws to simulate a diffusion-weighted MR signal is not suitable. Callaghan simulated MR signals from molecules restricted in 1- (1D), 2- (2D), and 3-dimensional solid spheres (1D and 2D solid spheres are line segments and disks, respectively) by using a propagator derived from the diffusion equation. The propagator is a solution of the diffusion equation with given boundary conditions in the case where the nonhomogeneous term is Dirac delta function. It is a function of the diffusion time, t, and the position at times 0 and t and written as follows:

$$P_s(\mathbf{r}|\mathbf{r}', t)$$

where r and r' are the positions at $t = 0$ and t, respectively.

The propagator is the conditional probability density that a molecule existing at r at $t = 0$ exists at r' at $t = t$. In other words, the propagator shows how a one-point source is spatially distributed after diffusion time t. **Fig. 1** shows a time-developing one-dimensional propagator restricted in the range ± 10 μm, that is, to a line segment of 20 μm in length. The left, middle, and right columns show the cases of $r = 0$, 5, and 10 μm at $t = 0$, respectively. The boundary condition is $\frac{\partial P_s}{dr} = 0$, which corresponds to the molecule being perfectly repulsed by barriers at $r = -a$ and a. In other words, the molecule is not absorbed at the barriers. One can infer from these figures that the point source at $t = 0$ spreads while being influenced by the boundary. Callaghan simulated the MR signal $S(q,t)$ using a propagator, assuming a pulsed-gradient spin echo (PGSE) with a pulse width of $\delta \rightarrow 0$and a diffusion time of t, as follows[4]:

$$S(q,t) = \iint \rho(r,0) P_s(r|r',t) exp[i2\pi q \cdot (r' - r)] dr dr'$$

Here, q is the q-vector, $\gamma/2\pi \cdot g$, g is the diffusion gradient vector, and $\rho(r,0)$ is the distribution at $t = 0$. The exponent in the exponential function is the phase difference caused by the diffusion gradient at $t = 0$ and t specified by the q-vector. Therefore, this integral shows the expected value of transversal magnetization with phase dispersion based on the probability density $P_s(r|r',t)$, which is the net MR signal from the system.

Fig. 2 shows the MR signal of a 1D restricted diffusion system based on Callaghan's analysis. The transversal axis shows the b-value, and the longitudinal axis shows the logarithm of the MR signal. The figure also shows the MR signal calculated from the well-known equation for diffusion-weighted signals when the diffusion coefficient is obtained from the Einstein-Smoluchowski equation as follows:

$$S \propto exp(-bD) = exp\left(-b\frac{\langle(\mathbf{r}' - \mathbf{r})^2\rangle}{2t}\right)$$

The expected value of the mean squared displacement can be calculated using the propagator as follows:

$$\langle(r' - r)^2\rangle = \iint \rho(r,0) P_s(r|r',t)(r' - r)^2 dr dr'$$

When the diffusion coefficient is held constant, the MR signal monotonically decreases as the b-value increases. On the other hand, the MR signal calculated by Callaghan's method tends to increase at higher b-values after decreasing once with certain conditions, as shown in this figure. Bar-Shir and colleagues[5] obtained similar results in experiments using thin glass tubes. The observed tendency is caused by phase dispersion in limited space. The local minima of the MR signal occur when the product of the system size and q is integral, and the phase diverges effectively the most (**Fig. 3**). When the diffusion coefficient is fixed, this observation is not predicted. The important point here is that the diffusion phenomena can be observed only through MR measurements.

A DWI shows the distance traveled by a water molecule within a voxel and its average direction of motion. It does not reveal the full trajectory of the water molecule's movement but rather the result (the position at the time of measurement). Although it is an average per voxel, it has information of a structure (several μm) much smaller than the size of the voxel being measured (the smallest is several hundred μm), which leads to the estimation of the microstructure in the tissue. This aspect is unique to DWI and is a significant difference between diffusion-weighted images and T2- or T1-

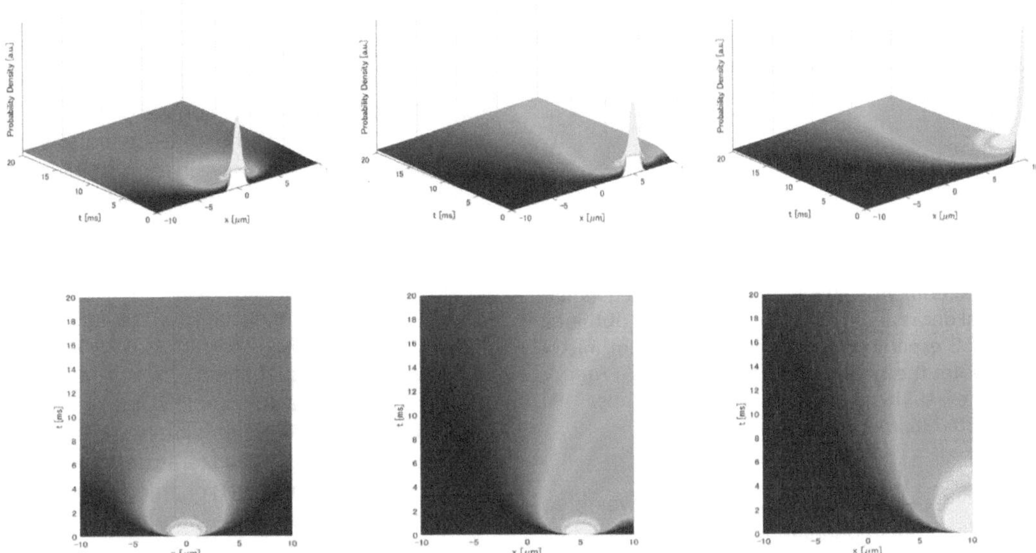

Fig. 1. Dynamic 1D-restricted diffusion. In this simulation, D = 3.0 × 10^{-3} $mm^2\ s^{-1}$, $\pm a$ = 10 μm, and t = 0 to 20 ms are assumed. From the left to right column, cases r = 0, 5, and 10 μm at t = 0 are shown.

weighted images. In routine images, no information with a size of less than a voxel exists, and the signal value shown by the north cell is the average of that of all the structures in the voxel.

More importantly, clinicians should be aware of the following issues when imaging, analyzing, and interpreting DWI, regardless how advanced the imaging technique used is.

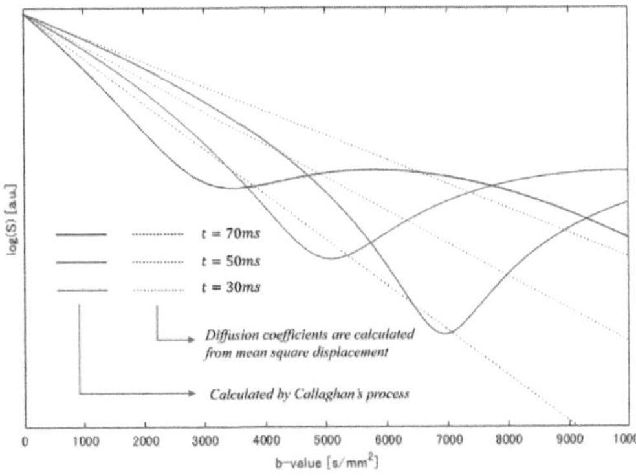

Fig. 2. b-value dependency of a 1D-restricted diffusion MR signal. In this simulation, D = 3.0 × 10^{-3} $mm^2\ s^{-1}$, $\pm a$ = 10 μm, and t = 0 to 20 ms are assumed. Solid lines show the simulation by Callaghan's method with a diffusion time t = 30 (*blue*), 50 (*magenta*), and 70 (*red*) ms. Dotted lines show the simulations by well-known equations for diffusion-weighted signals with the diffusion coefficient obtained from the Einstein-Smoluchowski equation (see text) and the same color coding. The simulation results calculated by Callaghan's method tend to increase at higher b-values after decreasing once.

First, the b-value is important in varying the contrast and quantitative values of DWI. However, the same b-value does not necessarily produce the same contrast and quantitative values. This problem is inherent to the definition of the b-value itself and not a result of the differences between vendors and scanners in different versions.

The definition of the b-value with the PGSE technique, which is widely used in clinical settings, is expressed as follows:

$$b = \gamma^2 G^2 \delta^2 \left(\Delta - \frac{\delta}{3}\right)$$

where γ is the gyromagnetic ratio, G is the amplitude of the gradients, δ is the time of the applied gradients, and Δ is the duration between paired gradients. G is determined by the hardware of each MR imaging scanner. Therefore, different diffusion times can be used to achieve the same b-value (**Fig. 4**). The importance of the diffusion time in MR images is described in detail in a later section.

Second, the quantitative values obtained from the diffusion-weighted image and its analysis are derived from the apparent signal values of the diffusion-weighted image. Therefore, the effect of the contrast due to each image acquisition method, especially relaxation, of the original images (ie, b = 0 images) cannot be completely eliminated. This is demonstrated, for example, by echo

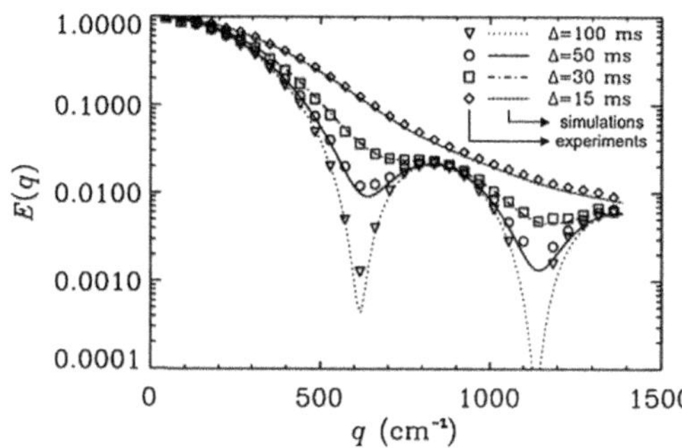

Fig. 3. Experimental (*symbols*) and simulated (*lines*) MR signal decay as a function of the q values obtained from PGSE experiments performed on 20 μm microtubes. Note: the system in the paper is 2D. (*From* A. Bar-Shir et al. Journal of Magnetic Resonance 194 (2008) 230–236, reprinted with permission.)

time (TE) dependence of DWI. Diffusion-weighted images and their quantitative values imaged at different TEs can be different from its original ones. Clinically, this is problematic, especially in the differential diagnosis of pathologic lesions, and very few clinicians are aware of it.

In many reports, especially clinical ones, diffusion times are less commonly referenced. However, the diffusion time is more important than the *b*-value when interpreting DWI and their quantitative metrics.

One of the emerging methods of diffusion MR imaging (dMRI) is used to probe the tissue microstructure by altering the diffusion time *t*, the time interval over which spin displacements are sampled. Although the diffusion coefficient, in general, depends on *t* except in the case of free diffusion (characterized by the absence of any barriers, with a Gaussian distribution) and *t*-dependence has long been a topic in dMRI biophysics,[6,7] only very recently was *t*-dependence confirmed in humans *in vivo* using clinical scanners. As *t* increases, *D* approaches its long-time limit D_∞. For sufficiently large *t*, *D* is almost constant, and the distribution becomes Gaussian. For this large *t*, each compartment can be regarded, in terms of the dMRI experiment, as equivalent to a completely uniform medium with a diffusion coefficient D_∞, all microstructural features being averaged. For a multicompartment system, multiexponential behavior is observed. In other words, the dependence on *t* is a signature of the microscopic features (such as cell size and packing density) that are not already averaged and therefore are quantifiable using dMRI.[8] **Figs. 5** and **6** illustrate $D(t)$ for simple 2D geometries obtained from a Monte-Carlo simulation of random walkers, as outlined in the literature.[9]

Along the *t* axis, at least 3 characteristic regimes have been described in the literature,[8,10] depending on the relationship between the characteristic length scale of the tissue microstructure and the diffusion length $\sqrt{D_0 t}$, that is, the typical distance traveled by a water molecule with free diffusivity D_0 during the diffusion time *t*.

1. Within a very small *t*, only a small portion of particles can reach a barrier; the other particles do not experience the effects of the barrier. Thus, the relevant parameter is the surface-to-volume ratio of the barriers (**Fig. 7**).[7] For biological tissues, meeting this short time limit with a clinical scanner is practically impossible. To date, this short-time regime has been probed mainly in preclinical studies using animal models of tumors that have relatively large cell sizes.[11]
2. At the other extreme, when *t* is sufficiently large, the Gaussian distribution becomes an effective

MPG pulses for DWI

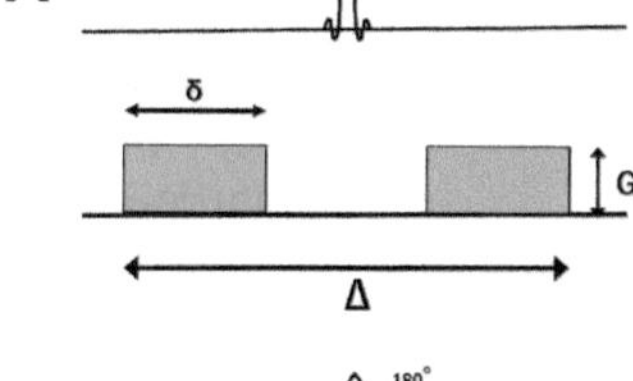

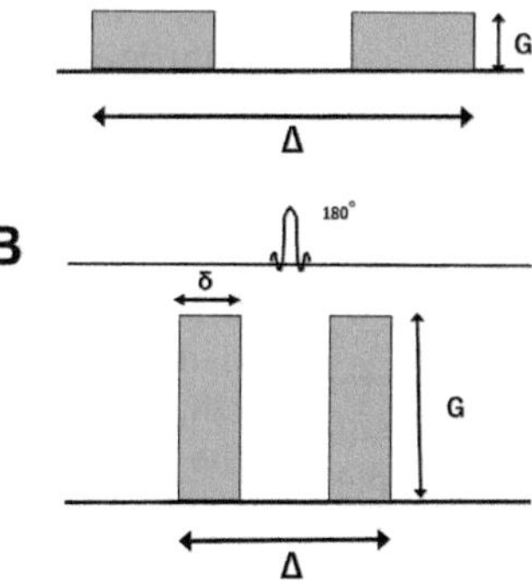

Fig. 4. Different diffusion times for the same b-values. Weak G requires a long diffusion time (*A*) to achieve the same *b*-values compared with a strong gradient MR scanner (*B*).

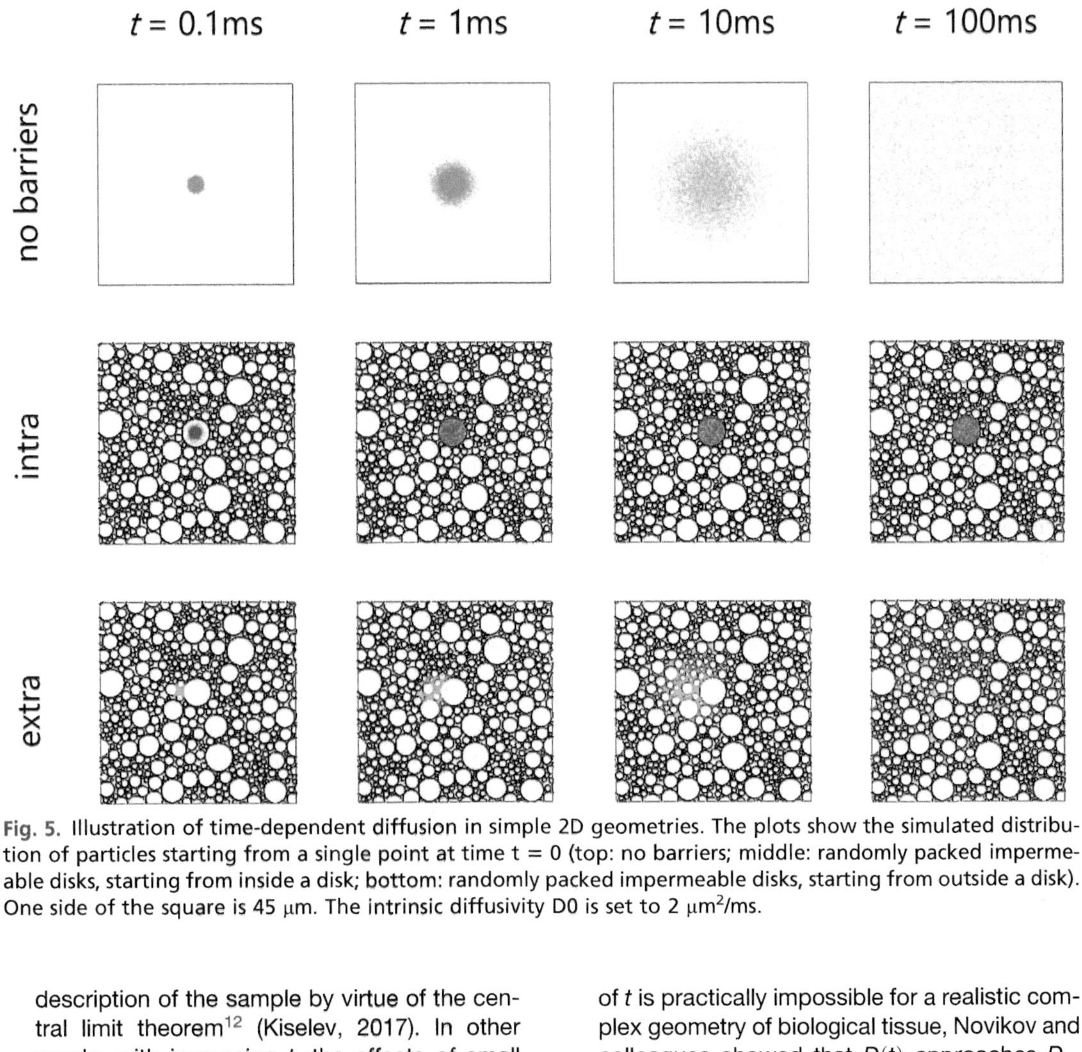

Fig. 5. Illustration of time-dependent diffusion in simple 2D geometries. The plots show the simulated distribution of particles starting from a single point at time t = 0 (top: no barriers; middle: randomly packed impermeable disks, starting from inside a disk; bottom: randomly packed impermeable disks, starting from outside a disk). One side of the square is 45 μm. The intrinsic diffusivity D0 is set to 2 μm²/ms.

description of the sample by virtue of the central limit theorem[12] (Kiselev, 2017). In other words, with increasing t, the effects of small local environments are "gradually forgotten."[8]

3. Between these extremes, $D(t)$ shows time-dependent behavior specific to the tissue microstructure. Although finding the exact analytical form of $D(t)$ applicable to all ranges of t is practically impossible for a realistic complex geometry of biological tissue, Novikov and colleagues showed that $D(t)$ approaches D_∞ according to a power law:

$$D(t) \simeq D_\infty + const \cdot t^{-\theta}, \tag{1}$$

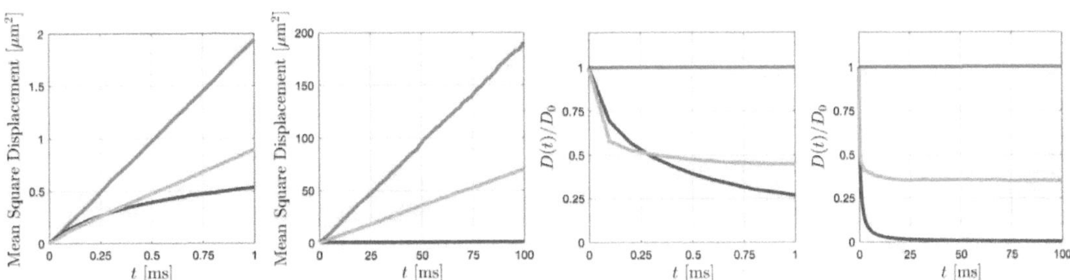

Fig. 6. Mean square displacement and diffusion coefficient of the same configuration as in Fig. 5 (*blue*: no barriers, *red*: inside disks, *yellow*: outside disks). The ensemble average over the voxel (initialized with a uniform distribution at $t = 0$) is shown.

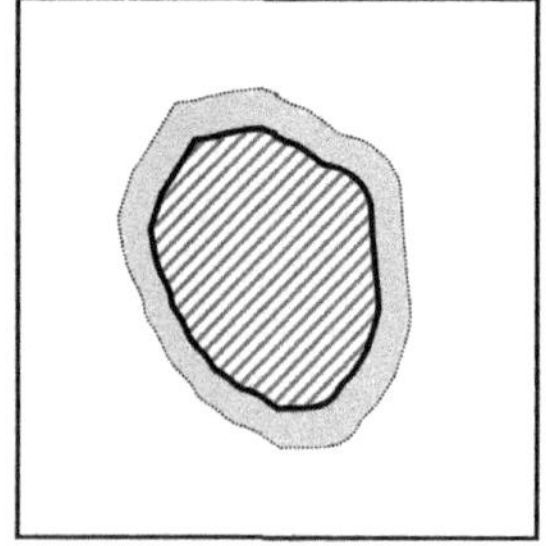

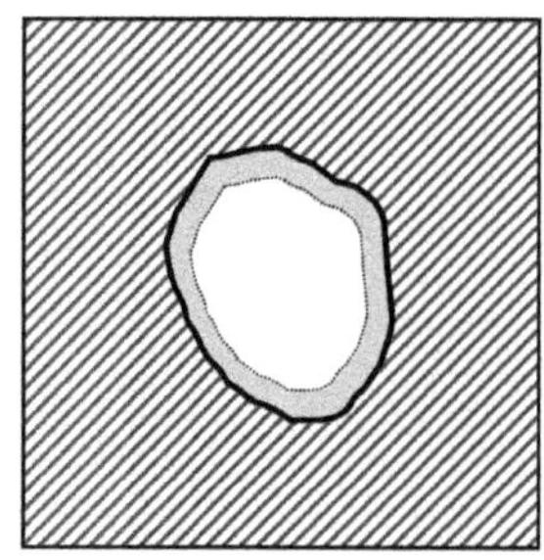

Fig. 7. Mitra's short-t limit. The same consideration applies to diffusion either inside (*right*) or outside (*left*) the cells, regardless of the pore shape. With very short t, only a small portion of particles (in the *gray-shaded area*) are affected by a barrier; the other particles (*white area*) do not experience any effect of the barrier (free diffusion). The fraction of the shaded area is proportional to the surface-to-volume ratio (height × surface/volume = $\sqrt{(D\_0\ t)} \times S/V$).

with the exponent $\theta = \frac{p+d}{2}$, where d is the number of dimensions and p is a structural exponent that takes discrete values defining mesoscopic structural disorder classes. For example, in the case of a one-dimensional short-range disorder (wherein barriers have finite correlation lengths), which is ubiquitous in nature, θ equals ½. This characteristic behavior has been confirmed for the axial diffusivity in the human brain[13,14] and correlated with the caliber variation along the axons (varicosities or beading).[15] Although the interpretation of $D(t)$ in terms of pathology remains to be established, the sensitivity to axon caliber variation should motivate investigations in future clinical studies because axonal beading is an early feature of neuronal degeneration.[16,17] Note that the $D(t)$ obtained by the usual PGSE obeys Eq[1] only for $\theta<1$. For $\theta \geq 1$, the $t^{-\theta}$ term is masked by the $\frac{1}{t}$ term.[18]

Reports of time-dependent diffusion imaging in humans with clinical scanners are rapidly increasing, both in neuronal[13,14,19] and nonneuronal[20–22] tissues. The recognition of t-dependence is critical not only for researchers but also for clinicians because it suggests that we can potentially improve the sensitivity and specificity of diagnostic imaging by controlling t so that the contrast between lesioned and healthy tissue or between different diseases is maximized.

Perhaps the most compelling example of the clinical implications of t-dependence is exhibited by acute infarction (Fig. 8), where the lesion contrast becomes weaker for smaller t,[23] realized by oscillating gradient spin echo (OGSE) (t = 4 ms) compared with the usual PGSE (t = 40 ms).[24] The dependence of the lesion contrast on diffusion time has also been observed within the PGSE (t = 22.3–47.3 ms).[25] This observation is exciting, as it implies that the drop in diffusivity in acute infarction reflects the alteration of the tissue microstructure, which can be quantified by altering t and may yield a novel-specific biomarker of neuronal damage in the future. Although neurite beading has been suggested as a candidate pathology underlying the observed behavior of $D(t)$,[24] the origin of the reduced

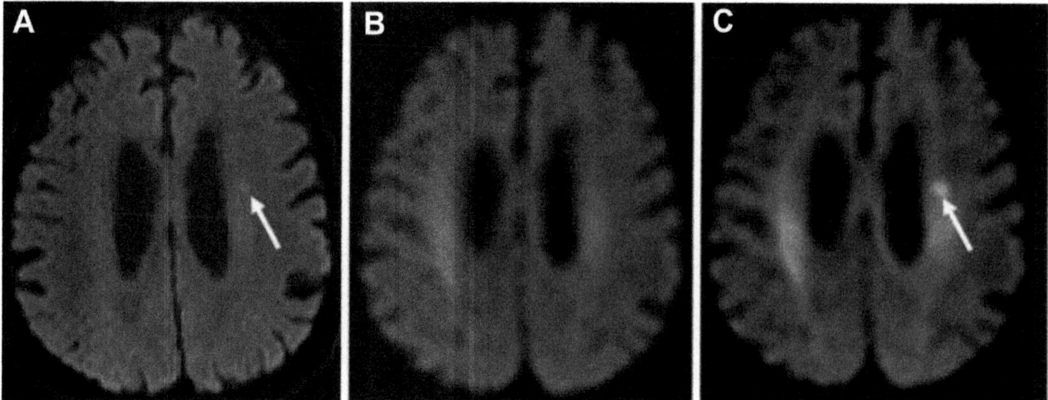

Fig. 8. Diffusion-weighted imaging of the brain of an 87-year-old patient, showing acute infarction (*arrow*). (*A*) DWI (*b*-value = 1000 s mm^{-2}, diffusion time = 22.3 ms), (*B*) DWI (b-value = 1500 s mm^{-2}, diffusion time = 8.5 ms), (*C*) DWI (*b*-value = 1500 s mm^{-2}, diffusion time = 47.3 ms). (Hori, M., Irie, R., Suzuki, M. *et al.* Teaching Neuroimages: Obscured Cerebral Infarction on MRI. *Clin Neuroradiol* **27**, 519–520 (2017); with permission. This article is available at SpringerLink with Open Access.)

diffusivity in acute infarction remains a matter of debate.[26]

Applications to tumors are also starting to emerge. Lemberskiy and colleagues[27] showed t-dependence in prostate cancer in the range $t = 20.8$ to 350 ms and a better differentiation of tumor grades at smaller t. The utility of a model of t-dependent diffusion incorporating tumor vasculature[28] has been examined in a large-cohort prospective study of prostate cancer.[29] Both Iima and colleagues[30] and Maekawa and colleagues[31] showed that the difference in D between an OGSE and a PGSE is greater in malignant tumors than in benign tumors and in head-and-neck and brain tumors, respectively.

In summary, time-dependent diffusion offers a new axis of measurement in the field of clinical dMRI, which promises to yield practical applications in the future.[32]

In the past, for example, reports on the usefulness of high b-values for imaging in cerebral infarction have been given, but the perceived advantages may have been mainly due to longer diffusion times.

As a future perspective, dMRI and measuring ADCs at different diffusion times would allow us to distinguish between spatially limited and viscosity-limited diffusion, which was previously difficult because the ADC is a unit of spatial extent per time; therefore, diffusion limitation by viscosity is unlikely to be sensitive to changes in the diffusion time at the time of measurement.[33]

CLINICS CARE POINTS

- The contrast and quantitative metrics of diffusion-weighted images depend on the diffusion time, which is an important factor. The lesions could be easily missing or misunderstood on diffusion-weighted images with inadequate diffusion time.

DISCLOSURE

M.Hori, this work was supported by Grants-in-Aid for Scientific Research "KAKENHI," the Japan Society for the Promotion of Science (grants 19K08161), and a research grant (2017-2020) from the Japanese Society of Neuroradiology. K. Kamiya has nothing to disclose. K. Murata is an employee of Siemens Healthcare, Japan.

REFERENCES

1. Stejskal EO, Tanner JE. Spin diffusion measurements: spin echoes in the presence of a time dependent field gradient. J Chem Phys 1965;42(1):5.
2. Wesbey GE, Moseley ME, Ehman RL. Translational molecular self-diffusion in magnetic resonance imaging. II. Measurement of the self-diffusion coefficient. Invest Radiol 1984;19(6):491–8.
3. Le Bihan D, Breton E, Lallemand D, et al. MR imaging of intravoxel incoherent motions: application to diffusion and perfusion in neurologic disorders. Radiology 1986;161(2):401–7.
4. Callaghan PT, Coy A, MacGowan D, et al. Diffraction-like effects in NMR diffusion studies of fluids in porous solids. Nature 1991;351:467–9.
5. Bar-Shir A, Avram L, Ozarslan E, et al. The effect of the diffusion time and pulse gradient duration ratio on the diffraction pattern and the structural information estimated from q-space diffusion MR: experiments and simulations. J Magn Reson 2008;194(2):230–6.
6. Latour LL, Svoboda K, Mitra PP, et al. Time-dependent diffusion of water in a biological model system. Proc Natl Acad Sci U S A 1994;91(4):1229–33.
7. Mitra PP, Sen PN, Schwartz LM. Short-time behavior of the diffusion coefficient as a geometrical probe of porous media. Phys Rev B Condens Matter 1993;47(14):8565–74.
8. Novikov DS, Fieremans E, Jespersen SN, et al. Quantifying brain microstructure with diffusion MRI: theory and parameter estimation. NMR Biomed 2019;32(4):e3998.
9. Fieremans E, Lee HH. Physical and numerical phantoms for the validation of brain microstructural MRI: a cookbook. Neuroimage 2018;182:39–61.
10. Sen PN. Time-dependent diffusion coefficient as a probe of geometry. Concepts Magn Reson Part A Bridg Educ Res 2004;23:1–21.
11. Reynaud O. Time-dependent diffusion MRI in cancer: tissue modeling and applications. Front Phys 2017;5:1–16.
12. Kiselev VG. Fundamentals of diffusion MRI physics. NMR Biomed 2017;30:e3602.
13. Fieremans E, Burcaw LM, Lee HH, et al. In vivo observation and biophysical interpretation of time-dependent diffusion in human white matter. Neuroimage 2016;129:414–27.
14. Lee HH, Papaioannou A, Novikov DS, et al. In vivo observation and biophysical interpretation of time-dependent diffusion in human cortical gray matter. Neuroimage 2020;222:117054.
15. Lee HH, Papaioannou A, Kim SL, et al. A time-dependent diffusion MRI signature of axon caliber variations and beading. Commun Biol 2020;3(1):354.
16. Roediger B, Armati PJ. Oxidative stress induces axonal beading in cultured human brain tissue. Neurobiol Dis 2003;13(3):222–9.
17. Takeuchi H, Mizuno T, Zhang G, et al. Neuritic beading induced by activated microglia is an early feature of neuronal dysfunction toward neuronal

death by inhibition of mitochondrial respiration and axonal transport. J Biol Chem 2005;280(11): 10444–54.

18. Novikov DS, Jensen JH, Helpern JA, et al. Revealing mesoscopic structural universality with diffusion. Proc Natl Acad Sci U S A 2014;111(14):5088–93.
19. Baron CA, Beaulieu C. Oscillating gradient spin-echo (OGSE) diffusion tensor imaging of the human brain. Magn Reson Med 2014;72(3):726–36.
20. Marschar AM, Kuder TA, Stieltjes B, et al. In vivo imaging of the time-dependent apparent diffusional kurtosis in the human calf muscle. J Magn Reson Imaging 2015;41(6):1581–90.
21. Sigmund EE, Novikov DS, Sui D, et al. Time-dependent diffusion in skeletal muscle with the random permeable barrier model (RPBM): application to normal controls and chronic exertional compartment syndrome patients. NMR Biomed 2014;27(5): 519–28.
22. Teruel JR, Cho GY, Moccaldi RTM, et al. Stimulated echo diffusion tensor imaging (STEAM-DTI) with varying diffusion times as a probe of breast tissue. J Magn Reson Imaging 2017;45(1):84–93.
23. Boonrod A, Hagiwara A, Hori M, et al. Reduced visualization of cerebral infarction on diffusion-weighted images with short diffusion times. Neuroradiology 2018;60(9):979–82.
24. Baron CA, Kate M, Gioia L, et al. Reduction of diffusion-weighted imaging contrast of acute ischemic stroke at short diffusion times. Stroke 2015;46(8):2136–41.
25. Hori M, Irie R, Suzuki M, et al. Teaching neuroimages: obscured cerebral infarction on MRI. Clin Neuroradiol 2017;27(4):519–20.
26. Blackband SJ, Flint JJ, Hansen B, et al. On the origins of diffusion MRI signal changes in stroke. Front Neurol 2020;11:1–7.
27. Lemberskiy G, Rosenkrantz AB, Veraart J, et al. Time-dependent diffusion in prostate cancer. Invest Radiol 2017;52(7):405–11.
28. Panagiotaki E, Walker-Samuel S, Siow B, et al. Noninvasive quantification of solid tumor microstructure using VERDICT MRI. Cancer Res 2014;74(7): 1902–12.
29. Johnston E, Pye H, Bonet-Carne E, et al. INNOVATE: a prospective cohort study combining serum and urinary biomarkers with novel diffusion-weighted magnetic resonance imaging for the prediction and characterization of prostate cancer. BMC Cancer 2016;16(1):816.
30. Iima M, Yamamoto A, Kataoka M, et al. Time-dependent diffusion MRI to distinguish malignant from benign head and neck tumors. J Magn Reson Imaging 2019;50(1):88–95.
31. Maekawa T, Hori M, Murata K, et al. Differentiation of high-grade and low-grade intra-axial brain tumors by time-dependent diffusion MRI. Magn Reson Imaging 2020;72:34–41.
32. Maekawa T, Kamiya K, Murata K, et al. Time-dependent diffusion in transient splenial lesion: comparison between oscillating-gradient spin-echo measurements and Monte-Carlo simulation. Magn Reson Med Sci 2020. https://doi.org/10.2463/mrms.bc.2020-0046.
33. Maekawa T, Hori M, Murata K, et al. Changes in the ADC of diffusion-weighted MRI with the oscillating gradient spin-echo (OGSE) sequence due to differences in substrate viscosities. Jpn J Radiol 2018; 36(7):415–20.

Intracranial Abnormalities with Diffusion Restriction

Steven P. Meyers, MD, PhD

KEYWORDS

• DWI • Restricted diffusion • Intracranial lesions • Abnormalities

KEY POINTS

- Diffusion-weighted imaging (DWI) is an MRI technique that can assess alterations in the normal random movement of water molecules in various tissues.
- Different pathologic disorders can result in various alterations in water diffusion.
- In addition to its routine use in the early diagnosis of acute brain ischemia, DWI can aid in the differential diagnosis of other pathologic conditions including infection, acute demyelination, metabolic encephalopathy, trauma, neoplasms, and tumorlike lesions.

Diffusion-weighted imaging (DWI) is a technique that can assess alterations in the normal random movement of water molecules in various tissues.[1–3] Multiple pathologic conditions can cause changes in this random movement of water, which can aid in making diagnoses. DWI has been routinely used for the evaluation of acute brain ischemia and infarction, as well as abscess formation.[4] Many other conditions can result in abnormal findings on DWI with either increased or decreased (restricted) diffusion.[4,5] For this article, the focus is on showing examples of common and uncommon disorders that can have phases with restricted diffusion secondary to cytotoxic and/or intramyelinic edema. These disorders include ischemia, infection, noninfectious demyelinating diseases, genetic mutations affecting metabolism, acquired metabolic disorders, toxic or drug exposures, neoplasms and tumorlike lesions, radiation treatment, trauma, and denervation.

ISCHEMIA

DWI has had an important role in the evaluation of acute ischemia and brain infarction in neonates, infants, children, and adults.[3–19] The locations and patterns of restricted diffusion in acute cerebral ischemia depend on patient age and mechanisms of hypoperfusion and are discussed in detail in this article.

Hypoxic Ischemic Injuries

Preterm neonates

Hypoxic ischemic injuries in preterm neonates vary depending on the duration and severity of the hypoxia as well as the neonate's gestational age.[6,7] Areas in the brain with maximal selective vulnerability to ischemia vary based on gestational ages.[6,7] In preterm neonates with episodes of severe hypoxia, restricted diffusion from cytotoxic edema is seen at sites with high metabolic demand, such as the ventrolateral thalami, basal ganglia, hippocampi, cerebellum, developing white matter, and corticospinal tracts[6–8] (**Fig. 1**).

In preterm neonates less than 32 weeks' gestational age, sites of selective vulnerability to hypoxia occur at locations of pre-oligodendrocytes in watershed vascular zones between the periventricular and subcortical white matter.[6,7] These watershed vascular zones progressively shift from a periventricular location to a more subcortical location.[6,7] Hypoxic injuries involving these

Department of Radiology/Imaging Sciences, University of Rochester Medical Center, University Medical Imaging, 4901 Lac de Ville Boulevard, Building D - Suite 140, Rochester, NY 14618, USA
E-mail address: Steven_Meyers@urmc.rochester.edu

Magn Reson Imaging Clin N Am 29 (2021) 137–161
https://doi.org/10.1016/j.mric.2021.02.004

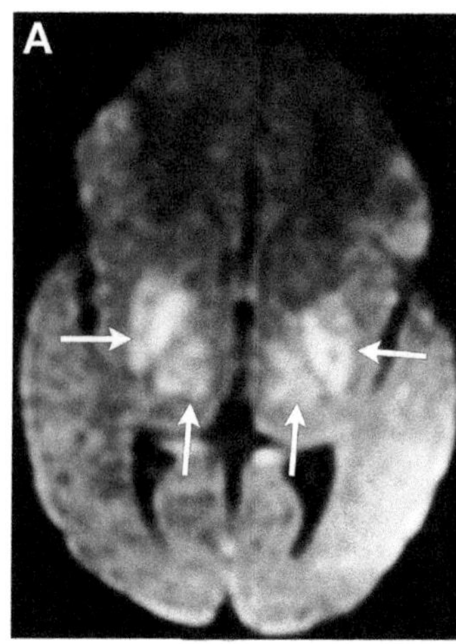

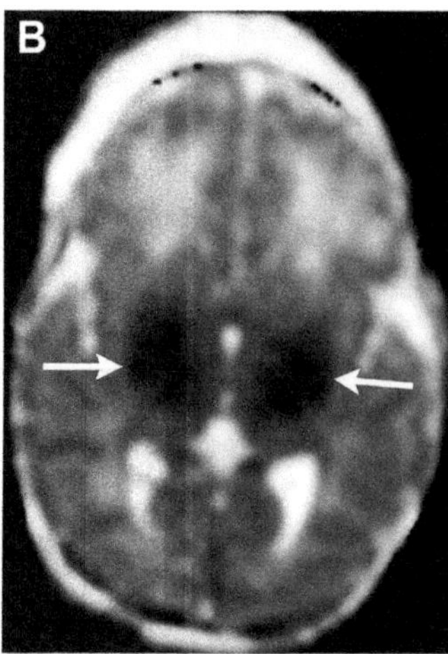

Fig. 1. A 4-day old preterm neonate with perinatal episode of severe hypoxic ischemic injury. Abnormal restricted diffusion involving the putamina and ventrolateral thalami is seen as high signal on axial DWI (*A*) and low signal on ADC (*B*) images (*arrows*).

watershed vascular zones are detected as areas with restricted diffusion[6,7] (**Fig. 2**).

Term neonates: hypoxic ischemic injuries

With severe hypoxic/hypotensive ischemic injuries involving term neonates, a central pattern of restricted diffusion from cytotoxic edema is seen in the ventrolateral thalami, putamina, lateral geniculate nuclei, posterior limbs of the internal capsules, dorsal mesencephalon, corticospinal tracts, and/or perirolandic cortex representing damage to sites with high metabolic demand.[6–10] Restricted diffusion at these locations can be seen within the first 24 hours after birth, and can become progressively greater over the next 4 to 5 days.[9,10] The apparent diffusion coefficient (ADC) values "pseudo-normalize" after the first week, and may be increased after the second week[6,7,9,10] (**Fig. 3**).

With moderate-severe hypoxic/hypotensive ischemic injuries involving term neonates, extensive diffuse injury with restricted diffusion can be seen involving the cerebral and cerebellar cortex, as well as involving the basal ganglia, thalami, and white matter. Restricted diffusion at these locations can be seen within the first 24 hours after birth, and can become more prominent over the next 4 to 5 days[9,10] (**Fig. 4**).

In term neonates with mild-moderate hypoxic injuries, zones with restricted diffusion from cytotoxic edema can be seen involving the cerebral cortex and subcortical white matter at watershed vascular boundary zones of the cerebrum and cerebellum within the first 24 hours.[7,9,10] ADC values eventually "pseudo-normalize" after 10 days, and may be increased after the second week[9,10] (**Fig. 5**).

Global hypoxic ischemic injuries in children and adults results in different degrees and locations of injuries that are related to the duration and severity of the hypoxia. Within the first 24 hours, ischemic changes from severe hypoxia can be seen as

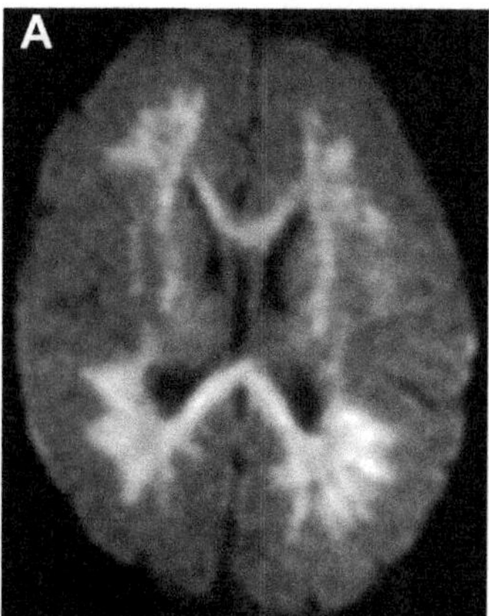

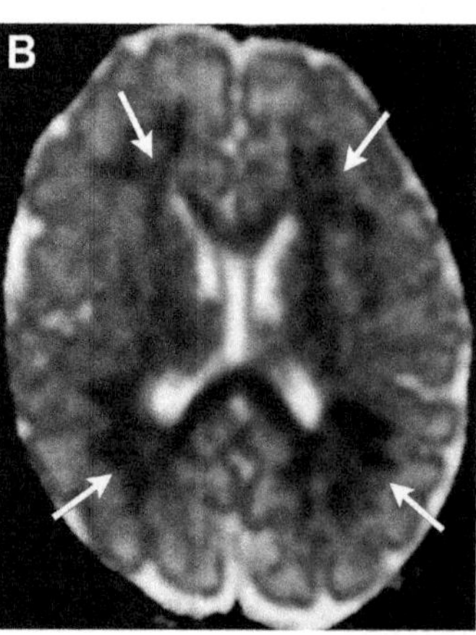

Fig. 2. Premature neonate with extensive white matter injury of prematurity as seen as large zones with restricted diffusion in the cerebral white matter on axial DWI (*A*) and ADC (*B*) images (*arrows*).

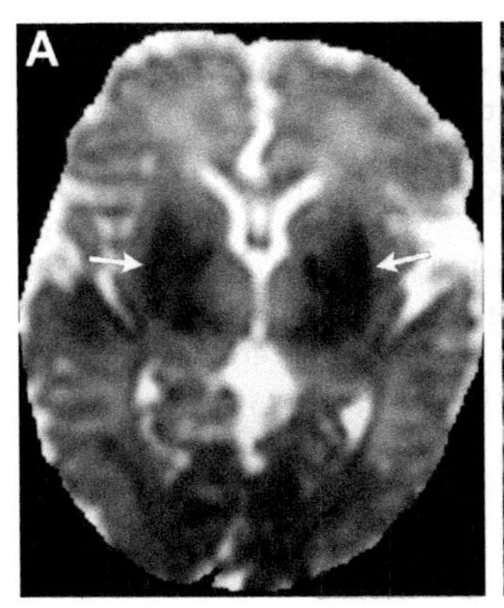
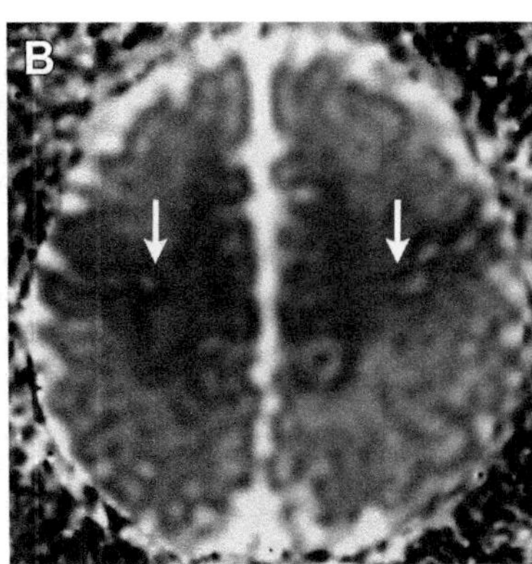

Fig. 3. Severe hypoxic injury in a 7-day-old term neonate. Restricted diffusion is seen in the putamina, thalami, and occipital lobes (*arrows*) on axial ADC (*A*) images, and perirolandic cortex (*arrows*) on axial ADC (*B*) images.

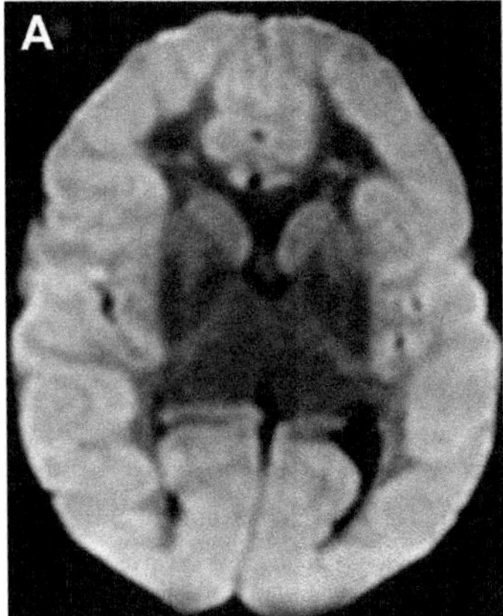
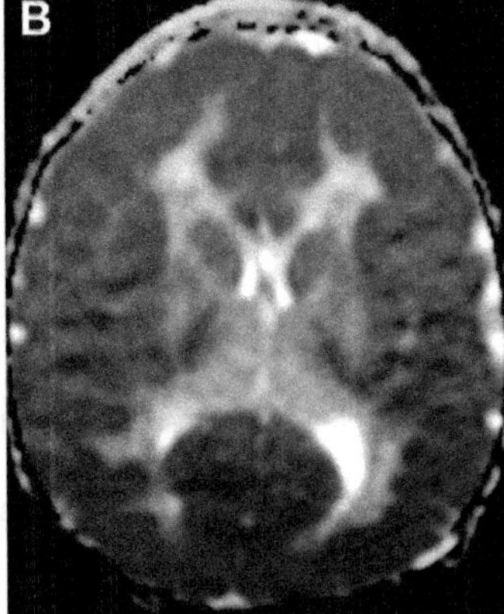

Fig. 4. Moderate-severe hypoxic injury in a neonate seen as zones with high signal on DWI (*A*) and low signal on ADC (*B*) images involving the cerebral cortex and subcortical white matter from restricted diffusion.

zones with restricted diffusion involving the basal ganglia, cerebral cortex, thalami, hippocampi, cerebellar hemispheres, and brainstem[7,9–11] (**Fig. 6**).

With mild-moderate hypoxic ischemic injuries in adults, zones with restricted diffusion can be seen at the arterial border (watershed) zones between the major cerebral arteries, and between the vascular distributions of the cerebellar arteries[7,9–11] (**Fig. 7**).

Arterial Infarction in Children and Adults

Cerebral and cerebellar infarcts most frequently result from stenosis or occlusion of arteries

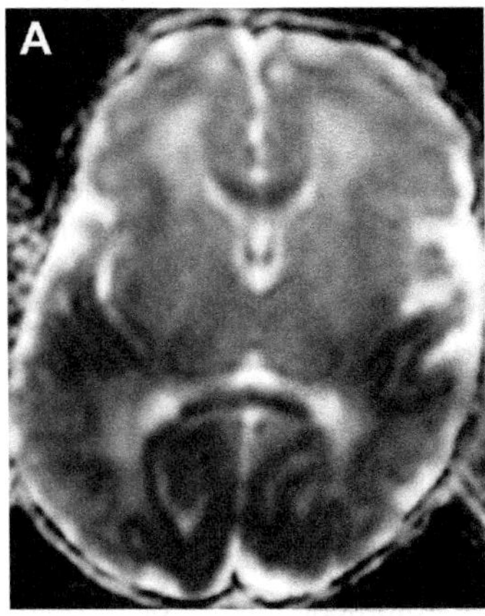
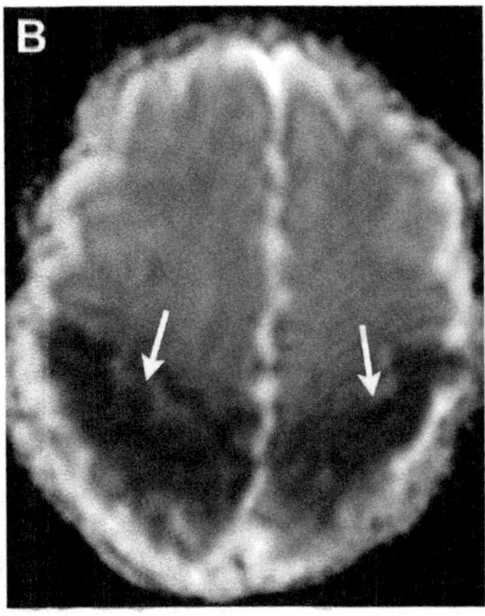

Fig. 5. Mild-moderate hypoxic injuries in a 3-day-old term neonate. Multiple zones of restricted diffusion with low signal are seen involving the cerebral cortex and subcortical white matter in the temporal and occipital lobes bilaterally (*A*), and both parietal (*arrows*) lobes (*B*) on axial ADC images.

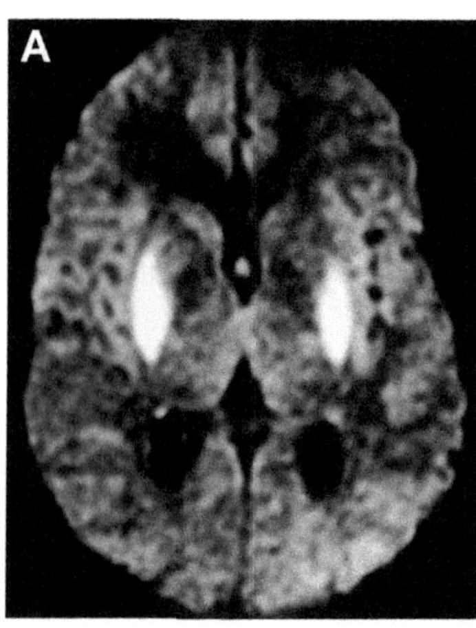

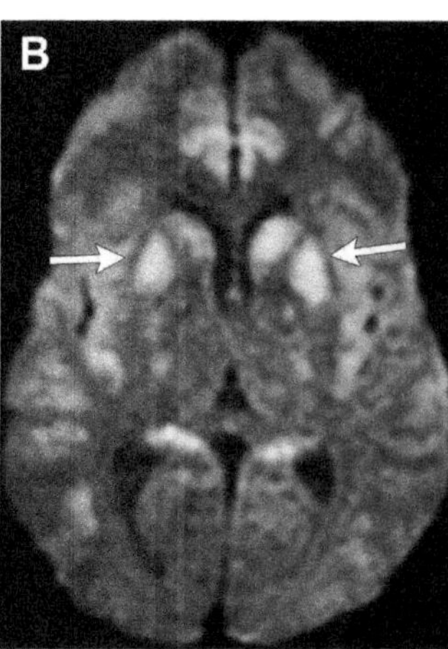

Fig. 6. A 16-year-old boy with severe hypoxic ischemic injury from cardiac arrest. Axial DWI shows restricted diffusion in the putamina (*A*). A 46-year-old resuscitated man after cardiac arrest complicated by global hypoxic brain injury with restricted diffusion in the caudate nuclei, putamina (*arrows*), and cerebral cortex on axial DWI (*B*).

producing focal or regional ischemia/infarction[12,13] (**Fig. 8**). Most strokes in adults are ischemic cerebral infarctions from arterial occlusions or stenosis of large or medium-sized arteries.[13] Other less frequent causes of stroke include cardioembolic disease, and small-vessel or lacunar infarctions[13–15] (**Fig. 9**). DWI may be useful for differentiating hemorrhagic transformations of strokes from other causes of intra-axial hemorrhage by demonstrating restricted diffusion in adjacent non-hemorrhagic infarcted brain tissue.[13–15]

Fig. 7. Acute cerebral infarct with restricted diffusion on DWI in the watershed vascular distribution zone between the distal branches of the right middle and anterior cerebral arteries resulting from occlusion of the right internal carotid artery and insufficient collateral blood flow from the anterior and right posterior communicating arteries.

Sinovenous Infarction in Children and Adults

Venous infarcts in neonates, children, and adults are rare, and represent a small percentage of all strokes. Venous infarcts can result from occlusion and/or thrombosis of the dural venous sinuses, superficial cortical veins, and/or deep veins which causes elevation of the venous pressure above the arterial perfusion pressure.[4,5,16–19] The most frequently occluded/thrombosed dural venous sinus is the superior sagittal sinus (SSS) followed by the transverse, straight, and cavernous sinuses.[16–19] DWI can show restricted diffusion in the intravenous thrombus in slightly less than 50% depending on the stage of clot formation.[4] Acute and subacute venous-related brain infarcts tend to have restricted diffusion in the subcortical white matter in the drainage territory of the occluded vein or dural venous sinus (**Figs. 10** and **11**). Zones of hemorrhage are frequently seen at sites of venous infarction.[4,5,16–19]

INFECTION

DWI has played an important role in the diagnosis and characterization of various types of infections involving the meninges and brain.[20–30] The patterns and locations of restricted diffusion can aid in the differential diagnosis of intracranial infections. Pathogens that cause infections involving the central nervous system (CNS) include bacteria, mycobacteria, fungi, viruses, prions, and parasites.

Meningitis refers to infections involving the pachymeninges, leptomeninges, or both.

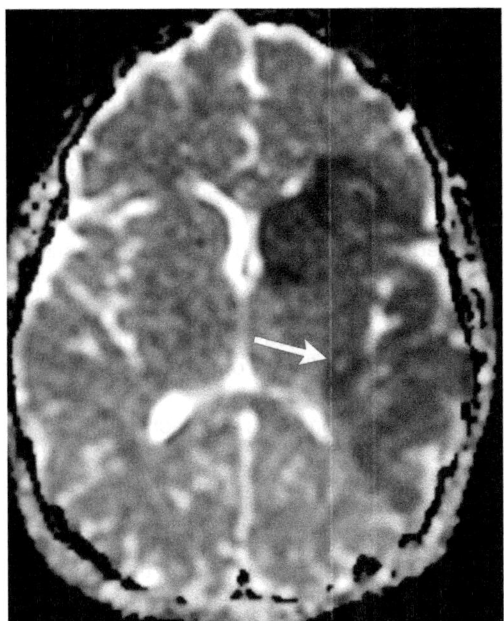

Fig. 8. A 14-year-old girl with an acute arterial infarction in the left cerebral hemisphere as seen as low signal on axial ADC (*arrow*), which resulted from dissection and occlusion of the left internal carotid artery.

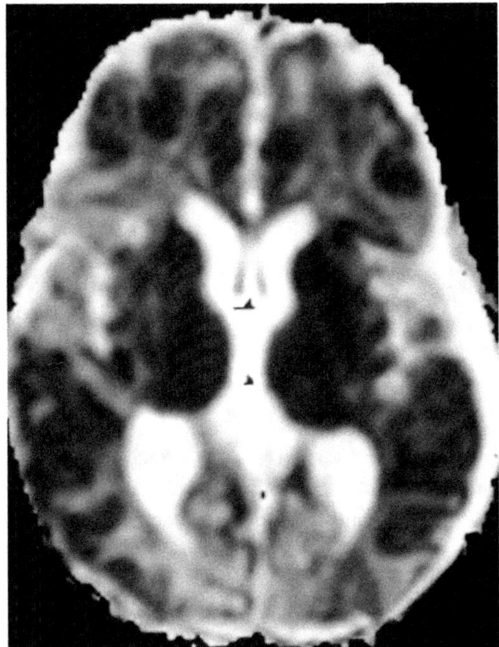

Fig. 10. A 2-month-old girl with sinovenous thrombus occluding the SSS and most of the straight and transverse venous sinuses resulting in extensive central and peripheral brain ischemia as seen as restricted diffusion on axial ADC.

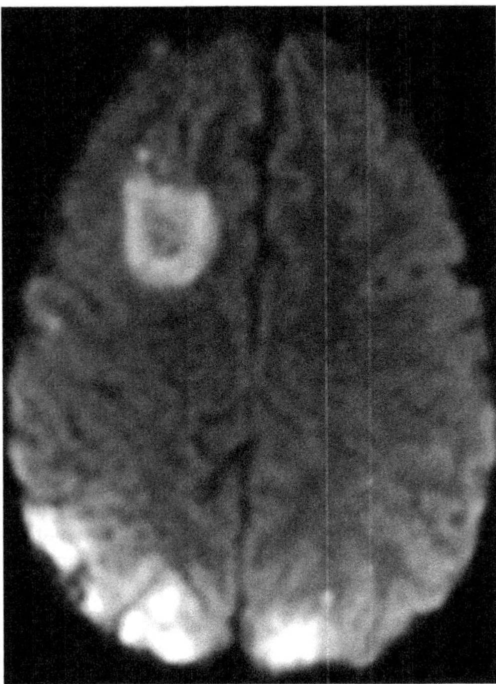

Fig. 9. A 12-year-old immunocompromised boy with fungal embolic infarcts in the brain as seen as zones with restricted diffusion on DWI.

Meningitis frequently results from bacteria, including mycobacteria, and can also result from infection by fungi and viruses.[20,21] With MRI, meningitis can be seen as contrast enhancement of

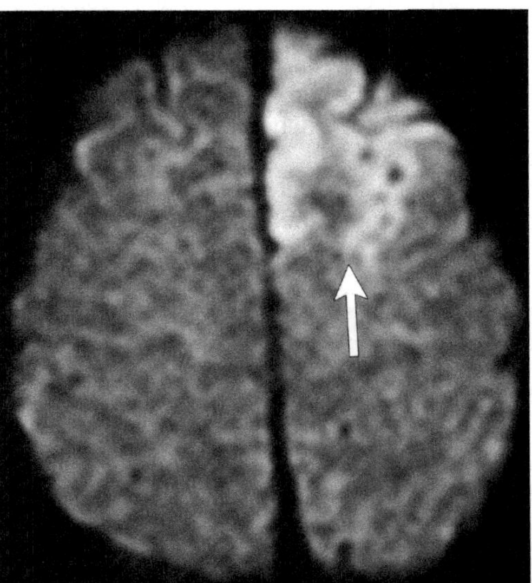

Fig. 11. A 49-year-old man with thrombosis of a cortical vein resulting in a venous infarct involving the upper anterior left frontal lobe as seen on axial DWI (*arrow*).

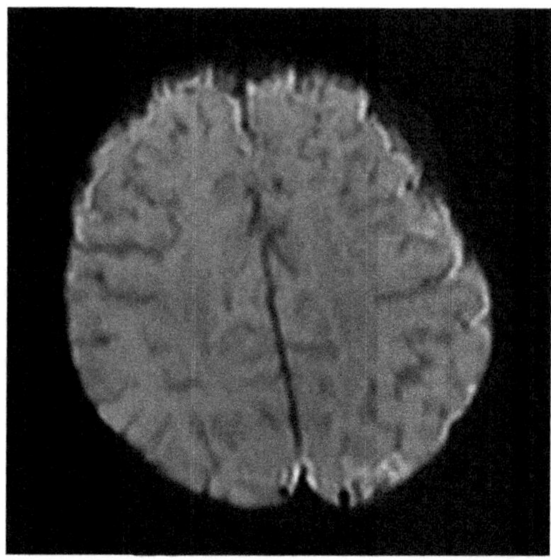

Fig. 12. A 3-month-old boy with bacterial meningitis from *Streptococcus pneumoniae,* as seen as zones with high signal from restricted diffusion on axial DWI involving the dura and leptomeninges.

thickened dura, with or without adjacent leptomeningeal contrast enhancement and corresponding restricted diffusion[21–27] (Fig. 12). Associated complications of meningitis include epidural and/or subdural abscesses with restricted diffusion (Fig. 13), as well as cerebritis, brain abscess, and ventriculitis, which can also show restricted diffusion.

Cerebritis represents intra-axial sites of acute brain inflammation resulting from infection by bacteria or fungi, and less frequently by parasites (Fig. 14A). Encephalitis refers to an infectious disease of the brain usually caused by viruses, and is typically associated with neurologic deficits.[27] Both cerebritis and encephalitis can have restricted diffusion depending on the stage and type of infection.[4,5,21,28] Brain abscesses account for 2% of intra-axial mass lesions.[25] Formation of brain abscesses can occur 2 weeks after cerebritis with liquefaction and necrosis centrally surrounded by a capsule and peripheral edema.[21,28] Brain abscesses are circumscribed lesions that contain a central zone of high signal on T2-weighted imaging (T2WI) surrounded by a thin rim (2–7 mm) with intermediate-low signal on T2WI, which shows ringlike Gd-contrast enhancement. The abscess contents typically have restricted diffusion related to the combination of the high protein content and viscosity of pus, necrotic debris, and bacteria[4,5,21,22,27,28] (Fig. 14B). The abscess wall is surrounded by peripheral poorly defined zones of high signal on T2WI representing edema.[4,5,21,28]

Ventriculitis represents infection involving the ventricles and can be seen as irregular zones with high signal on T2WI and fluid-attenuated inversion recovery (FLAIR) with associated restricted diffusion, and curvilinear and/or nodular Gd-contrast enhancement along the ependyma and periventricular brain parenchyma[21,23] (Fig. 14C).

Fungal Infections

Fungal brain infections usually occur in immunocompromised or diabetic patients with resultant granulomas involving the meninges and brain parenchyma.[21–23,25,28,30,31] Fungal infections of the CNS can occasionally occur in immunocompetent patients.[21–23,25,28,30,31] With MRI, fungal infections can be seen as localized zones of cerebritis, as well as irregular ring-enhancing brain lesions with low signal on T1WI and high signal on T2WI centrally.[21,30,31] Low signal on T2WI and gradient echo sequences at the walls of the lesions may occur from paramagnetic iron and magnesium within hyphae of the fungi. The MRI features of acute or chronic fungal abscesses are secondary to histologic features of acute and/or chronic inflammation with necrosis, as compared with the suppurative features associated with pyogenic

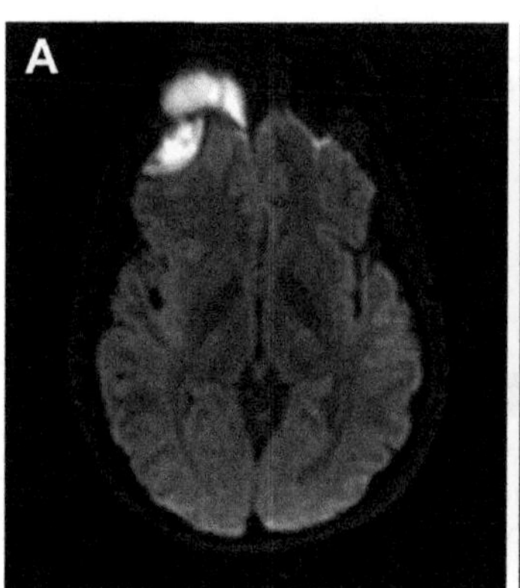

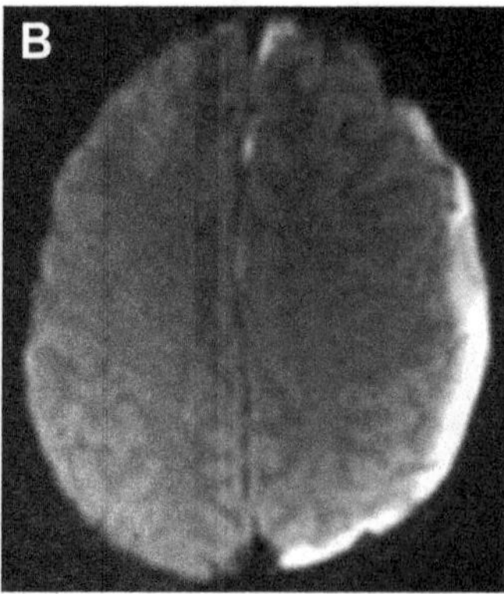

Fig. 13. An 8-year-old boy with frontal sinusitis complicated by an epidural abscess with restricted diffusion on axial DWI (*A*). An 18-year old woman with a subdural empyema on the left that has purulent material with restricted diffusion on axial DWI (*B*).

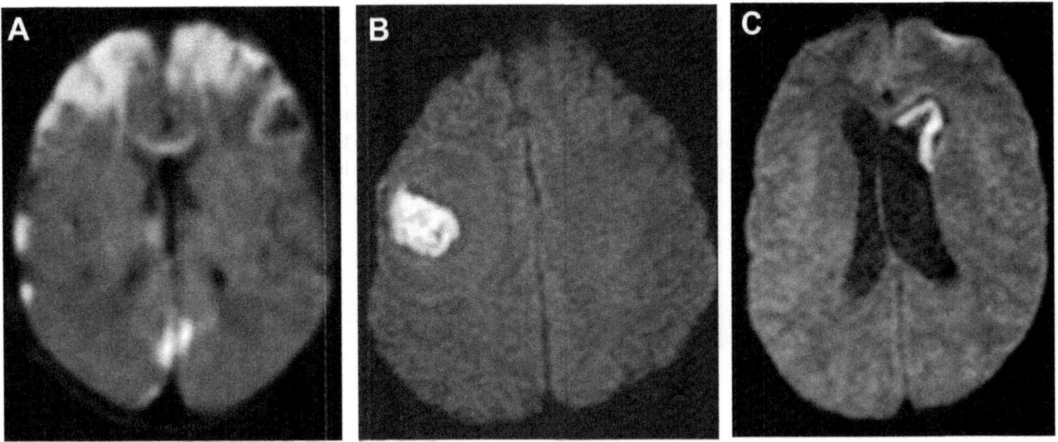

Fig. 14. A 7-day-old neonate with bacterial meningitis and cerebritis from *Escherichia coli* infection, which is seen as multiple zones of restricted diffusion involving the meninges and superficial brain parenchyma on axial DWI (*A*). A 56-year-old man with a pyogenic abscess in the right cerebral hemisphere with restricted diffusion on axial DWI (*B*). A 47-year-old woman with pyogenic ventriculitis/ependymitis with a curvilinear zone with diffusion restriction at the frontal horn of the left lateral ventricle on axial DWI (*C*).

abscesses.[31] Restricted diffusion can be seen at the periphery of the abscess cavity, and sometimes within the abscess cavity[21,30,31] (**Fig. 15**). *Aspergillosis* and *Mucormycosis* are commonly associated with invasion of blood vessels resulting in hemorrhagic brain lesions, cerebral infarcts, and/or mycotic aneurysms.[21,30]

Viral Infections: Acute Versus Chronic

Encephalitis refers to infections involving brain tissue that typically result from viruses.[28,32–34]

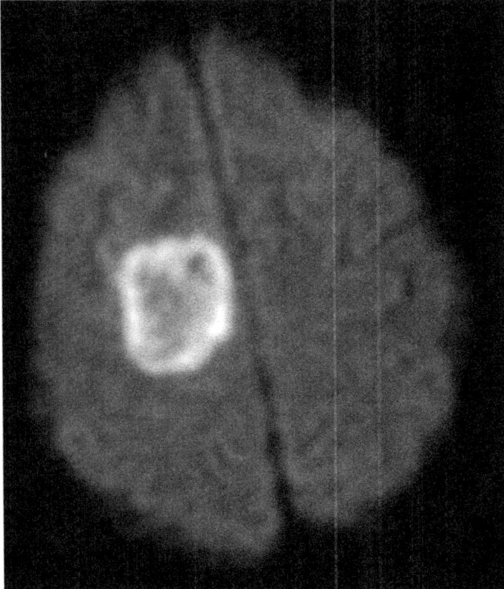

Fig. 15. A 16-year-old immunocompromised boy with Mucor fungal brain lesion/abscess in the right frontal lobe, which has heterogeneous mostly peripheral restricted diffusion on axial DWI.

Viruses can directly infect nerve cells (neurotropic), and secondarily involve the brain and meninges. Pathologic changes are often related to the variable host inflammatory responses relative to the degree of viral involvement.[33,34] Viral encephalitis can be primary or postinfectious.[32–34] With postinfectious encephalitis, a causative virus cannot be isolated and neuro-pathologic findings result from a secondary immune-mediated disorder.[32–34] Viral infections associated with high degrees of inflammation and necrosis tend to show more restricted diffusion than those viruses with lesser degrees.[32]

Herpes simplex (HSV) types 1 and 2 are common causes of encephalitis and can occur in immunocompetent or immunocompromised patients.[32–34] Restricted diffusion often occurs in the early stages of infection and can sometimes be more apparent than corresponding findings of abnormal increased signal on T2W and FLAIR images[32–34] (**Figs. 16** and **17**).

Cytomegalovirus (CMV) is the most common cause of fetal and neonatal brain infection.[32–35] In immunocompromised patients, reactivation of the latent virus can result in encephalitis, ependymitis, ventriculitis, necrotizing meningoencephalitis, and poly-radiculitis.[32–35] With MRI, high signal on T2WI, restricted diffusion and Gd-contrast enhancement can be seen along the ependymal lining of the ventricles.[33–35] Another finding associated with CMV are multiple punctate foci with high signal on T2WI and FLAIR with restricted diffusion in sub-ependymal and periventricular locations[35] (**Fig. 18**).

Varicella zoster virus (VZV) is the causative agent associated with varicella (chicken

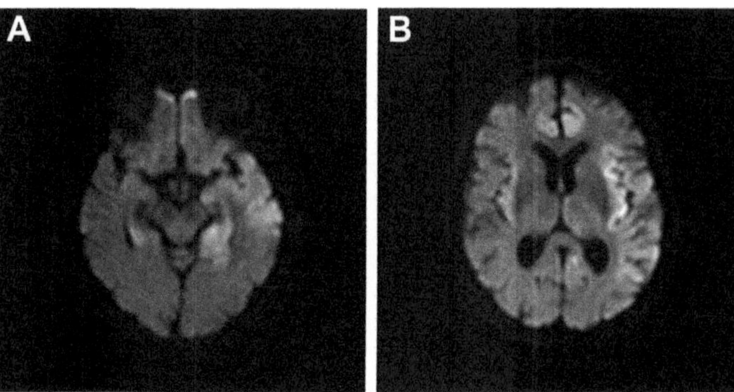

Fig. 16. A 62-year-old woman with acute HSV1 encephalitis. Axial DWI images (*A*, *B*) show asymmetric restricted diffusion involving the cerebral cortex and adjacent white matter of temporal lobes, cingulate, and insular portions of the frontal lobes.

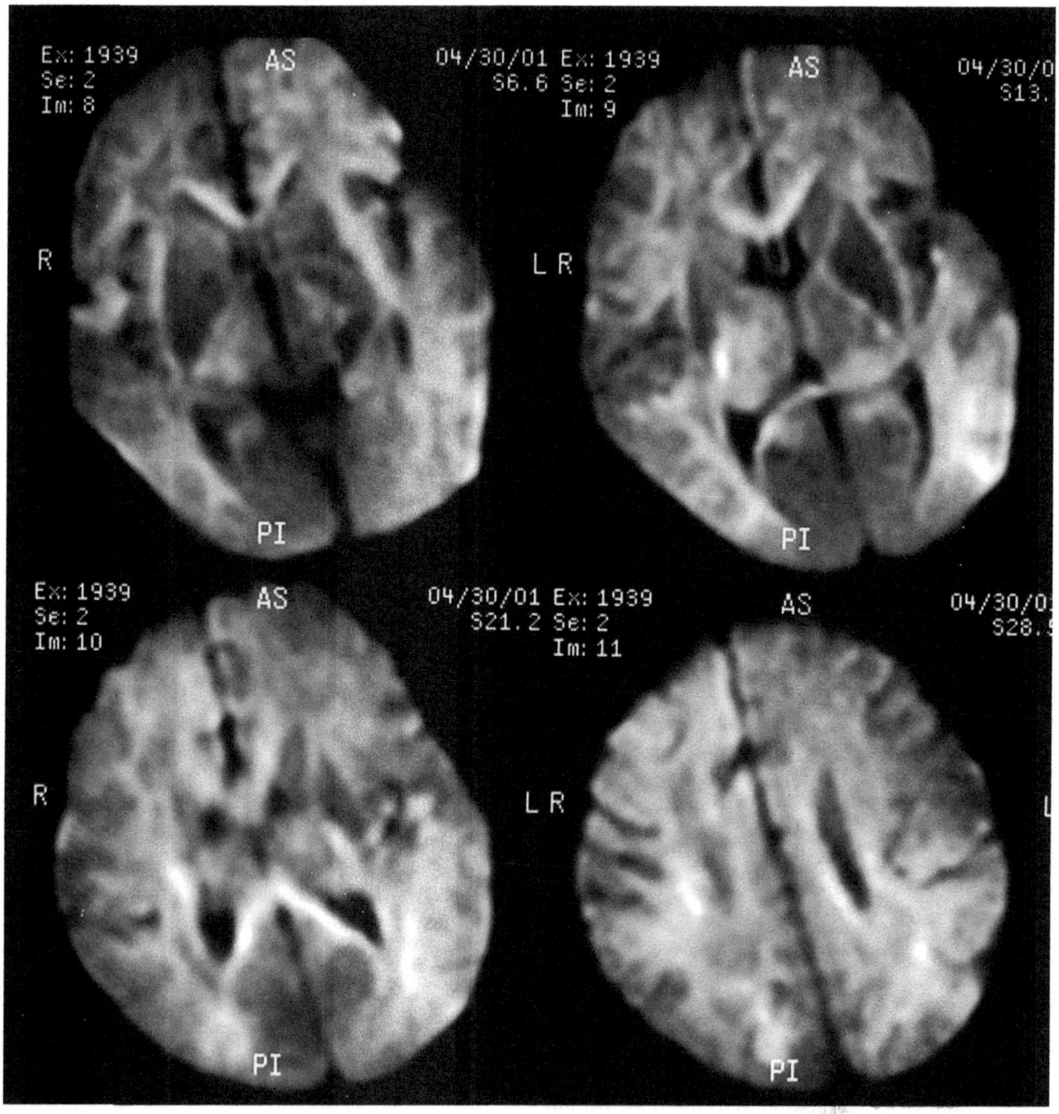

Fig. 17. A 1-week-old male neonate with HSV2 infection from delivery. Axial DWI shows irregular extensive zones with restricted diffusion within the brain.

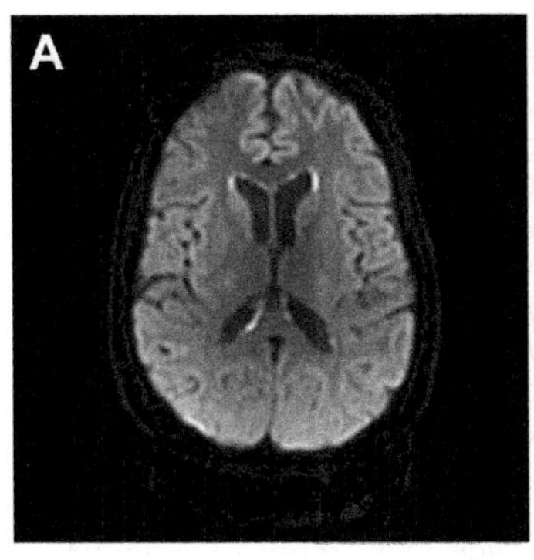

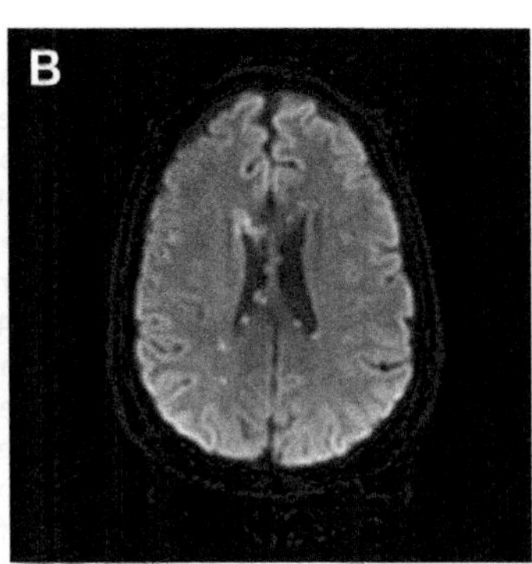

Fig. 18. A 33-year-old immunocompromised woman with CMV encephalitis. Axial DWI shows curvilinear restricted diffusion along the ependymal lining of the lateral ventricles (*A*) as well as multiple punctate foci involving ependymal, subependymal, and periventricular locations (*B*).

pox).[28,33,34] Varicella zoster can also occur in immunocompromised and older adult patients as a secondary disease of herpes zoster (shingles) from reactivation of latent virus within ganglionic neurons.[28,33,34] VZV meningoencephalitis is rare and is associated with direct infection of glial cells and/or media of arteries causing acute ischemia involving the cerebral cortex, subcortical white matter, and deep gray matter that can be detected with MRI as zones with increased signal on T2WI and FLAIR with restricted diffusion[28,33,34] (**Fig. 19**). Other viruses involving the brain and meninges can have phases with restricted diffusion including the Epstein Barr Virus, Human Herpes Virus 6, Flaviviruses (Japanese encephalitis, West Nile disease, Dengue, Zika virus), Chikungunya virus, Covid-19 Virus, Enteroviruses, Measles paramyxovirus, Influenza viruses, and JC Polyoma Virus.[32–44]

Fig. 19. A 67-year-old woman with VZV encephalitis with extensive restricted diffusion involving the cerebral cortex, subcortical white matter, and deep gray matter on axial DWI.

Immune-mediated encephalopathies associated with various viral infections include acute necrotizing encephalopathy (ANE) and mild encephalopathy with reversible lesions in the splenium (MERS).[35,44–49] In patients with ANE, zones increased signal on T2WI and FLAIR as well as restricted diffusion on DWI are seen in both thalami, cerebral white matter, putamina, internal capsules, dentate nuclei, and brainstem tegmentum[35,44–46] (**Fig. 20**A). Pathologic findings include necrosis of neuroglial cells, acute swelling of oligodendrocytes, vascular congestion, and perivascular hemorrhages, which are likely related excessive release of cytokines.[35,44,45] Patients usually have a poor prognosis.[35] In patients with (MERS), transient, nonenhancing solitary or symmetric, round or oval zones with increased signal on T2WI and FLAIR are seen located in the splenium of the corpus callosum.[35,47–49] Corresponding restricted diffusion is typically present from intramyelinic edema secondary to cytokine release from excessive release of excitatory neurotransmitters such as glutamate[35] (**Fig. 20**B). *MERS* can also result from other disorders such as pneumonia, seizures, trauma, hypoglycemia, and hyponatremia.[35,47–49]

Viral infections in immunocompromised patients

Immunosuppression is associated with active viral infections such as JC polyoma virus (JCV), HIV, Varicella zoster, Cytomegalovirus (CMV), and Herpes simplex.[22,33] In immunosuppressed patients with progressive multifocal encephalopathy (PML) related to JCV, asymmetric zones with increased signal on FLAIR and T2WI are present in cerebral and/or cerebellar white matter including the

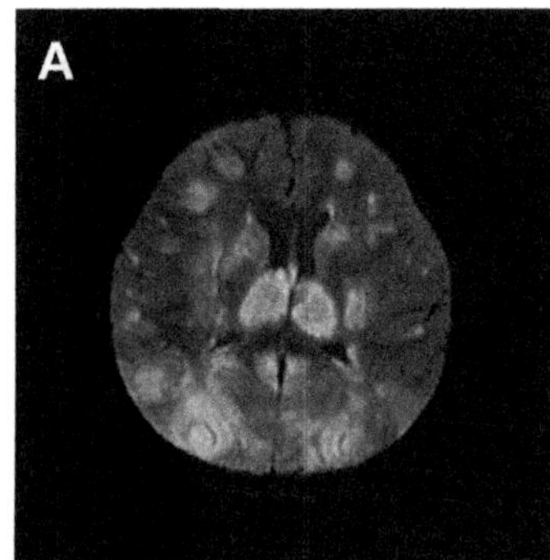

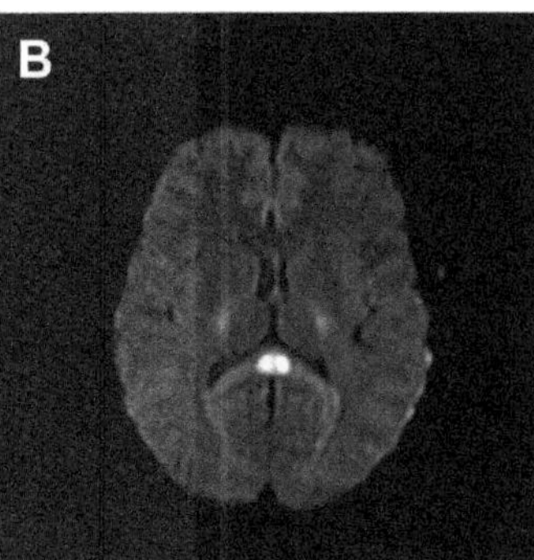

Fig. 20. ANE in a 2-year-old boy with influenza A infection associated with fever, dehydration, and rapid neurologic deterioration with seizures. Axial DWI shows restricted diffusion involving the thalami, basal ganglia, and cerebral white matter bilaterally (*A*). Diffusion restriction is also seen involving the insula and cerebral cortex secondary to seizures. MERS in a 20-year old woman after a viral illness. Axial DWI (*B*) shows a localized zone of restricted diffusion involving the splenium of the corpus callosum, which subsequently resolved on a follow-up MRI examination 6 weeks later.

subcortical U-fibers, as well as the middle cerebellar peduncles, pons and occasionally the basal ganglia and thalami.[22,34,35,50] Irregular zones of restricted diffusion may be present at the periphery of the PML lesions in the early stages of disease.[33–35,50] A complication of highly active anti-retroviral therapy is the PML-immune reconstitution inflammatory syndrome (PML-IRIS) that can occur from 1 week to 2 years after treatment.[22,33–35,50] Zones with abnormal increased signal on T2WI and FLAIR are seen in white matter with associated edema and transient marginal Gd-contrast enhancement[22,33–35,50–52] (**Fig. 21**A, B). High signal zones on DWI with or without restricted diffusion are often seen at the periphery of the lesions from inflammatory demyelination and swelling of the infected oligodendrocytes[22,33–35,50–52] (**Fig. 21**C).

Prion disease

Prions are small infectious proteinaceous structures, which do not contain DNA or RNA, and can replicate only when inside host cells.[33,53] Prions can cause progressive neurodegeneration resulting in spongiform encephalopathies. There are 2 major human prion diseases, which include sporadic Creutzfeldt Jakob disease (sCJD) representing 85% of cases, and familial Creutzfeldt Jakob disease (fCJD).[33,53] With MRI, increased signal on T2WI and restricted diffusion are seen involving the caudate nuclei and putamina without contrast enhancement[33,53] (**Fig. 22**A). Some patients have increased signal on T2WI and T2 FLAIR images with high signal on DWI involving cerebral cortex with or without signal alteration at the caudate nuclei and putamina[33,53] (**Fig. 22**B).

Parasites

Parasitic infections result when pathogens subsist and replicate at the expense and detriment of the host organisms. The 3 types of organisms that cause parasitic infections of humans include multi-cell helminths or worms (*Cysticercosis, Echinococcosis, Schistosomiasis*), single-cell protozoa (*Malaria, Toxoplasmosis, Giardia, Amebiasis,*

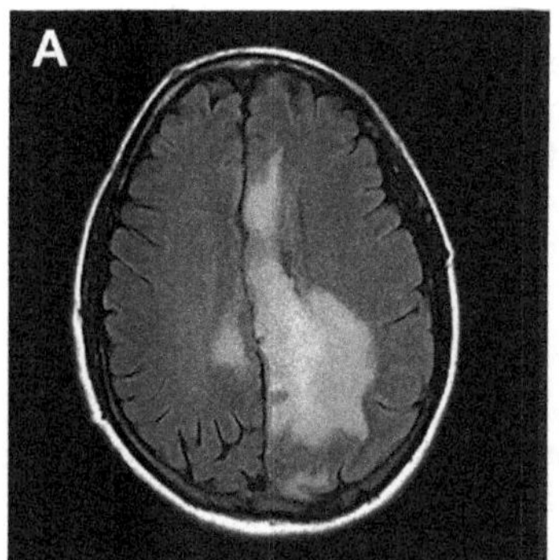

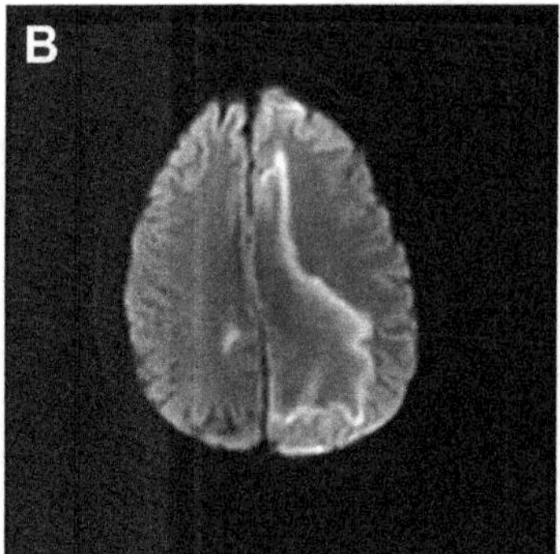

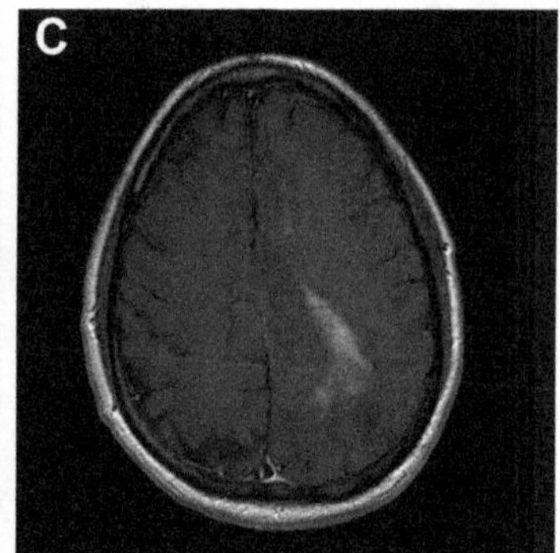

Fig. 21. A 47-year-old man with PML-IRIS after treatment with Rituximab for Waldenstrom macroglobulinemia. Axial T2-FLAIR (*A*) shows a large poorly defined zone with abnormal high signal involving the white matter of the left cerebral hemisphere, as well as a small zone in the right cerebral hemisphere, where there are also thin peripheral zones with diffusion restriction on axial DWI (*B*), as well as irregular zones with contrast enhancement on axial T1WI (*C*).

Trichomoniasis, Cryptosporidiosis) and ectoparasites that involve the skin.[21,54]

With *Cysticercosis,* the scolex can have variable signal, contrast enhancement and/or restricted diffusion.[55] Toxoplasmosis involving the brain can have variable findings on DWI that are likely related to which active stage of infection is predominant.[56]

Malaria results from infection by protozoan parasites from the genus *Plasmodium* and is the most lethal parasitic infection in the world.[57] Transmission of the parasite to humans occurs via bites from female mosquitoes *(Anopheles genus)* whose saliva contains the *Plasmodium* organisms. Cerebral malaria most commonly occurs in children and visitors to endemic regions such as sub-Saharan Africa and other tropical zones with altitudes less than 1500 m.[21,57] Aggregation of infected erythrocytes in cerebral blood vessels results in perivascular hemorrhage, myelin damage, and necrosis of white matter in 2% of cases.[21,56] Inflammatory reaction with cytokine release, vasodilation, and vascular engorgement can result in increased intracranial pressure.[21,57] MRI findings associated with cerebral malaria in children include diffuse cerebral edema, focal and/or poorly defined zones with high signal on T2WI and FLAIR in the cerebral white matter, basal ganglia, and/or thalami, with or without petechial hemorrhage at gray matter–white matter junctions.[21,57] Nearly 75% of children with cerebral malaria have 1 or more intra-axial zones of diffusion restriction.[57] Sites of restricted diffusion were bilateral cerebral white matter, corpus callosum, deep gray matter, cortical gray matter, and posterior fossa[57] (**Fig. 23**). There is limited literature related to the DWI findings of other types of parasitic infections.

NONINFECTIOUS DEMYELINATING DISEASES

Demyelinating disease can result from autoimmune disorders such as multiple sclerosis (MS); neuromyelitis optica spectrum disorders (NMOSD) with anti-AQP4 or anti–myelin oligodendrocyte glycoprotein (MOG) antibodies, acute disseminated encephalomyelitis (ADEM); or infectious, toxic-metabolic, post-radiotherapy, traumatic, and vascular processes.[58–61]

Autoimmune demyelinating diseases include classic MS, tumefactive demyelinating lesions (TDLs), Baló's concentric sclerosis, Marburg and Schilder variants, NMOSD, ADEM, and aggressive variants of acute hemorrhagic leukoencephalitis of leukoencephalopathy (Hurst disease).[58] MS is the most common acquired demyelinating disease characterized by peri-venular inflammation/demyelination with relative preservation of axons.[58] Lesions usually have high signal on T2WI and FLAIR, and sites of active demyelination show Gd-contrast enhancement in a pattern that can be nodular, ringlike or in a C-shape (incomplete ring) with or without restricted diffusion[58] (**Fig. 24**).

Variants of MS (eg, TDLs, Baló's, Marburg, and Schilder variants) are fulminant demyelinating disorders representing a much more aggressive immune-mediated destruction of myelin compared with the classic version of MS.[58–60] TDLs are defined as demyelinating lesions that are larger than 2 cm, and can be solitary or multiple.[58–60] With MRI, TDLs have high signal on T2WI and FLAIR, minimal perilesional edema, and mild localized mass effect[58–60] (**Fig. 25**). Postcontrast MRI often shows the lesion to have incomplete irregular ringlike enhancement at the leading margin of demyelination.[58–60] With DWI, high ADC values are seen centrally surrounded by irregular peripheral rims of diffusion

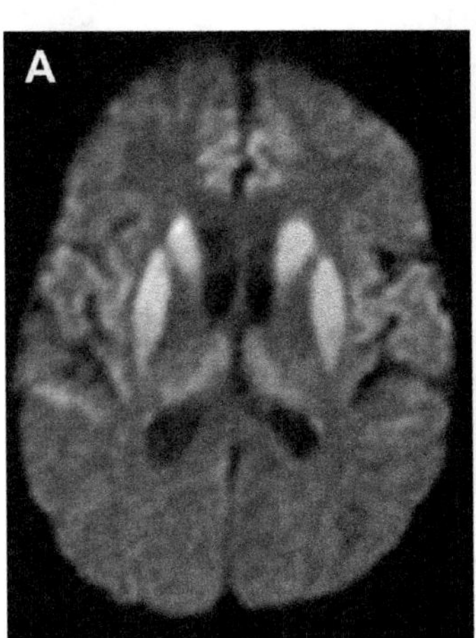

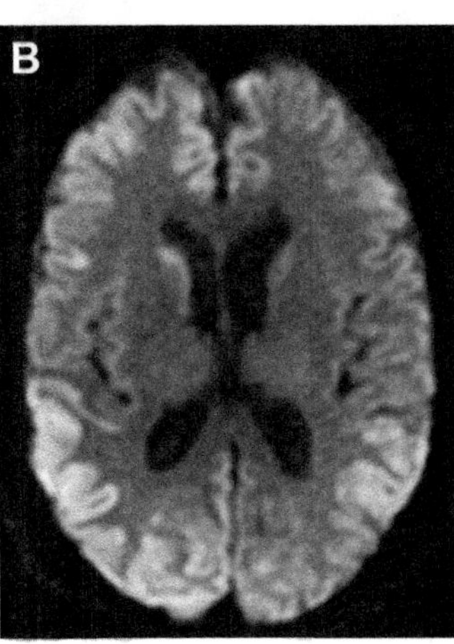

Fig. 22. A 60-year-old man with sCJD with restricted diffusion involving the caudate nuclei and putamina bilaterally on DWI (*A*). A 74-year-old man with sCJD with restricted on DWI involving the cerebral cortex bilaterally and right caudate (*B*).

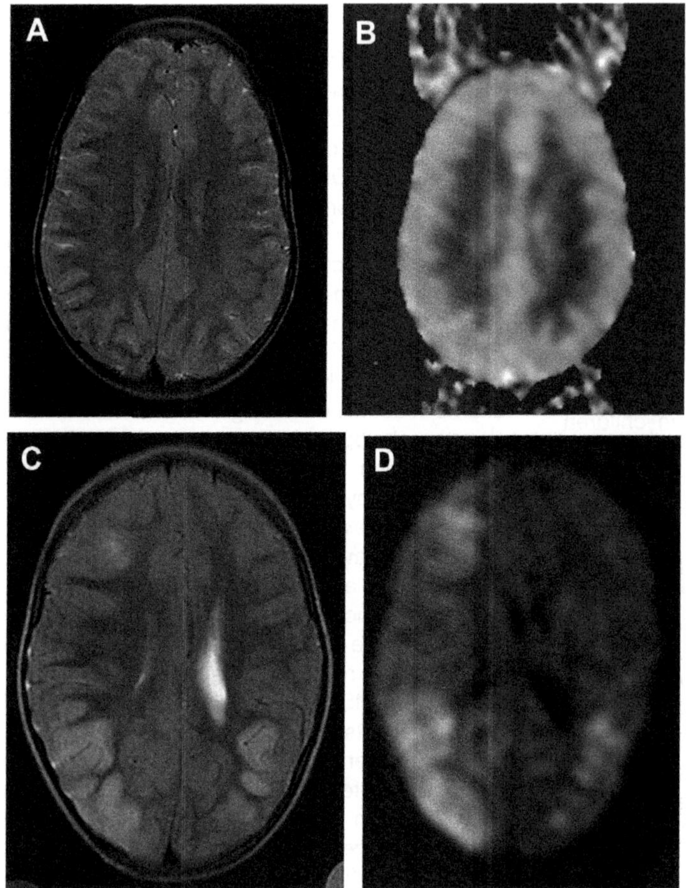

Fig. 23. Comatose child with cerebral malaria who has poorly defined zones with slightly increased signal on T2WI involving the cerebral white matter bilaterally (*A*) with corresponding diffusion restriction on axial ADC image (*B*). Another child with cerebral malaria who has asymmetric poorly defined bilateral zones with abnormal increased signal on axial T2WI involving the cerebral cortex and subcortical white matter (*C*) and corresponding diffusion-restricted diffusion on axial DWI image (*D*).

restriction.[58–60] The peripheral zones of restrictive diffusion correspond to active sites of demyelination.[58–60] MRI features of TDLs that are associated with high specificity in distinguishing from lymphoma and brain tumors include incomplete ringlike contrast enhancement, high central ADC values surrounded by a peripheral rim of restricted diffusion, and multiplicity of lesions.[60]

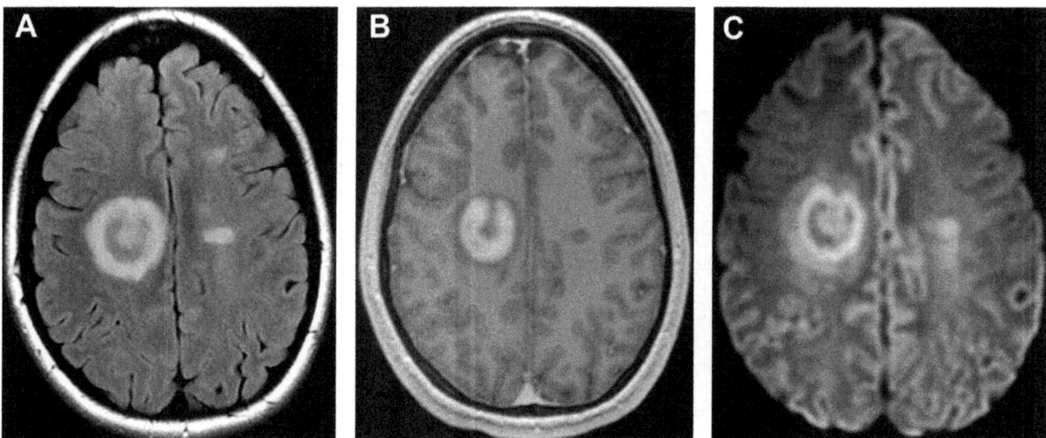

Fig. 24. A 30-year-old woman with MS with an acute demyelinating lesion in the right cerebral white matter that has a central zone with high signal surrounded by a C-shaped zone with intermediate signal and high-signal peripheral edema on axial FLAIR (*A*). The lesion shows a C-shaped zone of contrast enhancement (*B*) with corresponding restricted diffusion of axial DWI (*C*).

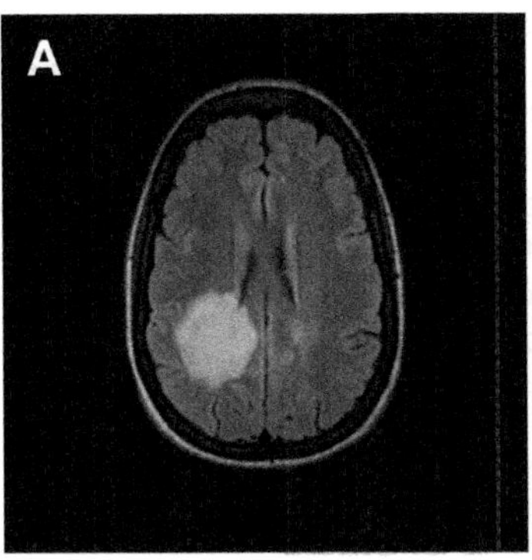

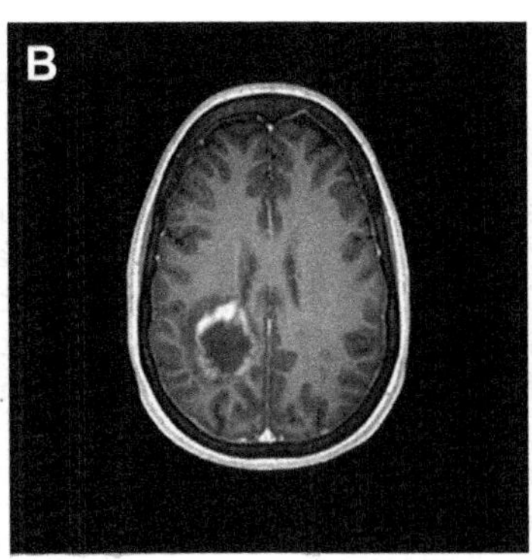

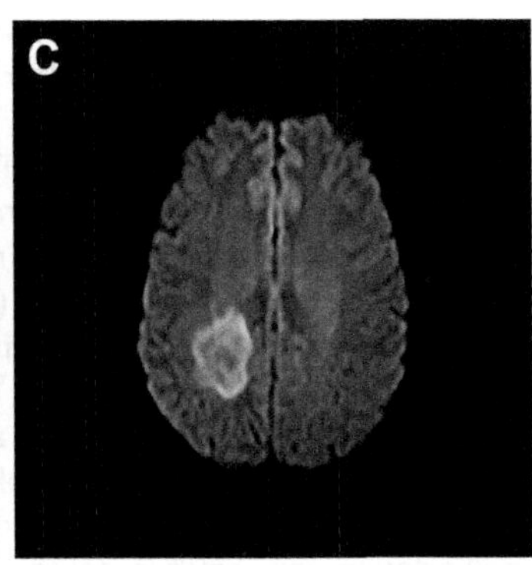

Fig. 25. A 34-year-old woman with MS with a tumefactive demyelinating lesion in the right cerebral hemisphere that has diffuse high signal on axial FLAIR (*A*), and a peripheral irregular zone of contrast enhancement on axial T1WI (*B*) that also shows restricted diffusion on axial DWI (*C*).

NMOSD consists of a group of 3 demyelinating disorders that are separated based on the presence or absence of immunoglobulin (Ig)G antibodies against aquaporin-4 (AQP4) and/or MOG.[58,61] With NMOSD, MRI findings can include longitudinally extensive transverse myelitis, optic neuritis, and demyelinating lesions in periventricular white matter, corpus callosum, midbrain, medulla, and corticospinal tracts.[58,61] Acute demyelinating lesions can have restricted diffusion. In addition, TDLs and "cloudlike-enhancing" lesions are more common with NMOSD than MS.[58,61]

ADEM is a monophasic immune-mediated demyelinating disease, which involves the white matter of the brain and/or spinal cord.[58,61] ADEM usually occurs in children younger than 15 years, and may be associated with a recent upper respiratory viral or bacterial infection, or vaccination.[58,61] Relapses within 3 months after onset can also occur.[58,61] Anti-MOG IgG antibodies are present in one-half of patients with ADEM.[58,61] With MRI, multiple bilateral asymmetric demyelinating lesions with increased signal on T2WI and FLAIR are often seen in the white matter of the brain.[58,61] ADEM lesions also tend to be more rounded and larger than with MS.[58,61] In the acute phase of ADEM, a peripheral rim of contrast enhancement and diffusion restriction can be seen at the advancing front of active demyelination[58,61] (**Fig. 26**).

Autoimmune encephalitis refers to a group of related diseases in which there are immune-mediated injuries involving the brain caused by specific auto-antibodies against auto-antigens.[62] Autoimmune encephalitis can be paraneoplastic and non-paraneoplastic. With the paraneoplastic type, host antibodies directed against antigens in neoplasms (small cell lung cancer, breast cancer, Hodgkin lymphoma, others) can also cross react with normal host neuronal cells resulting in inflammation.[62] With the non-paraneoplastic type, the immune-mediated attack on auto-antigens results from other nontumoral causes.[62] The MRI findings of autoimmune encephalitis depend on which sites of the brain where the immune-mediated

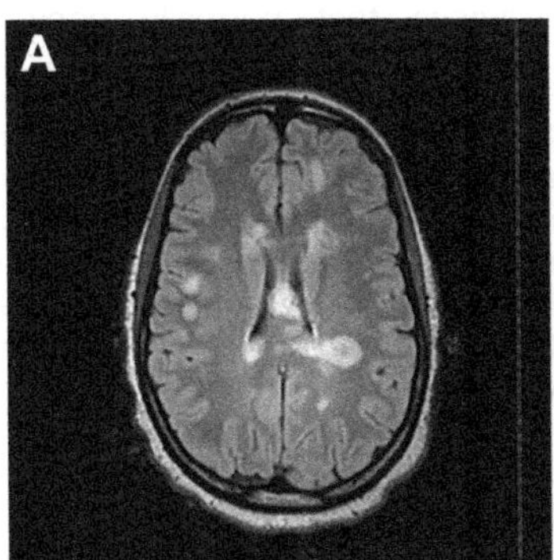

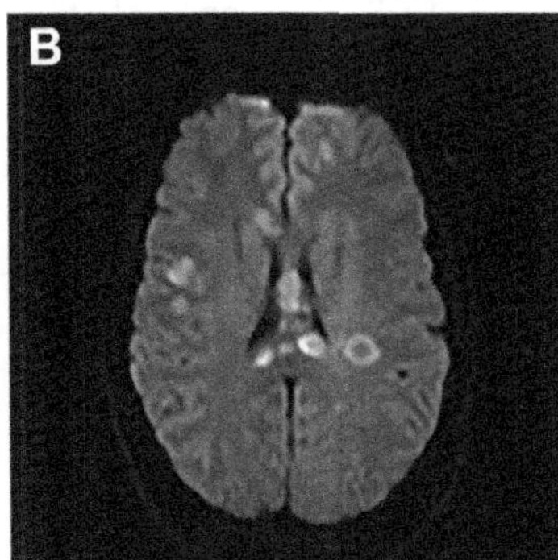

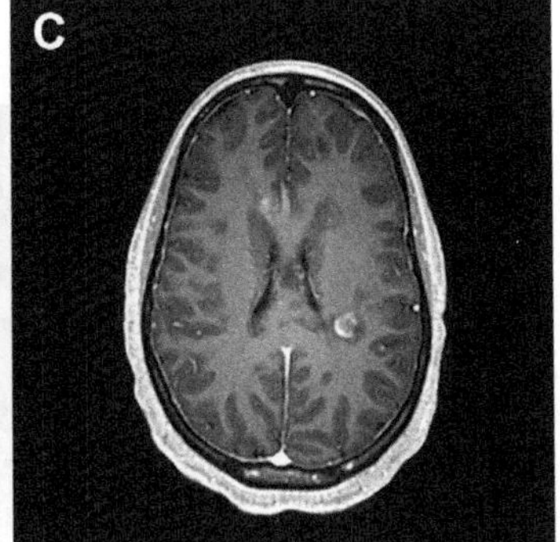

Fig. 26. A 1-year-old girl with MOG-Ab 1 ADEM. Axial FLAIR shows multiple demyelinating lesions with high signal in the corpus callosum, and subcortical and periventricular white matter (*A*), which have thin peripheral zones of restricted diffusion on axial DWI (*B*). Some of these lesions also have thin peripheral contrast enhancement on axial T1WI (*C*).

inflammation occurs. Common locations include the limbic system, cerebral and/or cerebellar cortex, and subcortical white matter.[62] Involved sites can have abnormal high signal on T2WI and FLAIR involving the limbic system, cerebral white matter, and/or brainstem, with or without restricted diffusion and contrast enhancement[62] (**Fig. 27**).

Susac syndrome is an autoimmune vasculopathy of small-vessels that results from autoreactive CD8-positive cells and anti-endothelial antibodies causing vasculitis involving the brain, retina, and cochlea.[58] This endotheliopathy of small arteries can result in acute small infarcts in the cerebral white matter including the corpus callosum observed as sites of restricted diffusion.[58] Ophthalmoscopy typically shows retinal infarcts from branch retinal artery retinal occlusions.[58]

The CNS can be affected by a variety of other HYPERLINK "https://www.sciencedirect.com/topics/medicine-and-dentistry/inflammatory-disease" \o "Learn more about Inflammatory Disease from ScienceDirect's AI-generated Topic Pages" inflammatory diseases including sarcoidosis, primary or secondary angiitis of the CNS (PACNS), and systemic vasculitis. Sarcoidosis is a multisystem, chronic, noncaseating granulomatous disease of uncertain cause, which can involve the CNS with symptoms in 5% to 15%.[63,64] Restricted diffusion rarely occurs in patients with sarcoidosis and can result from ischemic lesions related to leptomeningeal disease, small or large vessel vasculitis, emboli from cardiac involvement, and/or hypercoagulable states.[63,64]

Restricted diffusion can be seen at sites of acute ischemic stroke related to the primary or secondary vasculitis.[65,66] Systemic angiitis of the CNS can also result from infections, neoplasms, toxins, or drugs.[65,66] As with PACNS, restricted diffusion can be seen at sites of acute stroke.[65,66]

Hypereosinophilic syndrome occurs when there is abnormal accumulation of eosinophils in blood or various tissues that can result from parasitic infections, eosinophilic granulomatosis with polyangiitis (Churg Strauss syndrome), pneumonia, gastrointestinal disorders, medications, antibiotics, and myeloid malignancies.[67] Neurologic complications of hypereosinophilia include arterial thrombosis with acute cerebral infarction or border zone strokes cause by global hypoperfusion.[67]

Genetic Mutations Affecting Metabolism

CADASIL (Cerebral Autosomal-dominant Arteriopathy with Sub-cortical Infarcts and Leukoencephalopathy) is an inherited angiopathy of small and medium-sized arteries from mutations involving the *NOTCH3* gene on chromosome *19q12*. With MRI, multiple zones of high signal on T2WI and FLAIR are seen involving the subcortical and periventricular white matter, basal ganglia, thalami, and brainstem, usually without restricted diffusion unless there is a recent ischemic event.[58,65]

Mitochondrial encephalopathies result from mutations of nuclear and/or mitochondrial DNA that can impair oxidative phosphorylation and metabolism resulting in ischemia.[68–74] The MRI findings are variable depending on the specific mutation, metabolic defect, and patient age.[68] These disorders include MELAS (mitochondrial myopathy, encephalopathy, lactic acidosis, and strokelike episodes), Leigh syndrome, Kearns-Sayre syndrome, and Alpers syndrome. With MRI, high signal on T2WI and FLAIR can occur in the basal ganglia, thalami, cerebral and cerebellar cortex, and/or subcortical white matter with restricted diffusion depending on the timing of impaired oxidative metabolism[68–74] (**Fig. 28**). Findings typically do not correspond to a specific large arterial vascular territory.

Urea cycle disorders result from dysfunction of one of the enzymes that normally convert

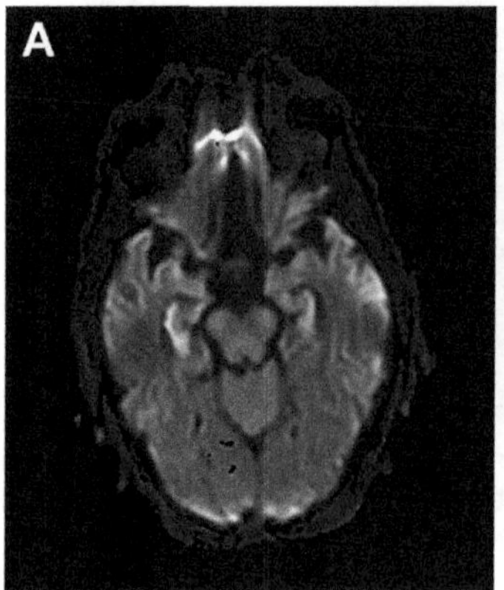

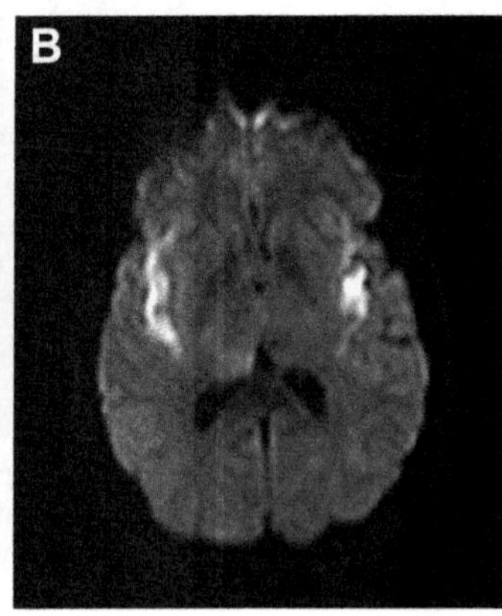

Fig. 27. A 63-year-old man with a paraneoplastic autoimmune encephalitis related to lymphoma who has restricted diffusion involving the hippocampi bilaterally on axial DWI (*A*). A 49-year-old man with postviral, non-paraneoplastic autoimmune encephalitis who has restricted diffusion involving the insular cortex bilaterally on axial DWI (*B*).

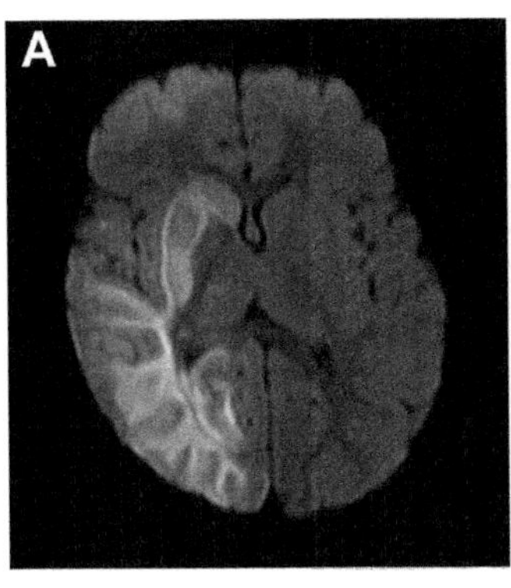

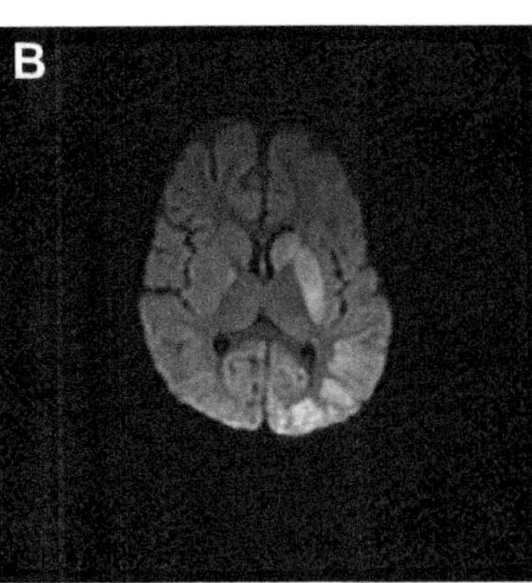

Fig. 28. A 1-year-old girl with MELAS who has restricted diffusion involving the right caudate, putamen, cerebral cortex, and white matter of the right temporal and occipital lobes on axial DWI (*A*). Axial DWI 2 weeks later shows new restricted diffusion involving the left caudate nucleus, putamen, and occipital cerebral cortex, and near-complete interval resolution of the DWI signal abnormalities involving the right cerebral hemisphere (*B*).

ammonia to urea.[75,76] The affected enzymes include ornithine transcarbamylase, carbamoyl phosphate synthetase 1, or arginosuccinate lyase. Patients typically present in the first week of life with difficulty feeding, emesis, hyperpnea, hypothermia, and lethargy.[75,76] The clinical findings are associated with elevated serum levels of ammonia, glutamine, and respiratory alkalosis.[75,76] With MRI, there is generalized cerebral edema with increased signal on T2WI and FLAIR involving the cerebral cortex, subcortical white matter, and lentiform nuclei.[75,76] Restricted diffusion can be seen at the involved sites secondary to cytotoxic edema[75,76] (**Fig. 29**).

Organic acidemias and aminoacidopathies are autosomal recessive metabolic diseases that result in abnormal accumulation of various organic acids and amino acids in the brain and other tissues.[77] These excess organic acids and amino acids can be detected in blood (acidemia) or urine (aciduria). These disorders cause toxic accumulation of metabolites resulting in mitochondrial dysfunction, ketoacidosis, and/or hyperammonemia, as well as alteration of normal myelin formation. The organic acidemias include glutaryl acidemia types 1 and 2, methylmalonic acidemia, propionic acidemia, isovaleric acidemia, multiple carboxylase deficiency, beta-ketothiolase deficiency, Canavan disease, and 5-oxoprolinuria.[77] In children with glutaric acidemia/aciduria type 1, restricted diffusion can be seen in the bilateral striatum with acute encephalopathy.[77] In neonates with methylmalonic acidemia, acute changes include diffuse increased signal on T2WI, and decreased diffusion, without or with infarctions of the globus pallidi.[77] In neonates and infants with propionic acidemia acute changes include diffuse increased signal on T2WI, and decreased diffusion. In older patients, increased signal on T2WI and FLAIR with restricted diffusion are often seen in the basal ganglia[77] (**Fig. 30**).

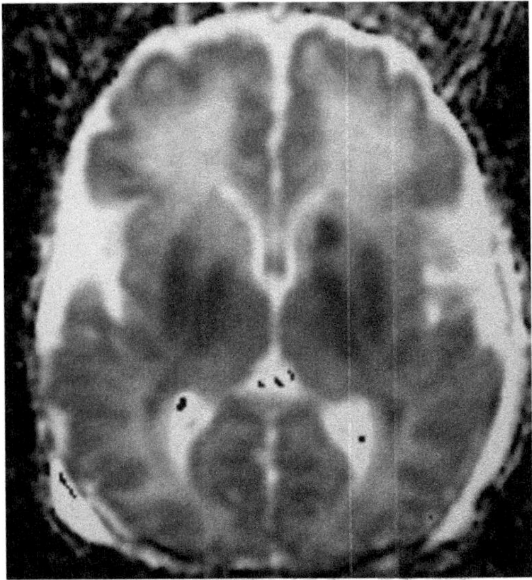

Fig. 29. A 9-day-old boy with ornithine transcarbamylase deficiency and hyper-ammonemia causing restricted diffusion in the left caudate nucleus, putamina, and thalami on axial ADC.

The aminoacidopathies are autosomal recessive diseases that result from deficient or dysfunctional enzymes or transporters necessary for normal metabolism of amino acids.[77] These diseases include maple syrup urine disease (MSUD), phenylketonuria, tyrosinemia, glycine encephalopathy, homocystinuria, and sulfite oxidase deficiency.[77] Restricted diffusion can be seen with metabolic decompensation related to ketoacidosis, hyper-excitatory neural effects, and ischemia (**Fig. 31**).

ACQUIRED METABOLIC DISORDERS

Severe hypoglycemia is defined as plasma glucose levels less than 40 mg/dL. Hypoglycemia (less than 20 mg/dL) for more than 4 hours results in irreversible brain injury.[78,79] Causes include

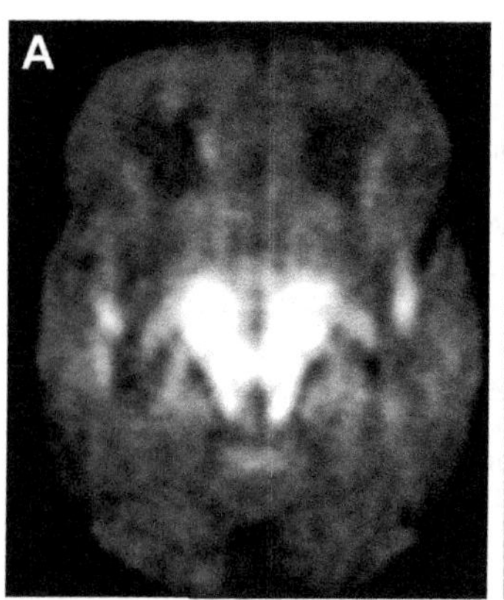

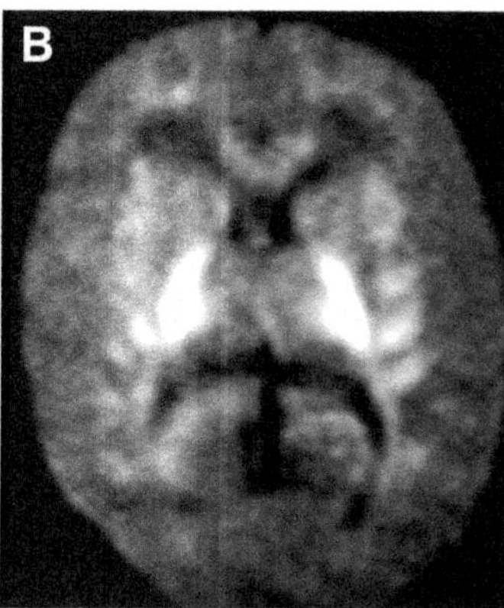

Fig. 30. A 1-week-old male neonate with methylmalonic acidemia and metabolic decompensation with acute toxicity. Restricted diffusion is seen in the brainstem, internal capsules, thalami and cerebral white matter on axial DWI (*A*, *B*).

overdose of insulin or other medications used by diabetic patients, insulin-secreting tumors, Addison disease, severe sepsis, and hepatic or renal failure.[49,70,78–80] Severe prolonged hypoglycemia can result in coma and death. Lack of adequate glucose can result in impaired oxidative brain metabolism leading to massive release of excitatory amino acid neurotransmitters such as aspartate causing cytotoxic edema involving neuronal and glial cells, which can progress to cell death.[49,70,78,79] Hypoglycemia is also associated with increased extracellular glutamate that can result in cellular apoptosis.[70] With MRI zones, with abnormal increased signal on T2WI, FLAIR, and restricted diffusion involving the brain (cerebral cortex, hippocampi, internal capsules, basal ganglia, cerebral peduncles, pons) can occur, which may be unilateral, bilateral symmetric or asymmetric[5,49,70,71,78–80] (**Fig. 32**). Timely correction of hypoglycemia can result in resolution of restricted diffusion within minutes. In neonates with severe hypoglycemia, restricted diffusion is

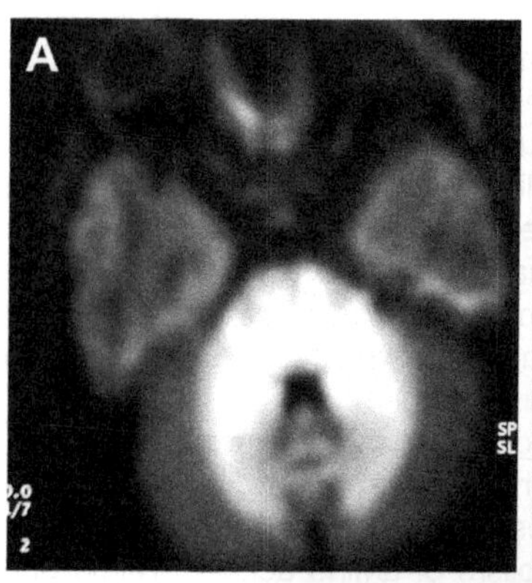

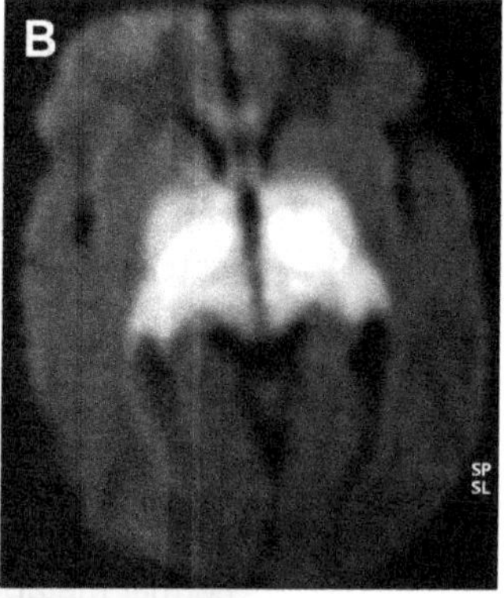

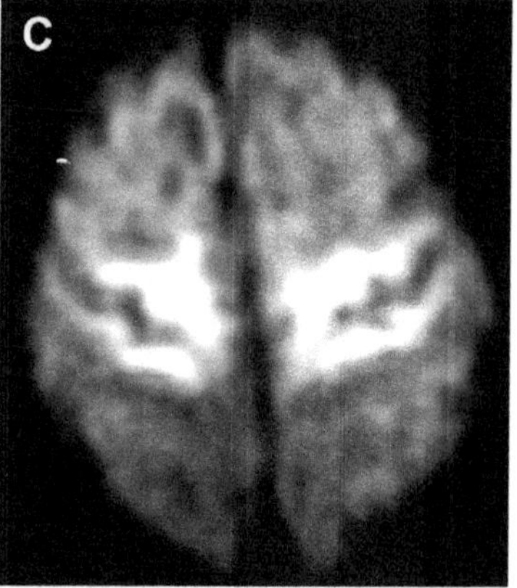

Fig. 31. A 2-week-old girl with MSUD and metabolic decompensation with restricted diffusion in the brainstem, middle cerebellar peduncles, cerebellar white matter, thalami, internal capsules, and pre- and post-central gyri on axial DWI (*A*, *B*, *C*).

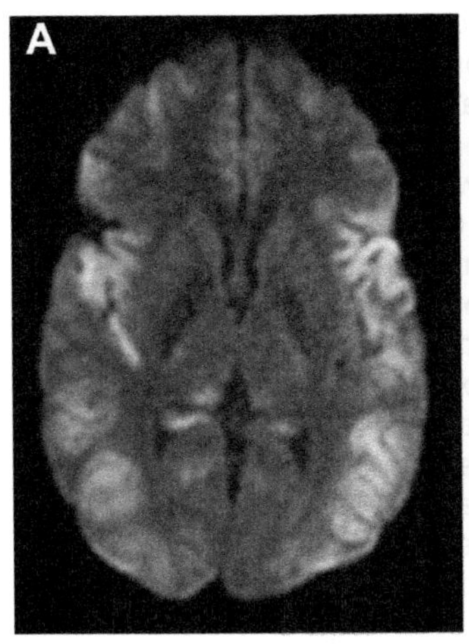

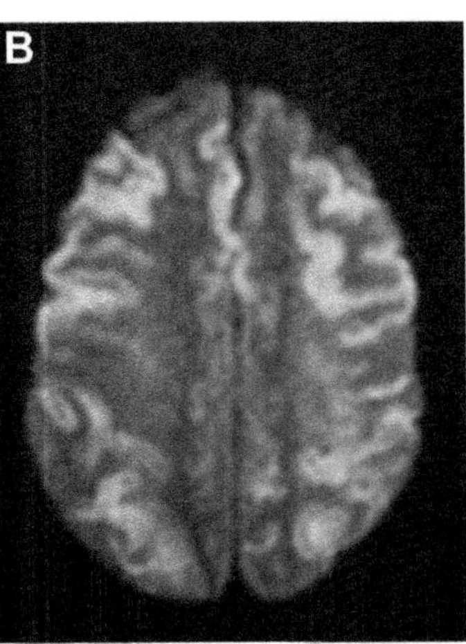

Fig. 32. DWI of a 42-year-old man with prolonged hypoglycemia shows restricted diffusion involving the cerebral cortex bilaterally (*A, B*).

often observed involving the parietal and occipital cerebral cortex as well as the corpus callosum, cortico-spinal tracts, and deep gray nuclei.[79]

Hyperammonemic encephalopathy occurs from elevated serum ammonia levels which can result from acute liver failure or with or without chronic liver disease, sepsis, portosystemic shunts, and drug toxicity.[49,70,78,80] Adverse effects from hyperammonemia occur from excess glutamine accumulation with associated impaired cerebral osmoregulation, and glutamate/NMDA receptor activation resulting in excitotoxic injury and energy deficit.[70,78] With MRI, symmetric zones with restricted diffusion can be seen in the cingulate and insular cerebral cortex bilaterally and basal ganglia[49,70,78,80] (**Fig. 33**).

Pontine and extra-pontine osmotic myelinolysis is an acute demyelinating disorder that can result from rapid correction of hyponatremia in chronically ill, malnourished or alcoholic patients.[49,58,80,81] Other comorbidities include diabetes mellitus, hepatitis, liver transplantation, chronic disease of the lungs, liver, and/or kidneys. Osmotic injury to the endothelium results in edema and release of toxins resulting in macrophage infiltration, loss of oligodendrocytes and myelin without initial destruction of axons or neuronal cell bodies.[49,58,80,81] Patients usually present with encephalopathy from hyponatremia followed by rapid resolution after correction of serum sodium levels.[80,81] With MRI, a poorly defined zone of high signal on T2WI and FLAIR is seen in the central portion of the pons with sparing of the cortico-spinal tracts and ventrolateral portions of the pons. In the acute phase, transient restricted diffusion and contrast enhancement can be seen[49,58,80,81] (**Fig. 34**). Extra-pontine sites of involvement include the cerebellum, middle cerebellar peduncles, midbrain, lateral geniculate bodies, cerebral white matter, extreme and external capsules, basal ganglia, and thalami.[80,81]

Seizures lasting more than 5 minutes are associated with abnormal neuronal homeostasis and cytotoxic edema, which can be detected with DWI[70,71,78,82] (**Fig. 35**). Seizures lasting more than 30 minutes are associated with irreversible

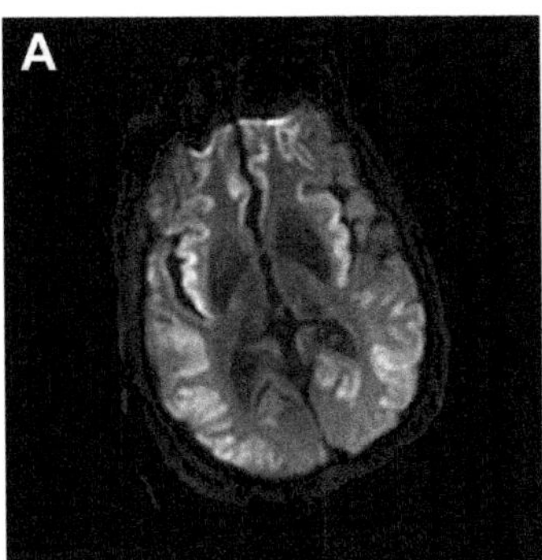

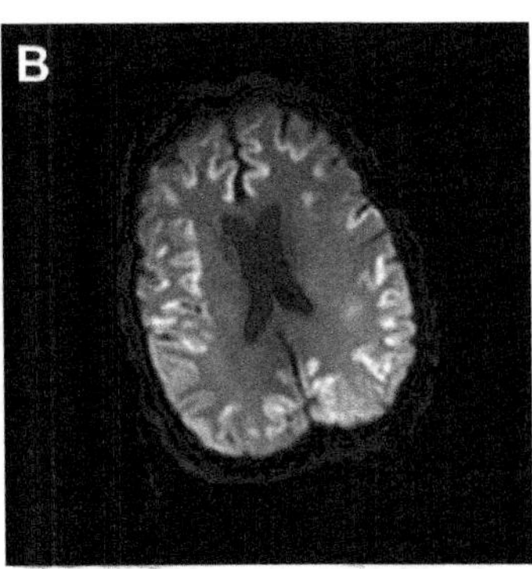

Fig. 33. DWI of a 57-year-old man with hyperammonemic encephalopathy related to liver failure shows symmetric zones with restricted diffusion involving the cerebral cortex bilaterally (*A, B*).

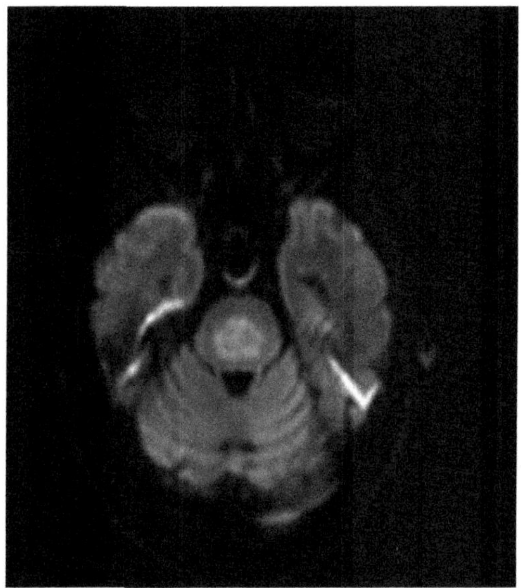

Fig. 34. A 58-year-old woman with osmotic myelinolysis involving the central portion of the pons that has restricted diffusion on axial DWI.

neuronal injury.[82] MRI abnormalities are often bilateral in patients with generalized seizures and status epilepticus; and unilateral for patients with partial complex seizures.[70,71,82]

TOXIC OR DRUG EXPOSURES

Carbon monoxide is a colorless and odorless gas, which often results from incomplete combustion of fuels.[49,58,80] Carbon monoxide has a 200-fold greater binding capability to heme protein compared with oxygen, and results in tissue hypoxia when inhaled. Acute toxic effects can be seen as restricted diffusion and increased signal on FLAIR and T2WI involving both globus pallidi, as well as the cerebral cortex, hippocampus, amygdala, white matter, midbrain, and cerebellum[49,80] (**Fig. 36**A). Several weeks after exposure to carbon monoxide, late effects include demyelination and necrosis of white matter that are seen as poorly defined zones of increased signal on T2WI and FLAIR with restricted diffusion[49,58,80] (**Fig. 36**B).

Alcohol is a widespread, commonly abused drug, which can cause direct and indirect functional and structural alterations in the brain.[49,83,84] A complication of chronic alcohol abuse is the nutritional deficiency of thiamine resulting in Wernicke encephalopathy (confusion, ocular paresis and nystagmus, and gait disturbances).[49,83,84] In the acute phases of Wernicke encephalopathy, contrast enhancement and restricted diffusion can be seen in the medial portions of the thalami, mammillary bodies, tectal plate, periaqueductal tissue, and floor of the fourth ventricle.[49,83,84]

Methanol is a colorless clear liquid, which is often used in solvents, antifreeze, windshield wiper fluid, paint removers, perfumes, and rubbing alcohol.[49,85] Ingested methanol is metabolized into highly toxic formaldehyde and formic acid, which results in severe metabolic acidosis with associated neurologic dysfunction that can lead to blindness, coma, and death if not treated promptly.[49,85] With MRI, bilateral symmetric necrosis of the putamina is commonly seen with increased signal on T2WI and FLAIR without or with associated hemorrhage.[49,85] Signal abnormalities can also be seen in the globus pallidi, subcortical white matter, cerebellum, brainstem, optic nerves.[49,85] Restricted diffusion can be seen at the involved sites in the acute phases.[49,85]

Ethylene glycol is a dihydroxyl alcohol and is a common component of antifreeze. Once ingested, this clear, colorless, and odorless fluid is rapidly absorbed, causing cerebral edema, seizures, severe encephalopathy, and Parkinsonian syndrome.[85,86] Ethylene glycol is metabolized by alcohol dehydrogenase and aldehyde dehydrogenase into glyoxylic acid, glycolaldehyde, glycolic acid and oxalic acid.[85,86] Glycolic acid causes a metabolic acidosis and oxalic acid binds soluble calcium forming calcium oxalate crystals that are

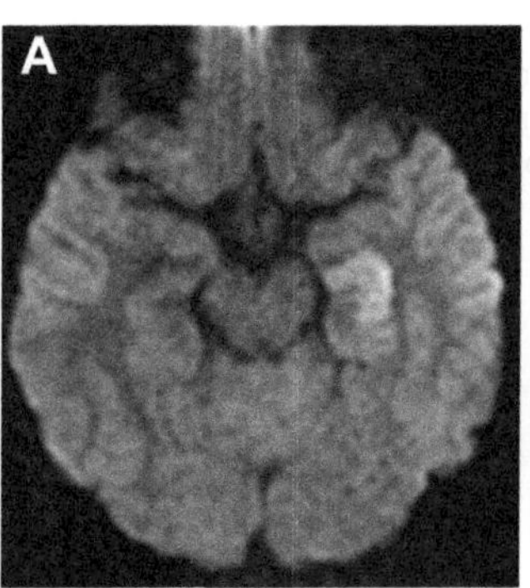

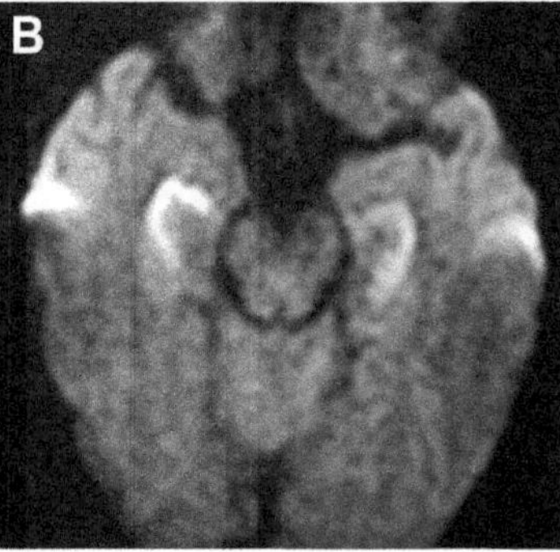

Fig. 35. DWI of a 12-year-old boy with recent partial complex seizure who has restricted diffusion involving the left hippocampus (*A*). DWI of a 48-year-old man with recent status epilepticus shows restricted diffusion involving both hippocampi (*B*).

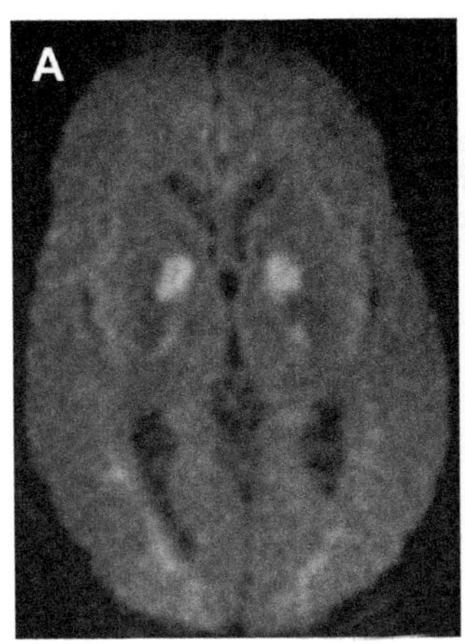

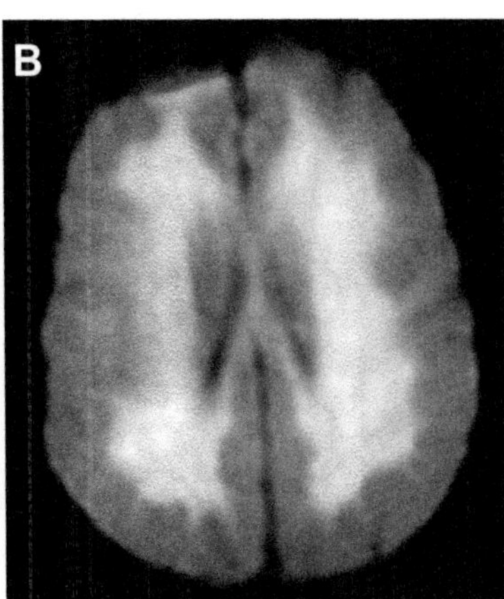

Fig. 36. A 42-year-old man with acute carbon monoxide toxicity who has restricted diffusion involving the globus pallidi on axial DWI (*A*). A 50-year-old woman with delayed demyelination and necrosis involving the cerebral white matter after carbon monoxide exposure, which is seen as extensive, poorly defined zones with restricted diffusion on axial DWI (*B*).

deposited in various tissue such the kidney, brain, liver, spleen, and lungs, with associated progressive multiorgan failure if not treated promptly.[85,86] Early treatment with bicarbonate, fomepizole and hemodialysis is required for optimal recovery.[85,86] With MRI, bilateral symmetric zones with abnormal increased signal on T2WI and FLAIR are seen in the basal ganglia, thalami, hippocampi, amygdala, brainstem, middle cerebellar peduncles, cerebral cortex, cerebral white matter including the corpus callosum, and internal capsules.[85,86] Corresponding restricted diffusion can be seen at the involved sites.[85,86]

Cocaine is a commonly abused drug that can be inhaled as powdered cocaine hydrochloride through nasal mucous membranes or as a vapor in the alkaloid combined form of cocaine hydrochloride with sodium bicarbonate or ammonia ("crack cocaine"). Cocaine blocks the reuptake of monoamines, which is associated with vasospasm, vasoconstriction, acute hypertension, tachycardia, enhanced platelet aggregation, and vasculitis.[80,84,87] Cocaine-induced vasospasm and vasculitis can be associated with intra-axial and/or subarachnoid hemorrhage, ischemic and hemorrhagic infarction. Cocaine can also produce a toxic encephalopathy from direct toxic effects after intravenous or inhalational use or secondary to contamination with levamisole.[80,84,87] With MRI, lesions with increased signal intensity on T2WI and FLAIR can be seen in the globus pallidi, splenium of the corpus callosum, and thalami, or related to infarcts in arterial territories or watershed vascular distribution zones in white matter.[80,84,87] Acute infarcts related to cocaine abuse typically have associated restricted diffusion.[80,84,87] In addition, multifocal leukoencephalopathy can be seen as poorly defined zones with increased signal on T2WI and FLAIR in the cerebral white matter, which can have restricted diffusion.[87] Intra-axial hemorrhage associated with cocaine abuse often occurs in the basal ganglia and thalami.[84]

Heroin is a drug derived from opium that has euphoric and analgesic effects when administered orally, intravenously, or by inhalation.[49,80,88,89] Intravenous heroin is associated with vasospasm, immune-mediated vasculitis, and embolism that can result in brain infarcts.[49,84] Inhalation of heroin vapors containing a lipophilic compound ("chasing the dragon") can cross through the blood-brain barrier and result in a toxic spongiform leukoencephalopathy.[49,84,88,89] Toxic leukoencephalopathy can also occur after intravenous heroin.[49,84,88,89] The onset of toxic leukoencephalopathy can occur soon after administration of heroin, or be delayed and/or progressive after exposure.[84] Inhalation of heroin vapor can result in symmetric abnormal increased signal on T2WI and FLAIR involving the cerebral and cerebellar white matter, middle cerebellar peduncles, brainstem, and/or internal capsules, without associated abnormal Gd-contrast enhancement. In the acute phase of spongiform leukoencephalopathy, restricted diffusion can be seen at the involved sites related to cytotoxic and intramyelinic edema[49,84,89] (**Fig. 37**).

Amphetamines and derivatives are frequently abused drugs that produce short-term periods of euphoria as well as increased alertness and energy.[80,84] These effects result from elevated levels of neurotransmitters, such as dopamine, norepinephrine, and serotonin.[84] Adverse effects include vasospasm and arteritis that can cause acute ischemia and stroke detected with MRI.[80,84] MDMA (3,4-methylenedioxymethamphetamine) is an amphetamine derivative (also referred to as "Ecstasy") that has stimulating and hallucinatory effects for 48 hours.[80,84] Adverse effects are related to elevated release of the vasoconstrictor 5-hydroxytryptamine, which can cause prolonged

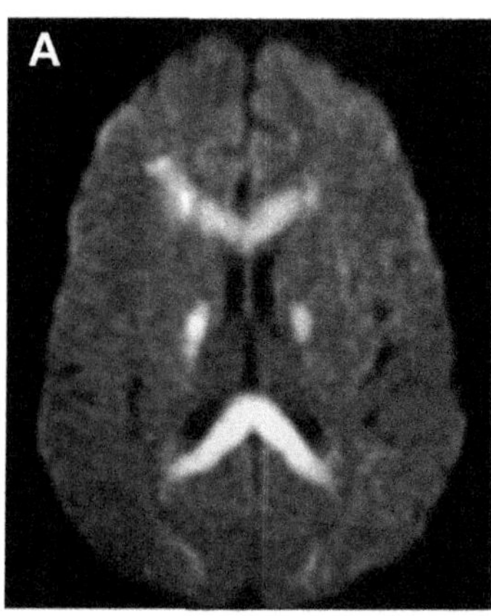
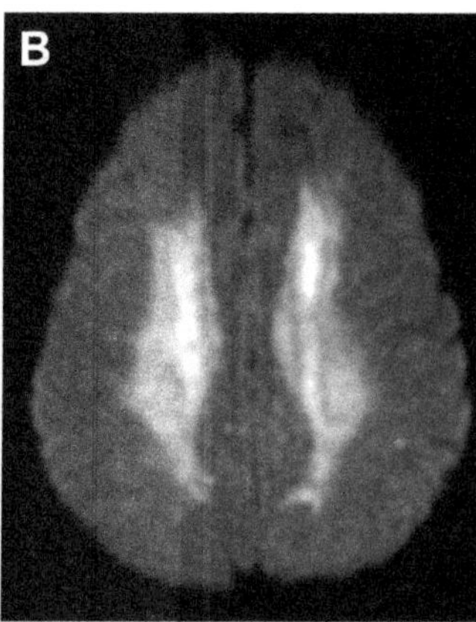

Fig. 37. Toxic leukoencephalopathy after inhalation of heroin vapor as seen as restricted diffusion involving the cerebral white matter including the internal capsules and corpus callosum on axial DWI (*A, B*).

vasospasm leading to acute ischemia involving the cerebral cortex and globus pallidi.[84]

Methotrexate is a chemotherapeutic medication that inhibits normal DNA replication by inhibiting the enzyme dihydrofolate reductase.[5,49,84,88,90] Methotrexate is commonly administered intravenously, and has also been given intrathecally for treatment of acute leukemia and lymphoblastic lymphoma within the CNS.[5,83,88,90] Adverse effects involving the brain include reversible cytotoxic and intramyelinic edema in the white matter seen with DWI that is related to dose, frequency, and route of administration.[5,83,88,90] Acute leukoencephalopathy can occur days to weeks after high dose and/or intrathecal administration.[5,49,84,88,90] Other chemotherapeutic drugs associated with delayed acute leukoencephalopathy include 5-fluorouracil, carmofur, and capecitabine[90]

TUMORS AND TUMORLIKE LESIONS

Intra-axial neoplasms can have varying diffusion characteristics based on the degree of tumor cellularity, nuclear to cytoplasmic ratios of neoplastic cells, regions of tumor hypoxia, tumoral cysts and/or necrosis, regions of viscous or mucinous degeneration, and relative proportion of the intracellular space to the extracellular space.[4,90,91] Reduced apparent diffusion coefficients in neoplasms have been shown to be related to the volume of the intracellular space relative to the extracellular space.[4,90,91] Malignant intra-axial tumors with high cellularity and high nuclear to cytoplasmic ratios often have low ADC values and include neoplasms such as embryonal tumors of the CNS (medulloblastoma, atypical teratoid/rhabdoid tumor, pineoblastoma), lymphoma, high-grade gliomas, as well as lower grade tumors such as central neurocytoma[4,90–92] (**Fig. 38**). Primary brain tumors or metastases with mucinous degeneration can also have restricted diffusion.[91]

Low ADC values can occur in extra-axial tumors such as meningiomas, lymphoma, and metastatic tumors.[93] Some meningiomas have restricted diffusion related to high cellularity and/or fibrous content. High-grade meningiomas tend to have lower ADC values compared with lower grade meningiomas, which can have prognostic value[93] (see **Fig. 38**F).

Epidermoid cysts are non-neoplastic, ectoderm-lined inclusion cysts that contain only squamous epithelium, desquamated skin epithelial cells, and keratin. These lesions result from persistence of ectodermal elements at sites of neural tube closure and suture closure. With MRI, epidermoid cysts typically have low-intermediate signal on T1WI, high signal on T2WI, and mixed low, intermediate and/or high signal on FLAIR.[94] These lesions characteristically have restricted diffusion and lack contrast enhancement[94] (**Fig. 39**).

RADIATION INJURY

Fractionated radiation therapy for tumors can result in increased extent of signal abnormality and contrast enhancement at the site of the treated neoplasm, which can be secondary to radiation necrosis or recurrent or worsening residual tumor.[95,96] DWI may be useful for some situations in distinguishing between radiation necrosis and recurrent tumor.[95,96] Cell necrosis and liquefaction associated with radiation necrosis can have facilitated diffusion, whereas recurrent tumors with high cellularity can have restricted diffusion.[95] In patients treated with stereotactic radiosurgery, DWI combined with contrast-enhanced perfusion imaging can show a 3-layer pattern for radiation necrosis with high specificity, which consists of an inner nonenhancing layer of

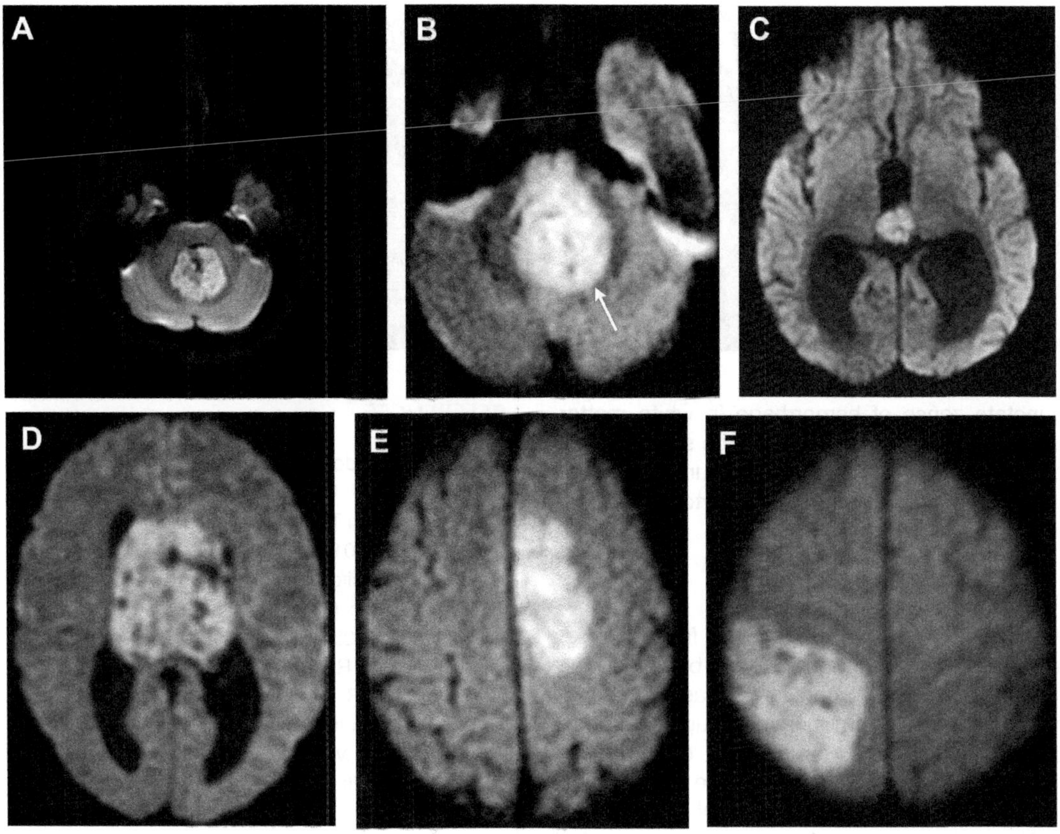

Fig. 38. Axial DWI shows restricted diffusion in tumors such as medulloblastoma involving the cerebellar vermis (*A*), atypical teratoid/rhabdoid tumor (*arrow*) (*B*), pineoblastoma (*C*), central neurocytoma involving the septum pellucidum (*D*), lymphoma (*E*), and malignant meningioma (*F*).

increased ADC from a liquefied center, a middle transitional nonenhancing layer with low ADC from high viscosity, and a peripheral contrast-enhancing layer from active inflammation.[96] This 3-layer pattern had high specificity in diagnosing radiation necrosis.[96]

TRAUMATIC BRAIN INJURIES

Diffuse axonal injury results from differences in linear and rotational accelerations of the superficial portions of the brain compared with the underlying deep brain structures.[88] In addition to

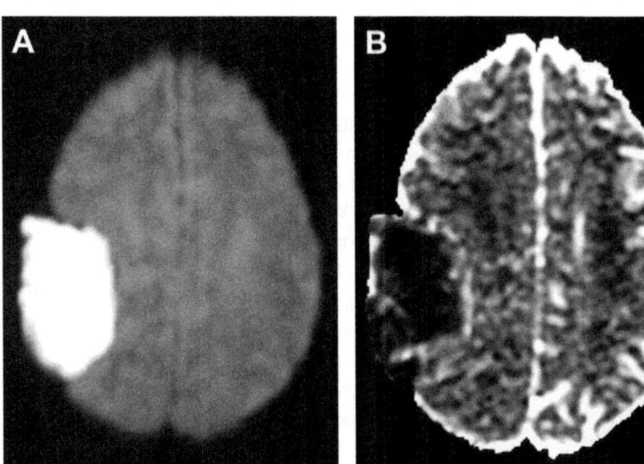

Fig. 39. A 39-year-old man with an epidermoid in the right side of the skull associated with intracranial and extracranial extension through eroded bone. The lesion has restricted diffusion on axial DWI (*A*) and ADC (*B*).

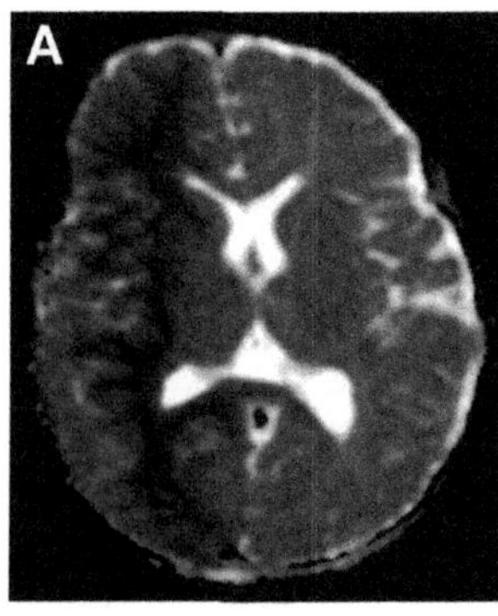

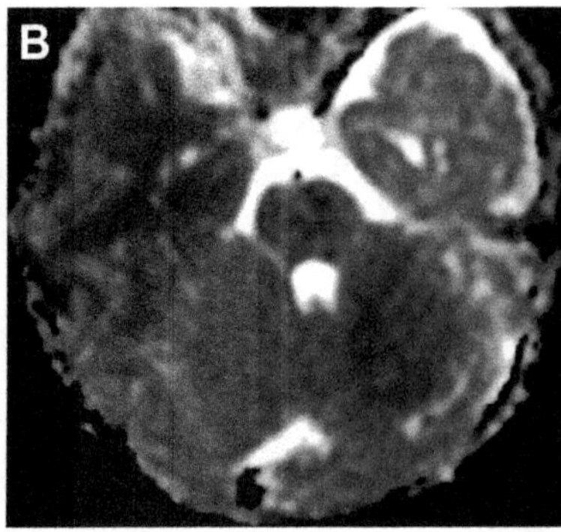

Fig. 40. A 9-month-old girl with a large recent infarct in the right cerebral hemisphere with restricted diffusion on axial ADC (*A*) associated with acute-phase crossed cerebellar diaschisis seen as restricted diffusion in the left cerebellar hemisphere on axial ADC (*B*).

punctate zones of hemorrhage in white matter, zones of restricted diffusion can be seen at some of the lesions secondary to traumatic axonal stretching, and intramyelinic and cytotoxic edema from membrane depolarization.[88]

DENERVATION

Wallerian degeneration results from injuries involving proximal portions and cell bodies of neurons, which causes progressive phases of axonal degeneration.[97] Such injuries include infarction, trauma, hemorrhage, neoplasms, or surgery.[97] Damage proximal to or involving the corticospinal tracts can result in increased signal on T2WI and FLAIR with corresponding transient restricted diffusion.[97] Wallerian degeneration can also result from disruption of the pontocerebellar tract with MRI findings of symmetric high signal on T2WI and FLAIR in both middle cerebellar peduncles, and restricted diffusion in the early phases.[97]

Crossed cerebellar diaschisis refers to the disruption of the cerebro-ponto-cerebellar pathway connecting the cerebral cortex to the contralateral middle cerebellar peduncle and cerebellar hemisphere via pontine nuclei.[98] Disruption of this pathway results from infarction, hemorrhage, neoplasm and/or seizures involving the affected cerebral hemisphere.[98] Disconnection of afferent associative, sensory, para-limbic and motor input into the cerebro-pontine-cerebellar pathway causes decreased synaptic cerebellar Purkinje function combined with hypo-metabolism.[98] In the acute phase, restricted diffusion and decreased perfusion can be seen in both a cerebellar hemisphere and contralateral cerebral hemisphere (**Fig. 40**). Progressive unilateral atrophy of a cerebellar hemisphere that is contralateral to a cerebral abnormality is typically seen.

DISCLOSURE

The author has no commercial or financial conflicts of interest, or funding sources.

REFERENCES

1. De Figueiredo E, Borgonovi A, Doring TM. Basic concepts of MR imaging, diffusion MR imaging and Diffusion Tensor imaging. Magn Reson Imaging Clin N Am 2011;19:1–22.
2. Yang E, Nucifora PG, Melhem ER. Diffusion MR imaging: basic principles. Neuroimaging Clin N Am 2011;21:11–25.
3. De Carvalho Rangel C, Cuz LCH, Takayasu TC, et al. Diffusion MR imaging in central nervous system. Magn Reson Imaging Clin N Am 2011;19:22–53.
4. Drake-Pérez M, Boto J, Fitsiori A, et al. Clinical applications of diffusion weighted imaging in neuroradiology. Insights into Imaging 2018;9(4):535–47.
5. Carney O, Falzon A, MacKinnon AD. Diffusion-weighted imaging in paediatric neuroimaging. Clin Radiol 2018;73:999–1013.
6. Chao CP, Zaleski CG, Patton AC. Neonatal hypoxic ischemic encephalopathy: multimodality imaging findings. RadioGraphics 2006;26:S159–72.
7. Huang BY, Castillo M. Hypoxic ischemic brain injury: imaging findings from birth to adulthood. Radiographics 2008;28:417–39.
8. Heinz ER, Provenzale JM. Imaging findings in neonatal hypoxia: a practical review. AJR Am J Roentgenol 2009;192:41–7.
9. Ghei SK, Zan E, Nathan JE, et al. MR imaging of hypoxic ischemic injury in term neonates: pearls and pitfalls. Radiographics 2014;34:1047–61.
10. Hayakawa K, Koshino S, Tanda K, et al. Diffusion pseudonormalization and clinical outcome in term neonates with hypoxic-ischemic encephalopathy. Pediatr Radiol 2018;48:865–74.
11. Muttikkal TJE, Wintermark M. MRI patterns of global hypoxic-ischemic injury in adults. J Neuroradiol 2013;40:164–71.
12. Kimchi TJ, Agid R, Lee SK, et al. Arterial ischemic stroke in children. Neuroimaging Clin N Am 2007;17:175–87.
13. Wessels T, Wessels C, Ellsiepen A, et al. Contribution of diffusion-weighted imaging in determination of stroke etiology. AJNR Am J Neuroradiol 2006;27:35–9.

14. Wessels T, Rottger C, Jauss M, et al. Identification of embolic stroke patterns by diffusion weighted MRI in clinically defined lacunar stroke syndromes. Stroke 2005;36:757–61.
15. Ha J, Le MJ, Kim SJ, et al. Prevalence and impact of venous and arterial thromboembolism in patients with embolic stroke of undetermined source with or without active cancer. J Am Heart Assoc 2019;8:e013215.
16. Ghoneim A, Straiton J, Pollard C, et al. Imaging of cerebral venous thrombosis. Clin Radiol 2020. https://doi.org/10.1016/j.crad.2019.12.009 [pii:S0009-9260(20)30002-30007].
17. Sadigh G, Mullins ME, Saindane AM. Diagnostic performance of MRI sequences for evaluation of dural venous sinus thrombosis. AJR Am J Roentgenol 2016;206:1298–306.
18. Leach JL, Fortuna RB, Jones BV, et al. Imaging of cerebral venous thrombosis: current techniques, spectrum of findings, and diagnostic pitfalls. Radiographics 2006;26(Suppl 1):S19–41.
19. Yildiz ME, Ozcan UA, Turk A, et al. Diffusion-weighted MR imaging of cortical vein thrombosis at 3T. Clin Neuroradiol 2015;25:249–56.
20. Riddell IVJ, Shuman EK. Epidemiology of central nervous system infection. Neuroimaging Clin N Am 2012;22:543–56.
21. Shih RY, Koeller KK. Bacterial, fungal, and parasitic infections of the central nervous system: radiologic-pathologic correlation and historical perspectives. Radiographics 2015;35:1141–69.
22. Shih RY, Koeller KK. Central nervous system lesions in immunocompromised patients. Radiol Clin N Am 2019;57:1217–31.
23. Mohan S, Jain KK, Arabi M, et al. Imaging of meningitis and ventriculitis. Neuroimaging Clin N Am 2012; 22:557–83.
24. Saberi A, Roudbary SA, Ghayeghran A, et al. Diagnosis of meningitis caused by pathogenic microorganisms using magnetic resonance imaging: a systematic review. Basic Clin Neurosci 2018;9:73–86.
25. Gasparetto EL, Cabral RF, Hygino da Cruz LC, et al. Diffusion imaging in brain infections. Neuroimaging Clin N Am 2011;21:89–113.
26. Lundy P, Kaufman C, Garcia D, et al. Intracranial subdural empyemas and epidural abscesses in children. J Neurosurg Pediatr 2019;22(24):14–21.
27. Parmar H, Ibrahim M. Pediatric intracranial infections. Neuroimaging Clin N Am 2012;22:707–25.
28. Rath TJ, Hughes M, Arabi M, et al. Imaging of cerebritis, encephalitis, and brain abscesses. Neuroimaging Clin N Am 2012;22:585–607.
29. Askoz A, Mukundan S, Lee TC. Imaging of Rickettsial, spirochetal, and parasitic infections. Neuroimaging Clin N Am 2012;22:633–57.
30. Mathur M, Johnson CE, Sze G. Fungal infections of the central nervous system. Neuroimaging Clin N Am 2012;22:609–32.
31. Gaviani P, Schwartz RB, Hedley-Whyte ET, et al. Diffusion-weighted imaging of fungal cerebral infection. AJNR Am J Neuroradiol 2005;26:1115–21.
32. Handique SK. Viral infections of the central nervous system. Neuroimaging Clin N Am 2011;21:777–94.
33. Koeller KK, Shih RY. Viral and prion infections of the central nervous system: radiologic-pathologic correlation. Radiographics 2017;37:199–233.
34. Maller VV, Bathla G, Moritani T, et al. Imaging in viral infections of the central nervous system: can images speak for an acutely ill brain? Emerg Radiol 2017;24: 287–300.
35. Moritani T, Capizzano A, Kirby P, et al. Viral infections and white matter lesions. Radiol Clin N Am 2014;52:355–82.
36. Renard T, Daumas-Duport B, Auffray-Calvier E, et al. Cytomegalovirus encephalitis: undescribed diffusion-weighted imaging characteristics. Original aspects of cases extracted from a retrospective study, and from literature review. J Neuroradiol 2016;43:371–7.
37. Jugpal TS, Dixit R, Garg A, et al. Spectrum of findings on magnetic resonance imaging of the brain in patients with neurological manifestations of dengue fever. Radiol Bras 2017;50:285–90.
38. Khatri H, Shah H, Roy D, et al. A case report on Chikungunya virus-associated encephalomyelitis. Case Rep Infect Dis 2018;4, 8904753.
39. Radmanesh A, Raz E, Zan E, et al. Brain imaging use and findings in COVD-19; a single academic center experience in the epicenter of disease in the United States. AJNR Am J Neuroradiol 2020. https://doi.org/10.3174/ajnr.A6610.
40. Rao A, Pimpalwar Y, Mukherjee A, et al. Serial brain MRI findings in a rare survivor of rabies encephalitis. Indian J Radiol Imaging 2017;27:286–9.
41. Lian ZY, Huang B, He SR, et al. Diffusion-weighted imaging in the diagnosis of enterovirus 71 encephalitis. Acta Radiol 2012;53:208–13.
42. Lian ZY, Li H, Zhang B, et al. Neuro-magnetic resonance imaging in hand, foot, and mouth disease: finding in 412 patients and prognostic features. J Comput Assist Tomogr 2017;41:861–7.
43. Chan DL, Young H, Palasanthiran P, et al. Fulminant subacute sclerosing panencephalitis: not only a disease of the past. J Paediatr Child Health 2018;54: 1264–7.
44. Dadak M, Pyl R, Lanfermann H, et al. Varying patterns of CNS imaging in influenza A encephalopathy in childhood. Clin Neuroradiol 2019. https://doi.org/10.1007/s00062-018-0756-3.
45. Britton PN, Dale RC, Blyth CC, et al. Influenza-associated encephalitis/encephalopathy identified by the Australian childhood encephalitis study 2013-2015. Pediatr Infect Dis 2017;36:1021–6.
46. Poyiadi N, Shahin G, Noujaim D, et al. COVID-19-associated acute hemorrhagic necrotizing

encephalopathy: CT and MRI features. Radiology 2020. https://doi.org/10.1148/radiol.2020201187.
47. Shi BC, Li J, Jang JW, et al. Mild encephalitis/encephalopathy with a reversible splenial lesion secondary to encephalitis complicated by hyponatremia. A case report and literature review. Medicine 2019;98:47.
48. Qing Y, Xiong W, Da-xiang H, et al. Statistical analysis of the apparent diffusion coefficient in patients with clinically mild encephalitis/encephalopathy with a reversible splenial lesion indicates that the pathology extends beyond the visible lesions. Magn Reson Med Sci 2020;19:14–20.
49. deOliviera AM, Paulino MV, VieiraAPF, et al. Imaging patterns of toxic and metabolic brain disorders. Radiographics 2019;39:1672–95.
50. Weldauer S, Wagner M, Enkirch SJ, et al. CNS infections in immunoincompetent patients. Clin Neuroradiol 2020;30:9–25.
51. Igra MS, Paling D, Wattjes MP, et al. Multiple sclerosis update: use of MRI for early diagnosis, disease monitoring and assessment of treatment complications. Br J Radiol 2017;90:20160721.
52. Wattjes MP, Wijburg MT, van Eijk J, et al. Inflammatory natalizumab-associated PML: baseline characteristics, lesion evolution and relation with PML-IRIS. J Neurol Neurosurg Pschiatry 2018;89:535–41.
53. Fragoso DC, Gonçalves Filho AL, Pacheco FT, et al. Imaging of Creutzfeldt-Jakob disease: imaging patterns and their differential diagnosis. Radiographics 2017;37:234–57.
54. Razek AAA, Watcharakorn A, Castillo M. Parasitic diseases of the central nervous system. Neuroimaging Clin N Am 2011;21:815–41.
55. Santos GT, Leite CC, Marchado LR, et al. Reduced diffusion in neurocysticercosis: circumstances of appearance and possible natural history implications. AJNR Am J Neuroradiol 2013;34:310–6.
56. Schroeder PC, Post MJD, Oschatz E, et al. Analysis of the utility of diffusion-weighted MRI and apparent diffusion coefficient values in distinguishing central nervous system toxoplasmosis from lymphoma. Neuroradiology 2006;48:715–20.
57. Moghaddam SM, Birbeck GL, Taylor TE, et al. Diffusion-weighted MR imaging in a prospective cohort of children with cerebral malaria offers insights into pathophysiology and prognosis. AJNR Am J Neuroradiol 2019;40:1575–80.
58. Sarbu N, Shih RY, Jones RV, et al. White matter diseases with radiologic-pathologic correlation. Radiographics 2016;36:1426–47.
59. Razek AAKA, Elsebaie NA. Imaging of fulminant demyelinating disorders of the central nervous system. J Comput Assist Tomogr 2020;44:248–54.
60. Mabray MC, Cohen BA, Villanueva-Meyer JE, et al. Performance of apparent diffusion coefficient values and conventional MRI features in differentiating tumefactive demyelinating lesions from primary brain neoplasms. AJR Am J Roentgenol 2015;205:1075–85.
61. Dutra BG, José da Rocha A, Nunes RH, et al. Neuromyelitis optica spectrum disorders: spectrum of MR imaging findings and their differential diagnosis. Radiographics 2018;38:169–93.
62. Kelley BP, Patel SC, Marin HL, et al. Autoimmune encephalitis: pathophysiology and imaging review of an overlooked diagnosis. AJNR Am J Neuroradiol 2017;38:1070–8.
63. Spurgeon E, Abbatemarco J, Prayson R, et al. Neurosarcoidosis flare with multifocal restricted diffusion: stroke, inflammation or both? J Stoke Cerebrovasc Dis 2018;27:e230–2.
64. Hodge MH, Williams RL, Fukui MB. Neurosarcoidosis presenting as acute infarction on diffusion-weighted MR imaging: summary of radiologic findings. AJNR 2007;28:84–6.
65. Bersano A, Kraemer M, Burlina A, et al. Heritable and non-hereditable uncommon causes of stroke. J Neurol 2020. https://doi.org/10.1007/s00415-020-09836-x.
66. Soun JE, Song JW, Romero JM, et al. Central nervous system vasculopathies. Radiol Clin N Am 2019;1117–31.
67. Tong LS, Wan JP, Cai X, et al. Global hypoperfusion: a new explanation of border zone strokes in hypereosinophilia. CNS Neurosci Ther 2014;20:794–6.
68. Saneto R, Friedman SD, Shaw DWW. Neuroimaging of mitochondrial disease. Mitochondrion 2008;8:396–413.
69. Bhatia KD, Krishnan P, Kortman H, et al. Acute cortical lesions in MELAS syndrome: anatomic distribution, symmetry, and evolution. AJNR Am J Neuroradiol 2020;41:167–73.
70. Pai V, Sitoh YY, Purohit B. Gyriform restricted diffusion in adults: looking beyond thrombo-occlusions. Insights into Imaging 2020;11:20.
71. Adam G, Ferrier M, Patsoura S, et al. Magnetic resonance imaging of arterial stroke mimics: a pictorial review. Insights into Imaging 2018;9:815–31.
72. Bonfante E, Koenig MK, Adejumo RB, et al. The neuroimaging of Leigh syndrome: case series and review of the literature. Pediatr Radiol 2016;46:443–51.
73. Yu M, Wang QQ, Liu J, et al. Clinical and brain magnetic resonance imaging features in a cohort of Chinese patients with Kearns-Sayre syndrome. Chin Med J 2016;129:1419–24.
74. Hayhurst H, Anangnostou ME, Bogle HJ, et al. Dissecting the neuronal vulnerability underpinning Alpers' syndrome: a clinical and neuropathological study. Brain Pathol 2019;29(1):97–113.
75. Bireley WR, Van Hov JLK, Gallagher RC, et al. Urea cycle disorders: brain MRI and neurological outcome. Pediatr Radiol 2012;42:455–62.

76. Yu D, Lu G, Mowshica R, et al. Clinical and cranial MRI features of female patients with ornithine transcarbamylase deficiency. Medicine 2019;98:33.
77. Reddy N, Calloni SF, Vernon HJ, et al. Neuroimaging findings of organic acidemias and aminoacidopathies. Radiographics 2018;38:912–31.
78. Koksel Y, Benson J, Huang H, et al. Review of diffuse cortical injury on diffusion-weighted imaging in acutely encephalopathic patients with an acronym: CRUMPLED. Eur J Radiol Open 2018;5:194–201.
79. Bathia G, Policeni B, Agarwal A. Neuroimaging in patients with abnormal blood glucose levels. AJNR Am J Neuroradiol 2014;35:833–40.
80. Godinho MV, Pires CE, Hygino da Cruz LC Jr. Hypoxic, toxic and acquired metabolic encephalopathies at the emergency room: the role of magnetic resonance imaging. Semin Ultrasound CT MR 2018;39:481–94.
81. Alleman AM. Osmotic demyelination syndrome: central pontine myelinolysis and extrapontine myelinolysis. Semin Ultrasound CT MR 2014;35:153–9.
82. Williams JA, Bede P, Doherty CP. An exploration of the spectrum of peri-ictal MRI change: a comprehensive literature review. Seizure 2017;50:19–32.
83. Bathla G, Hegde AN. MRI and CT appearances in metabolic encephalopathies due to systemic diseases in adults. Clin Radiol 2013;68:545–54.
84. Tamrazi B, Almast J. Your brain on drugs: imaging of drug-related changes in the central nervous system. Radiographics 2012;32:701–9.
85. Sharma P, Eesa M, Scott JN. Toxic and acquired metabolic encephalopathies: MRI appearance. AJR Am J Roentgenol 2009;193:879–86.
86. Malhotra A, Mongelluzzo G, Wu X, et al. Ethylene glycol toxicity, MRI brain findings. Clin Neuroradiol 2017;27:109–13.
87. Vosoughi R, Schmidt BJ. Multifocal leukoencephalopathy in cocaine users: a report of the literature. BMC Neurol 2015;208. https://doi.org/10.1186/s12883-015-0467-1.
88. Citton V, Burlina A, Baracchini C, et al. Apparent diffusion coefficient restriction in the white matter: going beyond acute brain territorial ischemia. Insights Imaging 2012;3:155–64.
89. Achamallah N, Wright RS, Fried J. Chasing the wrong dragon: a new presentation of heroin-induced toxic leukoencephalopathy mimicking anoxic brain injury. J Intensive Care Soc 2019;20:80–5.
90. Baehring JM, Fulbright RK. Diffusion-weighted MRI in neuro-oncology. CNS Oncol 2012;1:155–67.
91. Villanueva-Meyer JE, Mabray MC, Cha S. Current clinical brain tumor imaging. Neurosurgery 2017;397–415.
92. Tlili-Graiess K, Mama N, Arifa N, et al. Diffusion weighted MR imaging and proton MR spectroscopy findings of central neurocytoma with pathological correlation. J Neuroradiol 2014;41:243–50.
93. Surov A, Ginat DT, Sanverdi E, al at. Use of diffusion weighted imaging in differentiating between benign and malignant meningiomas. A multicenter analysis. World Neurosurg 2016;88:598–602.
94. Hoang VT, Trinh CT, Nguyen CH, et al. Overview of epidermoid cyst. Eur J Radiol Open 2019;6:291–301.
95. Shah R, Vattoth S, Jacob R, et al. Radiation necrosis in the brain: imaging features and differentiation from tumor recurrence. Radiographics 2012;32:1343–59.
96. Cha J, Lim ST, Kim H-J, et al. Analysis of the layering pattern of apparent diffusion coefficient (ADC) for differentiation of radiation necrosis from tumor progression. Eur Radiol 2013;23:879–86.
97. DeVetten G, Coutts SB, Hill MD, et al. Acute corticospinal tract Wallerian degeneration is associated with stroke outcome. Stroke 2010;41:751–6.
98. Zaidi SA, ul Haq MA, Bindman D, et al. Crossed cerebellar diaschisis: a radiological finding in status epilepticus not to miss. BMJ Case Rep 2013. https://doi.org/10.1136/bcr-2013-200478.

Diffusion-Weighted Imaging is Key to Diagnosing Specific Diseases

Aya Midori Tokumaru, MD, PhD[a,*], Yuko Saito, MD, PhD[b], Shigeo Murayma, MD, PhD[b,c]

KEYWORDS

- Diffusion-weighted imaging • Creutzfeldt-Jakob disease
- Neuronal intranuclear inclusion body disease • Hereditary diffuse
- Leukoencephalopathy with spheroids-CSF1R

KEY POINTS

- Persistent hyperintensities on DWI of the brain are important findings, because they are often disease specific.
- The first important step in the diagnostic work-up is to locate the regions with persistent hyperintensity on DWI.
- Common patterns of hyperintensities on DWI by disease are as follows:
  - Sporadic Creutzfeldt Jacob disease: Cortex and basal ganglia.
  - Neuronal intranuclear inclusion disease: corticomedullary junction.
  - Hereditary diffuse leukoencephalopathy with spheroids CSFR1R/adult onset leukoencephalopathy with axonal spheroids and pigmented glia: around the ventricles and deep white matter.

INTRODUCTION

Diffusion-weighted imaging (DWI) is an magnetic resonance (MR) imaging method that is an indispensable part of the examination. It has well-established roles in the detection of acute ischemic stroke and the differentiation from other processes that manifest with sudden neurologic deficits.[1] However, DWI also provides adjunctive information for other diseases, including neoplasms, infections, trauma, metabolic disorders, neurodegenerative diseases, and demyelinating processes.[2–7] This review covers diseases for which persistent signal abnormalities on DWI are the key to their diagnosis, with discussion on the associated neuroimaging findings, clinical manifestations, and pathologic backgrounds (**Table 1**).

Persistent hyperintensities on DWI of the brain are important findings, because they often show a disease-specific pattern. The first important step is to locate the regions with a hyperintense signal on DWI. If the region is within the cortex and the patient has subacute cognitive impairment progression, Creutzfeldt-Jakob disease (CJD) should be considered as the initial diagnosis.[5,8] Intranuclear inclusion body disease (NIID) should be suspected if DWI reveals persistent hyperintensities in the corticomedullary junction. If hyperintensities are found in the middle cerebellar peduncles (MCPs) in addition to the corticomedullary junction, NIID and fragile X-associated tremor/ataxia syndrome (FXTAS) should be suspected.[9–11] Hereditary diffuse leukoencephalopathy with axonal spheroids (HDLS)–

[a] Department of Diagnostic Radiology, Tokyo Metropolitan Geriatric Hospital and Institute of Gerontology, 35-2 Sakae-cho, Itabashi-ku, Tokyo 173-0015, Japan; [b] Brain Bank for Aging Research, Tokyo Metropolitan Geriatric Hospital and Institute of Gerontology, 35-2 Sakae-cho, Itabashi-ku, Tokyo 173-0015, Japan; [c] Brain Bank for Neurodevelopmental, Neurological and Psychiatric Disorders, United Graduate School of Child Development, Osaka University, 2-2, Yamadaoka, Suita-shi, Osaka-fu 565-0871, Japan
* Corresponding author.
E-mail address: tokumaru@tmghig.jp

Magn Reson Imaging Clin N Am 29 (2021) 163–183
https://doi.org/10.1016/j.mric.2021.02.001
1064-9689/21/

Table 1
Differential diagnosis of the brain identifying persistent hyperintensity in diffusion-weighted imaging

Cortex	Corticomedullary Junction	Subcortical ~ Deep WM	MCP	Congenital Metabolic Disorders	Others
• CJD • Postictal encephalopathy	• NIIID • FXTAS	• HDLS-CSF1R • ADLD • PML • AAR2 mutation–related leukodystrophy	• Prion Disease • NIID • FXTAS • ADLD • And so forth	• MSUD • PKU • Nonketotic hyperglycinemia • MAT I/III deficiency • MLD • LBSL • Canavan disease • Progressive cavitating leukoencephalopathy • And so forth	• Brain abscess • Epidermoid cyst • Brain tumor • Malignant lymphoma • Glioblastoma • Metastatic brain tumor • ETMR, C19MC-alterd), CNS embryonal tumor, NOS • AT/RT • Germinoma • Medulloblastoma • And so forth

Abbreviations: ADLD, autosomal dominant adult-onset leukodystrophy; AT/RT, atypical teratoma/rhabdoid tumor; CJD, Creutzfeldt-Jakob disease; CNS, central nervous system; ETMR, embryonal tumor with multilayered rosettes; FXTAS, fragile X-associated tremor/ataxia syndrome; HDLS-CSF1R, hereditary diffuse leukoencephalopathy with spheroid-CSF-R; LBSL, leukoencephalopathy with brainstem and spinal cord involvement and increased white matter lactate; MAT, methionine adenosyl transferase; MCP, middle cerebellar peduncle; MLD, metachromatic leukodystrophy; MSUD, maple syrup urine disease; NIID, neuronal intranuclear inclusion disease; NOS, not otherwise specified; PKU, phenylketonuria; PML, progressive multifocal leukoencephalopathy; WM, white matter.

colony-stimulating factor receptors (CSF1R)/adult-onset leukoencephalopathy with axonal spheroids and pigmented glia (ALSP) should be suspected if there are persistent hyperintensities around the ventricles and deep white matter on DWI, as well as thinning of the corpus callosum and calcification on computed tomography (CT).[12,13]

Although sporadic CJD (sCJD) is a rare disease, it is lethal, with rapidly progressing cognitive impairment, and should not be misdiagnosed. A probable diagnosis is justified when the expected neuroimaging patterns are demonstrated, and CJD-mimicking diseases are confidently ruled out. NIID is a pathologic entity usually diagnosed by postmortem histologic examination. Although NIID is a rare neurodegenerative disease, it is becoming clear that it occurs at a higher rate than was previously thought, because its diagnosis by skin/fat biopsy has become possible. Thus, the elucidation of the pathophysiologic condition of NIID has progressed, and recently there have been some reports on the genetic analysis of NIID. HDLS is a hereditary leukoencephalopathy, for which the pathophysiologic condition has been elucidated, with characteristic MR imaging and CT findings as the beginning of the diagnostic work-up, enabling an antemortem diagnosis.

This review reinforces what is known about the distinguishable imaging findings, and confirms that DWI features are important in the diagnostic work-up of these diseases.

CREUTZFELDT-JAKOB DISEASE

Prion diseases comprise a heterogeneous assortment of neurodegenerative diseases, characterized by the alteration of a naturally existing prion protein (PrP^{c}) to an abnormal degenerative protein, termed scrapie prion protein (PrP^{Sc}).[14] The incidence of prion disease in humans is approximately 1 to 2 per million individuals per year.[15] Human prion diseases can be classified as acquired, hereditary, or sporadic[16] (**Table 2**). The molecular biology of the prion protein is mainly affected by a polymorphism at codon 120 of the *PRNP* gene, which codes for either valine (V) or methionine (m), and 2 PrP^{Sc} profiles (type 1 and type 2), forming the basis of a molecular classification into 6 subtypes.[16] Sporadic CJD (sCJD), the largest group of prionic diseases, is the main focus of this review.

According to the considerable experience with the use of MR imaging in sCJD, characteristic MR imaging lesion patterns are known to correspond with specific sCJD subtyupes.[17–21] This article summarizes the clinical features and the diagnostic criteria, describing the usual and unusual findings on MR imaging. In addition, although the mechanisms of signal abnormalities on DWI have not been fully explained, the pathologic background is described here, along with example cases (**Figs. 1–3**).

Clinical Features

- Among prion diseases, sCJD has the highest frequency. The diagnosis of CJD remains a challenge, especially in its early stages, because it mimics several reversible or treatable disorders.
- Clinical symptoms vary depending on the molecular subtype[16–21] (**Table 3**). MM1 and MV1 are the most common sCJD subtypes, usually manifesting with the typical clinical findings of sCJD, which include rapidly progressing dementia, myoclonus, ataxia, visual disturbances/cerebellar dysfunction, and pyramidal and/or extrapyramidal features. Most patients develop akinetic mutism within an average of 3 to 6 months.

Diagnostic Criteria

- Although several diagnostic criteria have been proposed for sCJD, imaging findings have grown in importance in diagnosis since characteristic DWI findings were first revealed. On DWI, if hyperintensities are observed in the cortex or basal ganglia, sCJD should be the first disease considered for differential.[5,8,22]
- MR imaging abnormalities have been included as a preclinical test for sCJD in the diagnostic criteria published by the Centers for Disease Control and Prevention (CDC).[23]
- However, Vitali and colleagues[5] proposed diagnostic criteria for sCJD based on MR imaging findings that emphasized the importance of accurately distinguishing sCJD from on-priority rapid progressive dementia.

Typical Magnetic Resonance Imaging Patterns

- The most common MR imaging pattern in sCJD consists of cortical and basal ganglia involvement with hyperintensities on DWI, which are most typically found in patients with MM1 and MV1[5,24–26] (see **Fig. 1**). The perirolandic areas and hippocampi are usually spared.[18,26] Typically, none of the lesions show swelling, and they lack abnormal contrast enhancement.
- Cerebral atrophy progresses rapidly.
- Signal abnormalities on DWI can diminish with disease progression, which may reflect marked neuronal loss.[18]

Table 2
Spectrum of human prion disease

Acquired	Genetic (Hereditary), (10∼15%)	Sporadic (85%)
• The Kuru • Variant CJD • Iatrogenic CJD (dura mater, neurosurgery, depth electrode, corneal, human growth hormone, human gonadotropin)	• Familial CJD • Fatal familial insomnia • Gestmann-Sträussler-Scheinker disease • Others	• Classic form or Heidenhain variant: MM1/MV1 • Ataxic form: VV2, MV2 (Kuru-plaques variant) • Thalamic form (sporadic fatal insomnia: sFI, MM2-thalamic form): MM2 • Cortical form: MM2 (MM2-cortical form), VV1

Abbreviations: FFI, fatal familial insomnia; FI, sporadic fatal insomnia.

Unusual Magnetic Resonance Imaging Patterns

- Confluent hyperintensities in the posterior thalami (pulvinar area) and dorsomedial thalami on T2-weighted MR imaging, fluid-attenuated inversion recovery (FLAIR) imaging, and DWI (known as pulvinar and double hockey stick signs, respectively) are the most sensitive radiologic hallmarks of variant CJD.[27]
- In the idiopathic CJD, the pulvinar sign according to current criteria was identified in the MV2 subtype only.[17]
- MM2-type thalamic variant CJD is the most difficult subtype to diagnose because MR imaging is generally negative.[28]
- Predominant subcortical signal abnormality with limited cortical hyperintensities on DWI is seen in the MV2 (see **Fig. 2**) or VV2 subtype of sCJD.[17]
- CJD with V180I mutation is a rare hereditary type. MR imaging reveals cortical swelling,

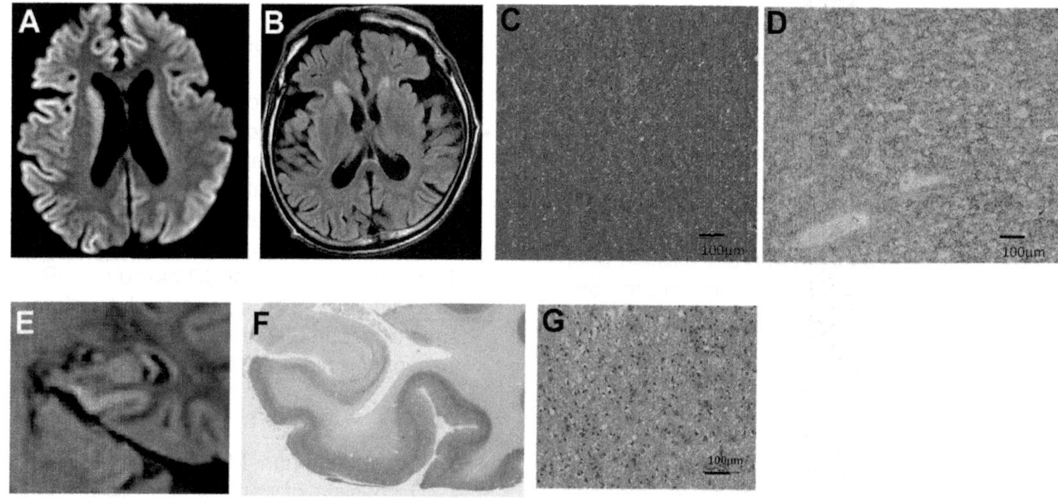

Fig. 1. Usual MR imaging pattern of sCJD. A man in his 70s with sporadic CJD (type MM1), with progressive cognitive impairment and intermittent myoclonus. Electroencephalography showed periodic synchronous discharge. There are more widespread high-intensity signals in the cortical ribbon and bilateral caudate nuclei on axial DWI (*A*) than on fluid-attenuated inversion recovery (FLAIR) imaging (*B*). The perirolandic area is relatively spared. Hematoxylin-eosin (H&E) staining of a specimen from the frontal cortex (*C*, bar = 100 μm) shows widespread neuronal loss, marked gliosis, and diffuse vacuole formation (5∼20 μm). Staining for PrP^{Sc} using 3F4 antibody (*D*) shows PrP^{Sc} accumulation, corresponding with a high-intensity signal area on DWI. Coronal DWI (*E*) shows high-intensity signals in the parahippocampal gyrus, with relative sparing of the hippocampus. Staining for PrP^{Sc} using 3F4 antibody (*F*) shows PrP^{Sc} accumulation in the entorhinal cortex and parahippocampal gyrus, corresponding with a high-intensity signal area on DWI. H&E staining of a microscopic specimen from the entorhinal cortex (*G*, bar = 100 μm) shows widespread neuronal loss, marked gliosis, and diffuse vacuole formation (5–35 μm).

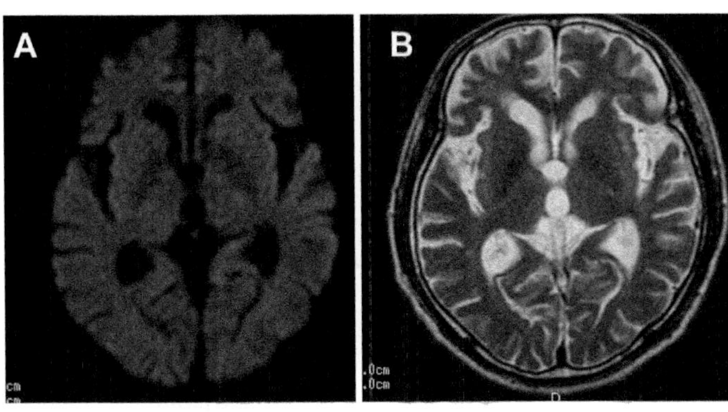

Fig. 2. Unusual MR imaging pattern of sCJD. A man in his 70s with sporadic CJD (type MV2) with progressive cognitive impairment. Axial DWI (*A*) shows no abnormal signals in the cortex, thalamus, and basal ganglia. Axial T2-weighted image (*B*) shows no abnormal signals in the cortex, thalamus, and basal ganglia, with frontal-predominant atrophy.

which is an unusual finding in sCJD[29,30] (see **Fig. 3**).

- Hyperintensity in the globus pallidus on T1-weighted images has been reported.[31,32]
- Few reports have described DWI hyperintensities involving the cerebellum.[33,34]

Physiochemical and Pathologic Basis for Diffusion-Weighted Imaging Abnormalities in Creutzfeldt-Jakob Disease

- The mechanism of persistent DWI hyperintensities in sCJD remains unclear. However, the vacuolization of neuropils (a network of neurons and glial cell molecules that exist along blood vessels) is thought to be associated with hyperintensities on DWI.[35,36] In general, if the vacuole diameter is less than 14 to 16 μm, the diffusion of water (observed on normal DWI) is restricted.[36] The vacuoles produced in sCJD are 5 to 25 μm in diameter, limiting diffusion.[35] However, persistent hyperintensities on DWI in CJD cannot be explained by vacuolization alone. One theory is that the DWI hyperintensities reflect the deposition of prion proteins.[37] However, rather than a single cause, it is thought that sCJD-PrP^{Sc} accumulation, vacuolization, astrocytic gliosis, and neuronal cell loss, which are all neuropathologic findings of sCJD, combine (depending on the stage or condition of the disease) to contribute to persistent DWI hyperintensities (see **Fig. 1**).

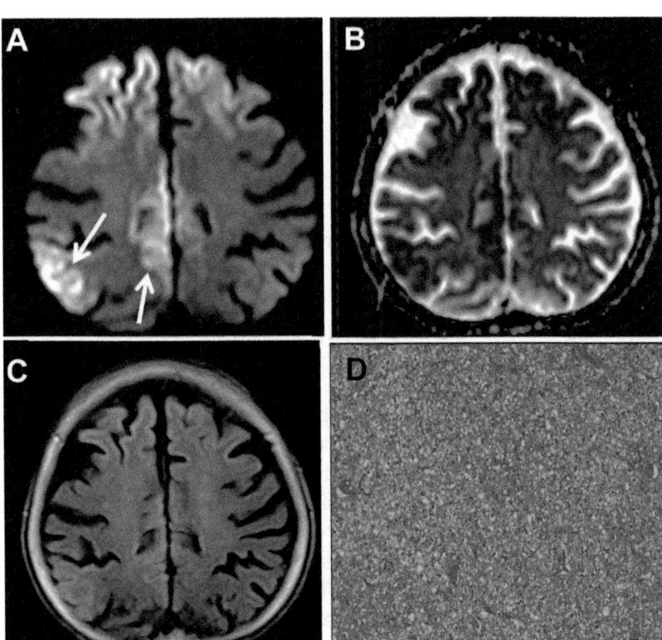

Fig. 3. Genetic CJD with V180I mutation. A woman in her 80s with gradual progressive cognitive impairment. Axial DWI (*A*) shows widespread high-intensity signals in the cortical ribbon, with swelling (*arrows*). The perirolandic areas are spared. An apparent diffusion coefficient (ADC) map (*B*) shows diffusion restriction at in the cortical ribbons. Axial FLAIR (*C*) shows slight high-intensity signals in the cortex. H&E staining of a microscopic specimen from the frontal cortex (*D*, bar = 100 μm) shows widespread neuronal loss, marked gliosis, and diffuse vacuole formation (5–20 μm).

Table 3
Clinical, paraclinical, and magnetic resonance imaging findings of the main molecular subtypes of idiopathic prion diseases

Prion Diseases by Group	Molecular Subtypes	Main Clinical Features	CSF Analysis	EEG	MR Imaging Lesion Profile
Idiopathic					
Sporadic	MM1	Classic sCJD	14-3-3 protein levels increased	PSWCs	BG ± frontal lobes, parietal lobes, cingulate gyri, hippocampus, and thalamus spared
	MV1	Classic sCJD	14-3-3 protein levels increased	PSWCs	Cortex, insula, BG
	VV2	Atypical sCJD Ataxic variant	14-3-3 protein levels not increased	Absence of PSWCs	BG and thalamus
	MM2 cortical	Progressive dementia	—	Atypical	Cortex, BG, thalamus
	MV2	Progressive dementia, ataxia,	—	Atypical	BG, thalamus, pulvinar sign
	VV1	Progressive dementia	—	Atypical	Cortex, cingulate gyri, insula, temporal lobe, BG, and thalamus spared
sFI	MM2 thalamic	Thalamic variant, presenile dementia, sleep disturbances, inability to initiate and maintain sleep, enacted dreams	14-3-3 protein levels not increased	Absence of PSWCs	In general negative (hypoperfusion or hypometabolism on SPECT and PET)

Abbreviations: BG, basal ganglia; EEG, electroencephalogram; PSWCs, periodic sharp wave complexes; SPECT, single-photon emission computed tomography.

Differential Diagnosis

- The differential diagnoses according to the localization of abnormal lesions on MR imaging are summarized in **Table 4**.[38–45]
- It is important to rule out these conditions because many of them are reversible and treatable if accurately diagnosed in a timely manner.
- Conditions with predominant cerebral cortex involvement, such as hypoglycemic encephalopathy,[38,39] hypoxic-ischemic encephalopathy, hyperammonemia, and encephalitis, show widespread DWI hyperintensities in the cortex and basal ganglia (**Figs. 4-6**).[40–45]
- Postictal state can induce signal abnormalities in areas such as the cortex, basal ganglia, thalamus, and cerebellum (either alone or in combination)[42,43,45] that may be difficult to differentiate from sCJD (see **Figs. 5** and **6**; **Fig. 7**).

NEURONAL INTRANUCLEAR INCLUSION DISEASE

NIID is a slowly progressive neurodegenerative disorder, pathologically characterized by localized neuronal loss and the presence of eosinophilic intranuclear inclusions in neurons and glia cells, the peripheral nervous system, and visceral organs.[46–50] Because characteristic MR imaging findings and skin/fat biopsies are now used for diagnosis, the prevalence of NIID seems to be higher than was previously thought.

Table 4
Differential diagnosis of sporadic Creutzfeldt-Jakob disease

Predominant Cerebral Cortex Involvement	Predominant Basal Ganglia Involvement	Thalamic Involvement
• Posticteric state • Hypoglycemic encephalopathy • Hypoxic-ischemic encephalopathy • Encephalitis (autoimmune mediated, infectious) • Hyperammonemia • Mitochondrial disorders	• Extrapontine osmotic demyelination • Encephalitis (EB virus, paraneoplastic, and so forth) • Hypoxic striatal necrosis	• Variant CJD • Wernicke encephalopathy • Wilson disease • Deep venous infarct • And so forth

Abbreviation: EB, Epstein-Barr.

Clinical Features

- The clinical features of NIID vary; disease onset occurs at all ages (in infants to the elderly), and both sporadic and familiar cases have been reported.[46–50]
- The clinical manifestations are summarized in **Table 5**.[46–49]
- Most adult-onset NIID is diagnosed at the age of 50 to 70 years. The disease duration ranges from 1 to 19 years.
- Core symptoms in typical NIID are memory loss, cognitive dysfunction, and disorientation. Abnormal behavior has also been noted as an initial symptom. Autonomic and peripheral nerve disturbances, bladder and rectal disturbances, and orthostatic hypotension are also common symptoms. Some cases of peripheral neuropathy without apparent cognitive dysfunction have also been reported.
- Twenty percent of patients with NIID present with subacute encephalitic or strokelike episodes.[47,49]

Genetic Cause

- Recently, noncoding CGG repeat expansions[51] and a large GGC repeat expansion within the human-specific NOTCH2NLC gene has been reported as the cause.[52]

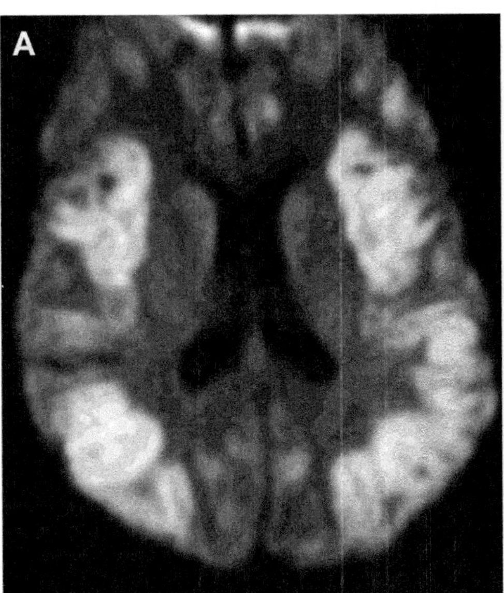

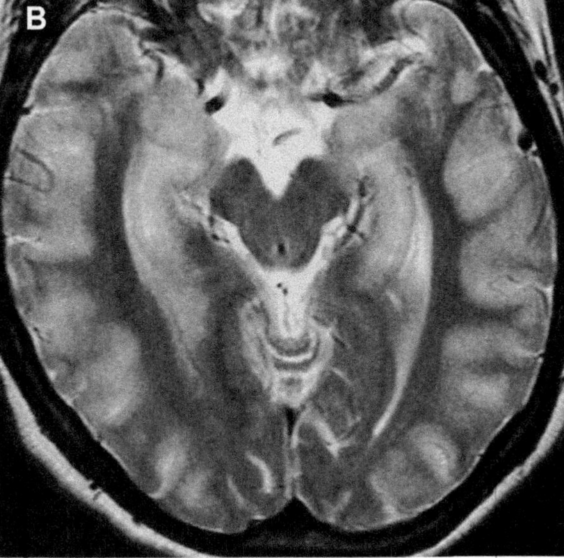

Fig. 4. A woman in her 20s with hypoglycemic encephalopathy who underwent an MR imaging examination because of a disturbance in consciousness. Her blood sugar level was 28 mg/dL. DWI (*A*) and T2-weighted MR imaging (*B*) show high-intensity signals in the bilateral cortices, with swelling including the hippocampus.

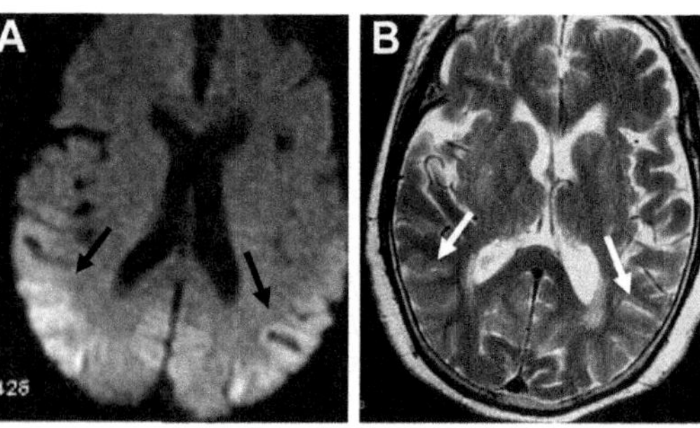

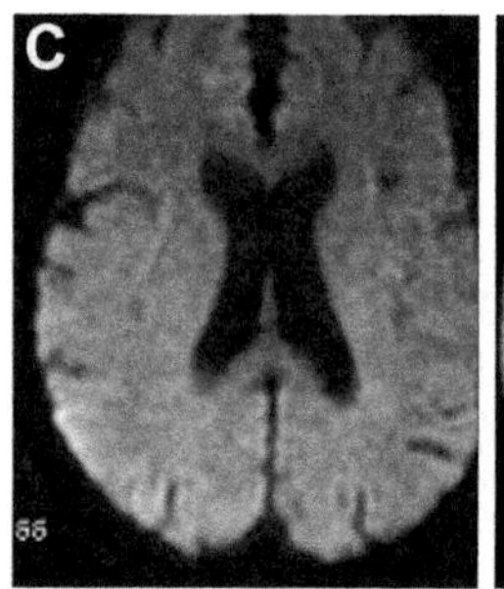

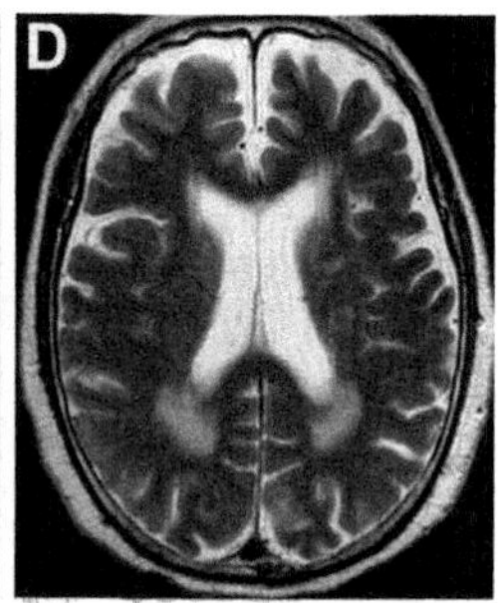

Fig. 5. A woman in her 70s with status epilepticus, in the posticteric stage. DWI (*A*) and T2-weighted images (*B*), taken as an emergency MR imaging examination, show high-intensity signals in the bilateral temporooccipital cortex, with swelling (*arrows*). These findings disappeared on the follow-up scans taken a month later (*C, D*).

MRI Findings

- Characteristic MRI findings are provided in **Table 6** (**Figs. 8–13**).[46,47,50,53]
- Persistent hyperintensities on DWI in the corticomedullary junction are the strongest and earliest indicators of NIID (see **Figs. 8** and **9**). High-intensity along the corticomedullary junction correspond to pathological spongiform changes (see **Fig. 12**).
- During the advanced stage of the disease, T2-weighted and FLAIR images show diffuse hyperintensities in the white matter, corresponding to pathologic diffuse myelin pallor changes (see **Fig. 8**).
- Abnormal FLAIR high-intensity signals in the paravermal area and MCP, as well as cerebellar atrophy, are also characteristic (see **Figs. 9** and **10**). A high-intensity signal in the pons is also recognized as a characteristic finding.
- It is noteworthy that 20% of patients with NIID show focal brain edema on MRI with the emergence of encephalitic and/or stroke-like symptoms. The lesions, including those in the cortex, show high-intensity signals on T2-weighted or FLAIR images. These lesions may or may not show high-intensity signals on DWI and are enhanced by gadolinium in some cases (see **Figs. 11** and **12**).

Pathologic Features

- In NIID, spherical and eosinophilic nuclear inclusions are found in neurons and glial cells. A moderate to severe loss of myelinated fibers is observed in cerebral white matter. Spongiform changes can be accentuated at the corticomedullary junction (see **Figs. 8**, **10**, **12**, and **13**). Such accentuations might correspond with persistently hyperintense DWI lesions.

Proposed Diagnostic Flowchart for Neuronal Intranuclear Inclusion Disease

- Although international diagnostic criteria have not yet been formulated, Sone and colleagues[47] proposed a diagnostic flowchart centered on MR imaging and skin biopsy findings. When evaluating patients with cognitive

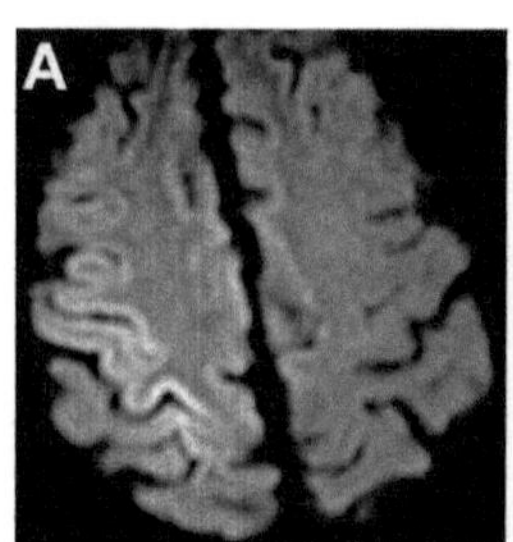

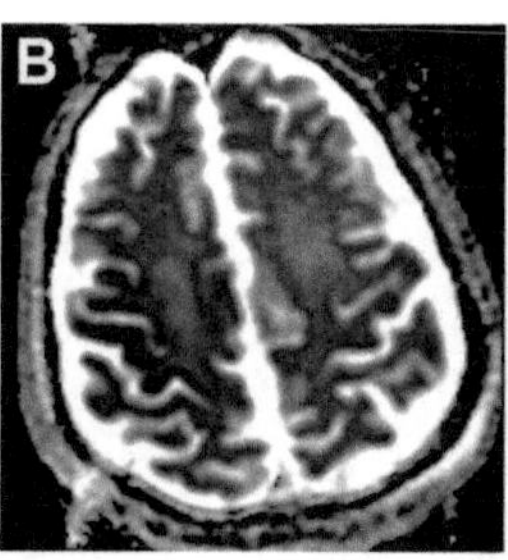

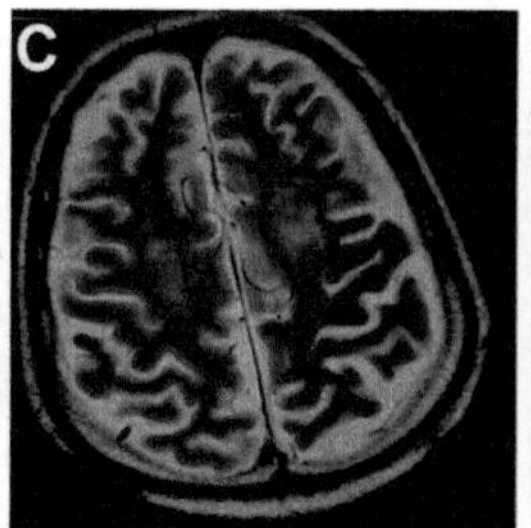

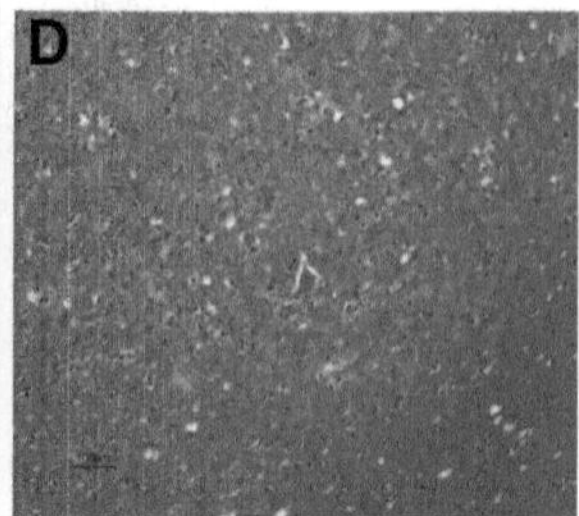

Fig. 6. Posticteric encephalopathy of a man in his 70s. The MR imaging was performed 4 hours after a status epilepticus. DWI (*A*) shows high-intensity signals in the right cerebral cortex, including the precentral gyrus. An ADC map (*B*) shows diffusion restriction in the right frontal cortex. A T2-weighted image (*C*) shows no obvious signal abnormalities or swelling at this stage. H&E staining of a microscopic specimen from the precentral gyrus (*D*, bar = 100 μm) shows ischemic changes in neurons, marked gliosis, and spongiform changes.

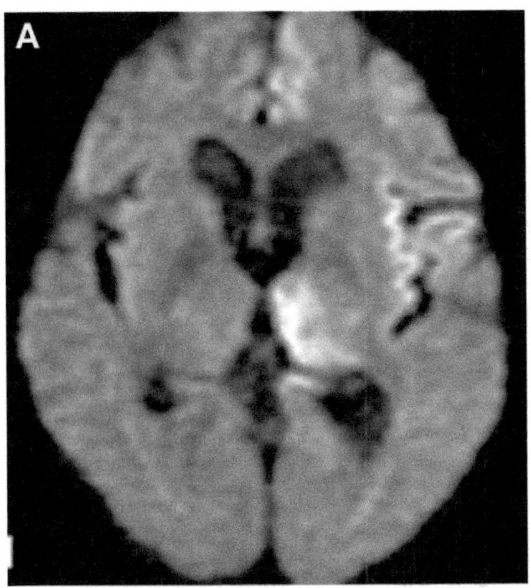

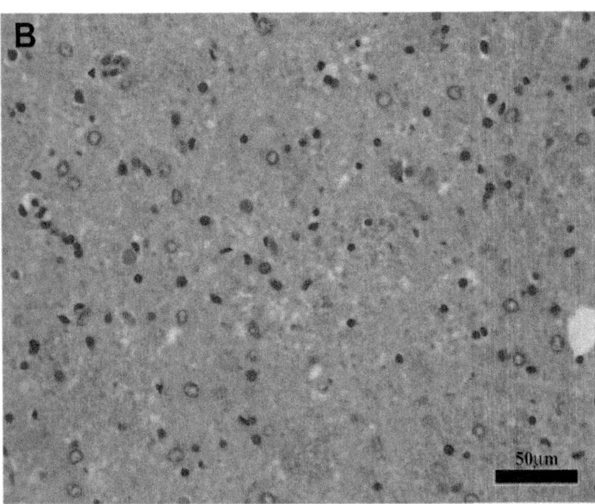

Fig. 7. A woman in her 70s with status epilepticus, in the posticteric state. DWI (*A*) taken 2 hours after an epileptic attack shows high-intensity signals in the left medial thalamus, left anterior frontal cortex, and left insula. H&E staining of a microscopic specimen from the dorsomedial thalamus (*B*, bar = 50 μm) shows abundant gliosis with spongiform changes.

dysfunction, MR imaging is first performed. If DWI hyperintensities are observed in the corticomedullary junction, a skin biopsy is performed. If positive intranuclear inclusions are found, then the NIID and FXTAS remain to be differentiated. FXTAS can be excluded if a genetic test for the *FMR1* CGG mutation is positive. It is recommended that differentiation is performed by skin biopsy in patients with a family history; in weakness-dominant patients, a skin biopsy should be performed after the nerve conduction tests.

Table 5
Clinical features of neuronal intranuclear inclusion disease

Age at Onset (y)	39–71
Age at Diagnosis (y)	51–70s
Disease duration (y)	1–19
Sex (Male/Female)	No obvious difference
Clinical Manifestations	
Cognitive Dysfunction/ Dementia (%)	>90
Peripheral Neuropathy (%)	>30
Autonomic Nervous System: Syncope, Miosis, Bladder Dysfunction (%)	15∼90
Tremor (%)	30
Epilepsy (%)	10∼20
Encephalitic or strokelike episode (%)	>20

Differential Diagnosis

- Because the pathophysiologies of FXTAS and NIID have substantial overlap, distinguishing these disorders based on the clinical presentation, imaging findings, and family history is not feasible (**Figs. 14** and **15**).[49,53–60] Moreover, the pathologic changes are also similar, because FXTAS and NIID both usually present with intranuclear eosinophilic inclusions (see **Fig. 15**).
- To exclude FXTAS, an analysis of the CGG repeat length of the *FMR1* gene is necessary.[58,59]

Pitfalls

- Hyperintensities on DWI in the corticomedullary junction are a characteristic finding in NIID. However, there are a small number of cases in which DWI signal abnormalities in the corticomedullary junction are not clear, especially in the early stage of the disease, or at the time when diffuse white matter lesions become clear (see **Fig. 13**).

FRAGILE X-ASSOCIATED TREMOR/ATAXIA SYNDROME

FXTAS is a trinucleotide repeat disorder caused by mutations in the *FMR1* gene, which is located on

Table 6
Summary of magnetic resonance imaging findings of neuronal intranuclear inclusion disease

Cerebrum	Cerebellum	Brainstem
• High-intensity signal along the corticomedullary on DWI • Diffuse high-intensity signal of cerebral white matter on FLAIR image • Atrophy • Focal brain edema/high-intensity signal on T2-weighted image/FLAIR	• High-intensity signal in the medial part of cerebellar hemisphere beside the vermis on FLAIR image • High-intensity signal in the middle cerebellar peduncle on FLAIR image • Atrophy	• High-intensity signal in the pons

band 27.3 on the long arm of the X chromosome (Xq27.3).[59–62] Fragile X syndrome, which occurs in childhood and is associated with severe mental retardation, is caused by an expansion of the CGG repeat in the *FMR1* gene, with a length exceeding 200 CGGs. FXTAS, which occurs in middle age and is associated with tremor, ataxia, and parkinsonian symptoms, and the CGG repeat, ranges in length from to 50 to 200 CGGs. It is challenging to distinguish FXTAS from NIID by skin biopsy, and this remains an urgent issue in clinical settings. It is also difficult to distinguish FXTAS from NIID on imaging alone.

Clinical Features

- Occurs mostly in men more than 50 years of age.

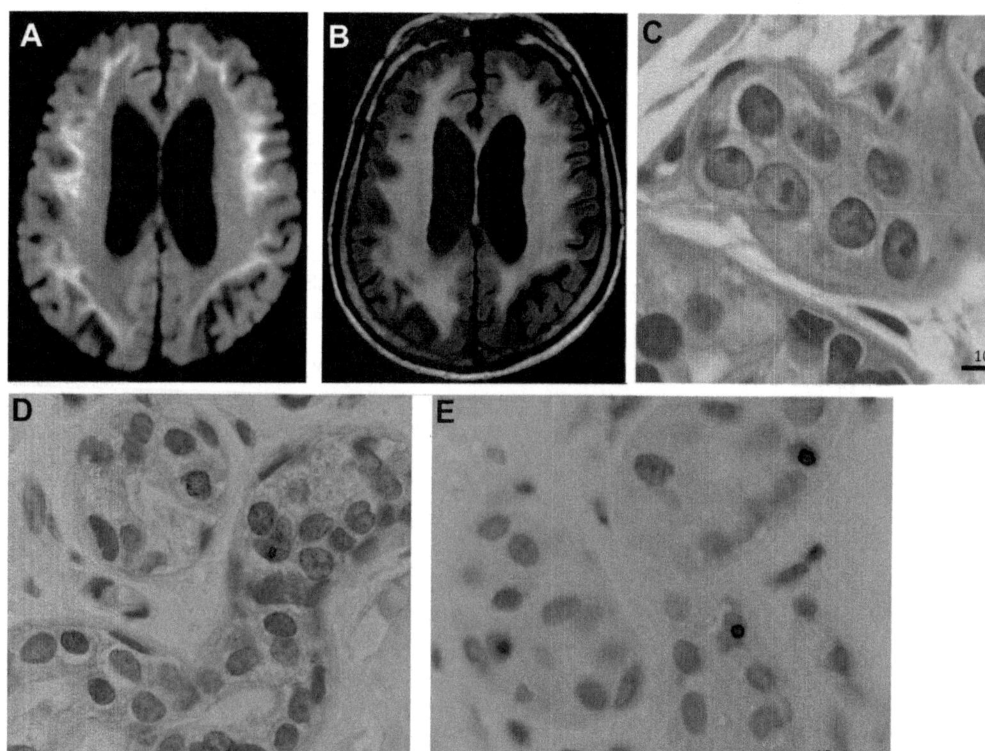

Fig. 8. Typical MR imaging findings of NIID. A man in his 70s with NIID, with progressive cognitive impairment. DWI (*A*) shows high-intensity signals along the corticomedullary junction. FLAIR (*B*) image shows diffuse high-intensity signals in the bilateral cerebral hemispheres. H&E staining of a skin biopsy specimen (*C*) shows eosinophilic nuclear inclusion. The nuclear inclusion stained with antiubiquitin antibody (*D*) and anti-p62 antibody (*E*).

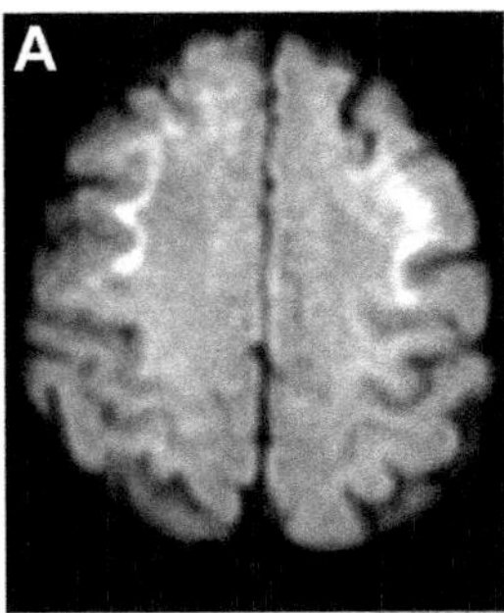

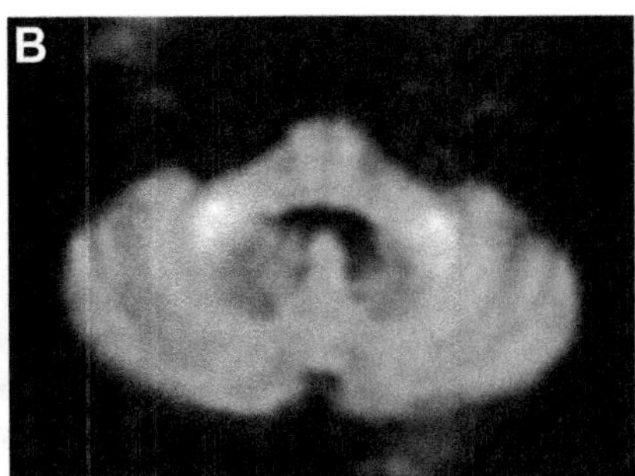

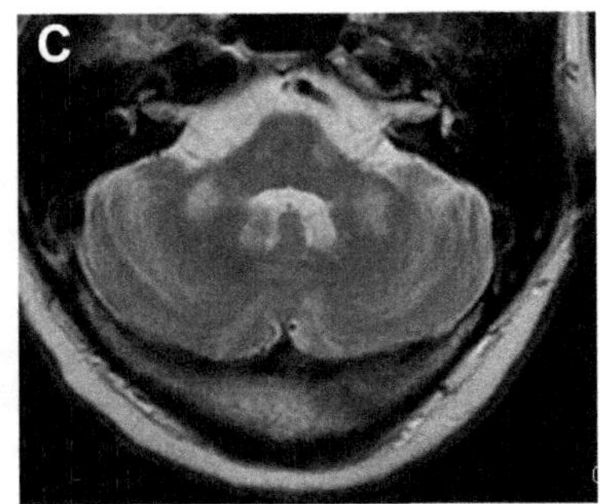

Fig. 9. Cerebellar findings of NIID. A woman in her 60s with tendency to fall. DWI (*A*) shows high-intensity signals along the corticomedullary junction. DWI (*B*) and T2-weighted (*C*) axial images show diffuse high-intensity signals in the bilateral MCPs.

- A definitive diagnosis is possible through genetic test. It is necessary to prove that there is an *FMR1* gene mutation (permutation of the CGG repeat length to 50–200).
- It is said to occur in 40% of men and 8% to 16% of women who carry the *FMR1* mutation. In female carriers, premature ovarian dysfunction may be the only symptom, and, in some cases, central nervous system disorders may not be present.
- With more CGG repeats, the onset is earlier and the symptoms are more severe.
- Core symptoms of FXTAS include cognitive dysfunction, disordered gait, parkinsonian symptoms, tremor, tumbling, peripheral neuropathy, and autonomic neuropathy. Attention should be paid to the tendency to fall as the initial symptom.[56,57,59,62]
- FXTAS may be initially diagnosed as essential tremors. If tremor is accompanied by ataxia or parkinsonian symptoms, it is important to consider FXTAS for the differential diagnosis of Parkinson syndrome.[54,55,57,59,62]
- It is important to obtain a family history. Because it is mediated by the X chromosome, it is essential to determine whether the patient's grandchildren have intellectual disabilities, or whether the patient's daughter has a history of early menopause or infertility.

Magnetic Resonance Imaging Findings

- The MCP sign is characteristic, and can prompt the diagnosis (see Fig. 14). FLAIR, T2-weighted images, and DWI show high-intensity signals in both MCPs.[56,57] The MCP sign is observed in 60% of male patients, and positive rate is low (approximately 13%) in female cases. If an adult male with Parkinson syndrome with a tremor has a positive MCP sign, FXTAS should be the first differential diagnosis.
- High-intensity signals may appear on T2-weighted and FLAIR images, even in the brain stem, white matter around the ventricles, and corpus callosum.
- DWI high-intensity signals along the corticomedullary junction have been noted.
- A thin corpus callosum and cerebellar atrophy have also been reported. In a detailed analysis using voxel-based morphometry,

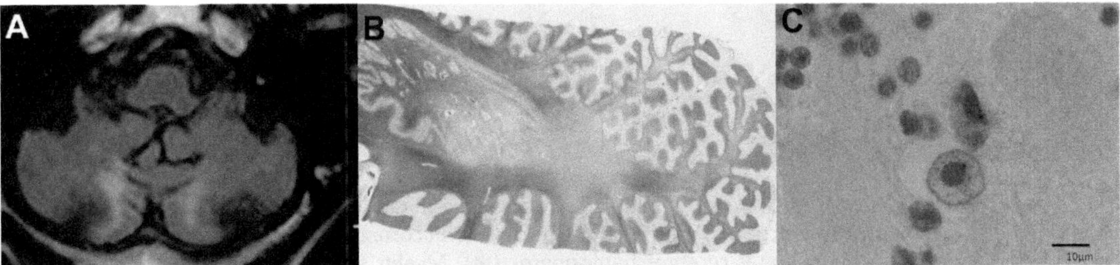

Fig. 10. Cerebellar findings of NIID. A man in his 60s with progressive cognitive impairment. FLAIR axial image (*A*) shows bilateral high-intensity signals in the medial cerebellar hemisphere (the paravermal area). Myelin sheath staining (*B*) shows decreased stainability in the cerebellar hemisphere. In the degenerative glial cells, ubiquitin-positive intranuclear inclusion is recognized (*C*).

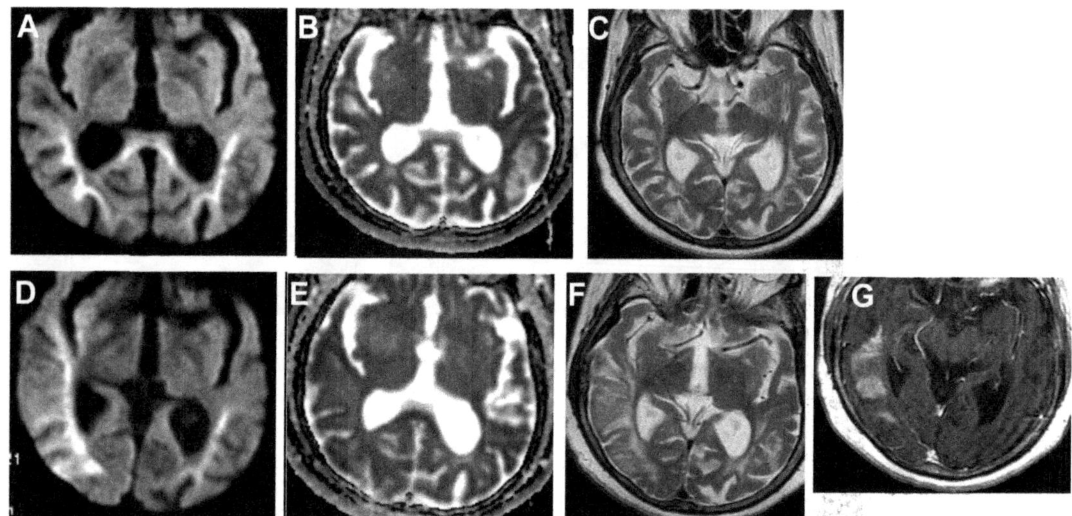

Fig. 11. Cortical involvement of NIID. A woman in her 60s with gradually progressive motor dysfunction and cognitive decline. At the first MR imaging examination, axial DWI (*A*) shows high-intensity signals in the corticomedullary junction. An ADC map (*B*) shows no obvious diffusion restriction. T2-weighted MR imaging image (*C*) shows high-intensity signals in the white matter. Brain atrophy is also noted. One month after the first examination, she presented with an acute headache and rapidly deteriorating consciousness. At the emergency MR imaging examination, DWI (*D*) shows high-intensity signals in wider area of temporo-occipital cortex and the corticomedullary junction, without diffusion restriction on ADC map (*E*). T2-weighted axial image (*F*) shows high-intensity signals in the same area. Postcontrast T1-weighted image (*G*) shows enhancement by gadolinium-based contrast agent.

atrophy in the cerebellar vermis and anterior hemisphere was observed, and correlated positively with the disease severity and negatively with the number of CGG repeats.[11,60,61,63,64]

- Studies using diffusion tensor imaging and functional MR imaging have also been conducted,[62] suggesting the possibility that neuroimaging analysis of various aspects can contribute to the pathologic elucidation of patients with FXTAS and presymptomatic carriers.

Differential Diagnosis

- FXTAS may be similar to NIID in terms of clinical features, neuroimaging, and pathology

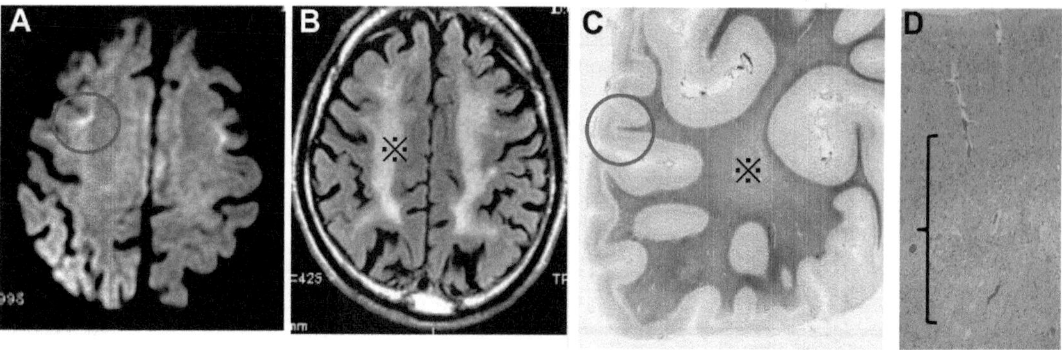

Fig. 12. A man in his 60s with NIID. Histopathologic correlations with DWI. Axial DWI (*A*) shows high-intensity signals in the corticomedullary junction (*circled*) and occipito-parietal cortex. FLAIR (*B*) axial image shows diffuse high-intensity signals in the bilateral cerebral hemispheres (※). Myelin sheath staining (*C*) shows markedly decreased stainability in the corticomedullary junction (*circled*), with evident spongiform changes in the cortex and corticomedullary junction ({) on H&E staining (*D*), which might correspond with the persistent high-intensity signal on DWI. Moderate to severe loss of myelinated fibers (*C*, ※) is observed in the cerebral white matter, possibly corresponding with the diffuse high-intensity signal on FLAIR images (*B*, ※).

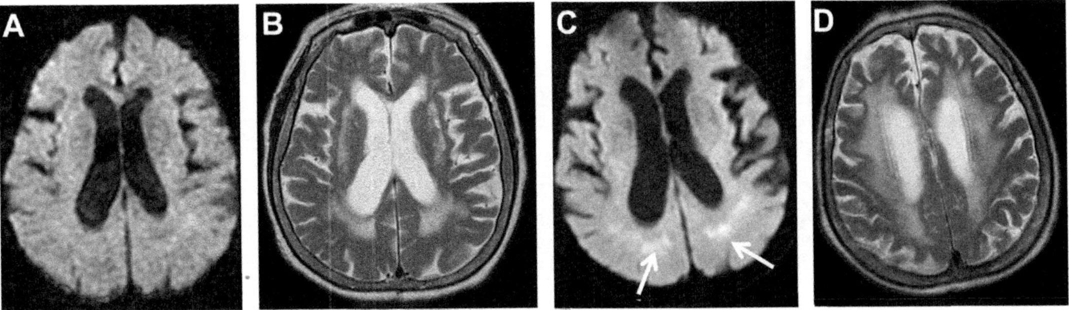

Fig. 13. Pitfall example. A woman in her 80s who presented with progressive cognitive impairment, with NIID proved by skin/fat biopsy. Axial DWI (*A*) shows no obvious abnormal signals at her initial examination. T2-weighted axial image (*B*) shows diffuse high intensity in the white matter. DWI (*C*) 8 years after the initial examination, when a recurrent consciousness disorder appeared, shows high-intensity signals in the bilateral subcortical area (*arrows*). T2-weighted image (*D*) shows exacerbated diffuse high-intensity signals in the bilateral hemispheres.

(see **Figs. 8**, **10**, **12**, and **15**); however, unlike in NIID, the appearance of MCP lesions may precede the supratentorial lesions in FXTAS.[47,49,53,65]

Pitfalls

- The MCP sign on MR imaging is an important finding of FXTAS. However, there are multiple disorders that can cause MCP signs[11] (**Box 1**).

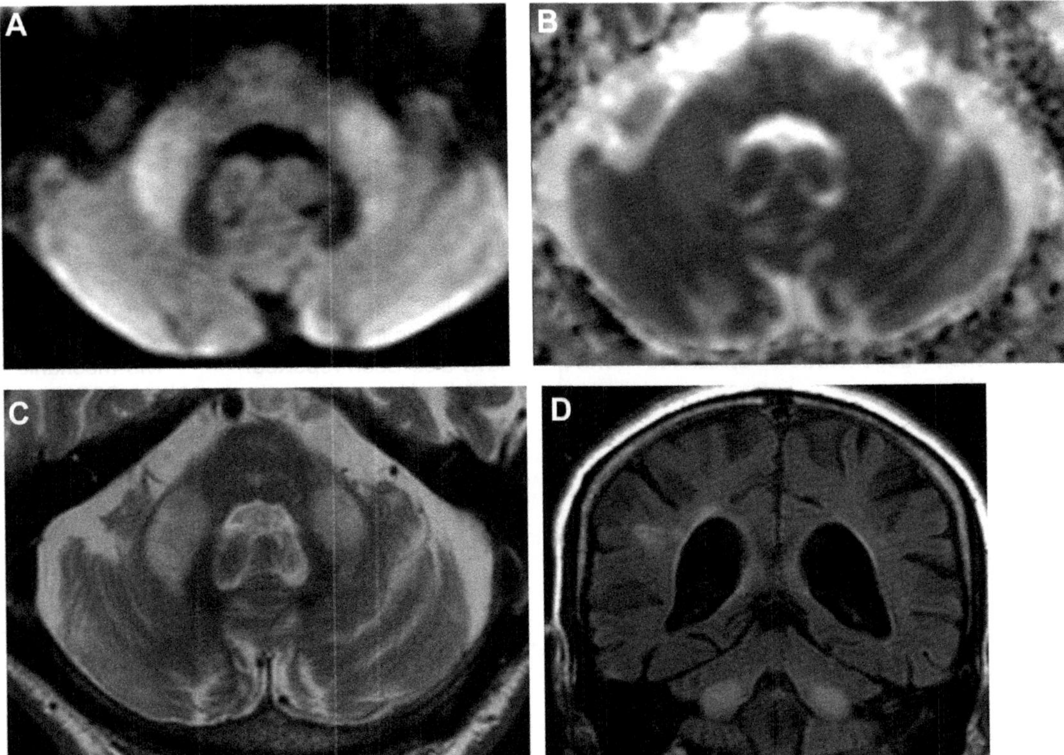

Fig. 14. A 70-year-old man with FXTAS, who presented with progressive motor ataxia and cognitive decline (CGG repeat size on the *FMR1* gene is 84). DWI (*A*) shows bilateral high-intensity signals in the MCPs, with mild high intensity on the corresponding ADC map (*B*). T2-weighted axial image (*C*) and coronal FLAIR image (*D*) show bilateral high-intensity signals in the MCPs, with swelling. Coronal FLAIR image (*D*) shows high-intensity signals in the cerebral white matter. Atrophy is also noted. (*Courtesy of* Dr. Ryo Kurokawa and Kouhei Kamiya, Dept of Radiology, The University of Tokyo. Figures are adapted from reference 81 with permission.[78])

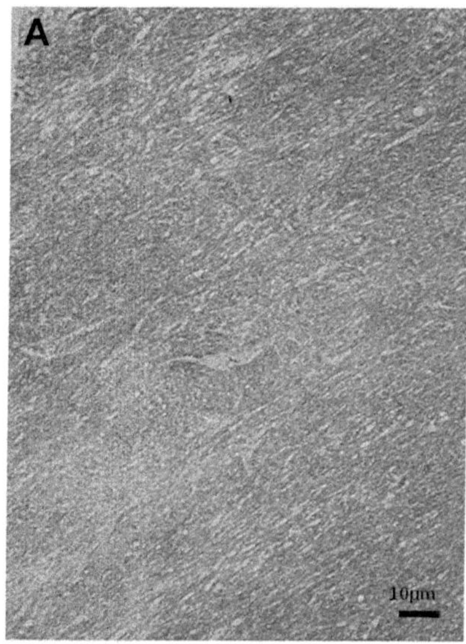

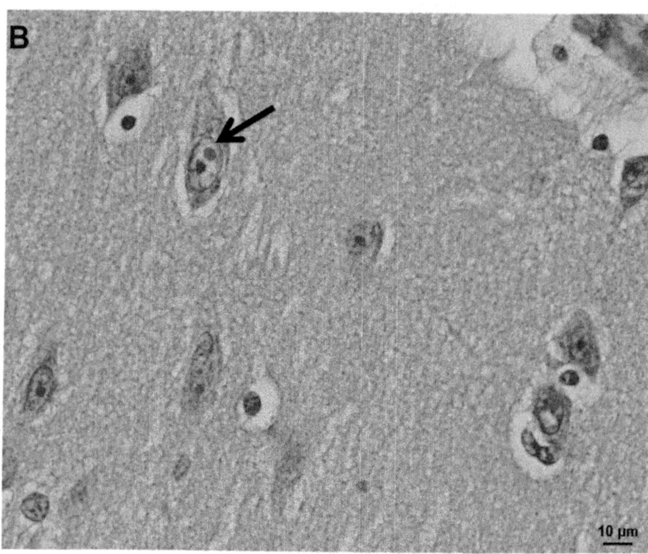

Fig. 15. Neuropathology of FXTAS. Klüver-Barrera staining (*A*) shows low stainability in the middle cerebellar peduncle. H&E staining (*B*) shows eosinophilic intranuclear inclusions in hippocampal neurons (*arrow*). Nuclear inclusions in the astrocytes of the hippocampus are stained with anti-p62 antibody. (*Courtesy of* Dr. Ayako Shioya, Dept of Pathology and Laboratory Medicine, National Center Hospital for Neurology and Psychiatry).

HEREDITARY DIFFUSE LEUKOENCEPHALOPATHY WITH AXONAL SPHEROIDS–COLONY-STIMULATING FACTOR RECEPTORS/ADULT-ONSET LEUKOENCEPHALOPATHY WITH AXONAL SPHEROIDS AND PIGMENTED GLIA

HDLS-CSF1R/ALSP is a rare neurodegenerative disorder with various clinical presentations. The disease is caused by mutations in the protein tyrosine kinase domain of CSF1Rs, encoded by the *CSF1R* gene on chromosome 5q32. The *CSF1R* gene is considered to be the cause of the autosomal dominant disorder, but sporadic cases have also been reported.[13,66–71] The mechanism of disease onset is unknown. Since *CSF1R* was first identified in 2011, at least 54 cases of kindreds have been reported, and this disorder may be present at a higher rate than was previously thought.[13,69–71]

Clinical Features

- HDLS-CSF1R/ALSP is an important differential disease of juvenile dementia. It frequently occurs in middle-aged and elderly people, but the onset age varies from childhood to old age. The mean age at onset is 44.3 years, and the disease gradually progresses. The mean disease duration, from symptom onset to death, is 5.8 years.
- The core symptoms comprise personality changes, cognitive impairments, parkinsonism, seizures, and depression.[13,66–70]

Box 1
Diseases that can cause middle cerebellar peduncle signs

- FXTAS
- NIID
- Wallerian degeneration associated with infarction
- MSA-C
- PML
- Osmotic demyelination syndrome
- Adult-onset autosomal dominant leukodystrophy
- GSS
- Malignant lymphoma
- Toluene, heroin
- Methotrexate-induced cerebellar leukoencephalopathy
- and so forth

Abbreviations: GSS, Gerstmann-Sträussler-Scheinker disease; MSA-C, multiple system atrophy with cerebellar ataxia; PML, progressive multifocal leukoencephalopathy.

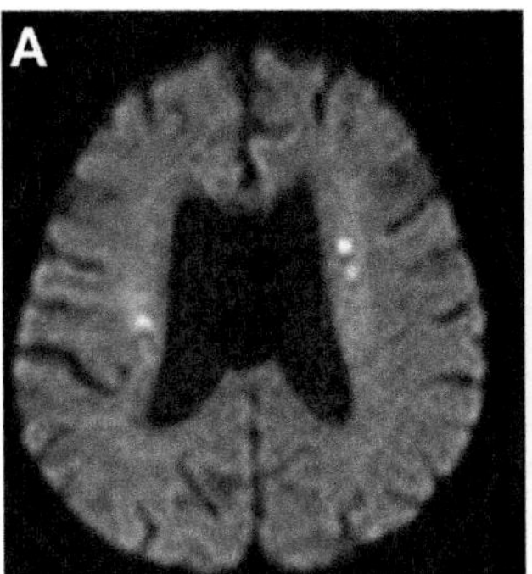

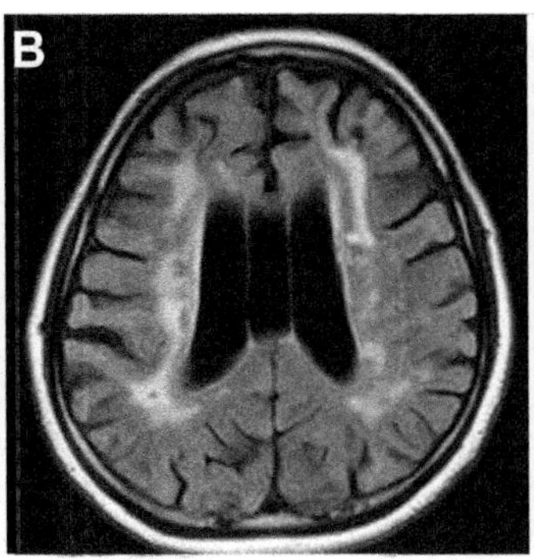

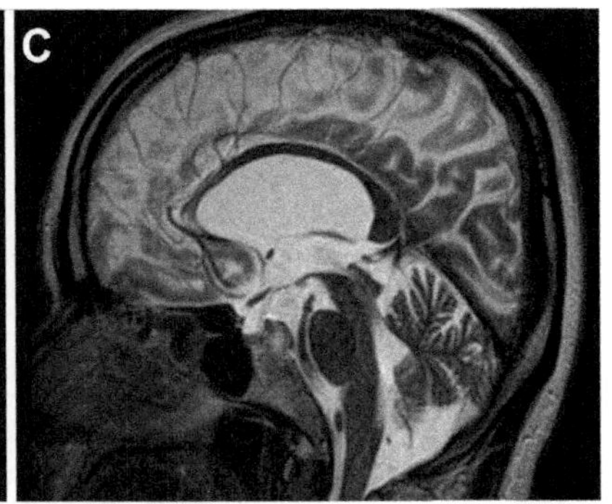

Fig. 16. MR imaging of a patient with HDLS. T2-weighted image (*A*) and DWI (*B*) show white matter hyperintensities, along with brain atrophy, particularly in the corpus callosum (*C*), and frontal and parietal lobes include spotty hyperintensity on DWI. (*Courtesy of* Dr. Takashi Abe, Dept of Radiology, Nagoya University.)

Neuroimaging Findings

- Persistent DWI hyperintensities in the white matter are a diagnostic clue for HDLS-CSF1R/ALSP (**Fig. 16**).[13,66,69–71] The apparent diffusion coefficient may be decreased, but there are many cases in which this is not confirmed.
- Progressive cerebral atrophy, especially in the frontal and parietal lobes, and white matter hyperintensities on T2-weighted images, FLAIR, and DWI are frequent findings (see **Fig. 16**).[13,66,69–73]
- Corpus callosal atrophy is a hallmark of HDLS-*CSF1R*/ALSP and may be accompanied by high intensity on T2-weighted images (see **Fig. 16**; **Fig. 17**).
- White matter lesions may extend through the corticospinal tract, from the cerebrum to the brain stem and spinal tract (**Figs. 18** and **19**).
- U-fiber preservation is at a high rate in HDLS-*CSF1R*/ALSP. The diagnostic utility of this finding is limited because it is also found in other leukoencephalopathies.
- CT findings are also important. Microcalcifications in the white matter around the anterior horn of the lateral ventricle and in the subcortical white matter of the parietal lobe are highly disease specific; a sagittal view of the calcification around the anterior horn of the lateral ventricle has a stepping-stone appearance (see **Fig. 17**).[71] Because the calcification is minute, setting a thin slice is desirable. There are also reports of cases in which calcification was detected around the ventricles and white matter on CT at birth. In such cases, TORCH (toxoplasmosis, other agents, rubella, Cytomegalovirus, and Herpes simplex). syndrome is an essential differential diagnosis.
- HDLS-CSF1R/ALSP calcification may not reflect secondary calcification that follows degeneration. It is also reported at birth, and its localization is close to the place where microglia aggregate during fetal development.[74]
- In HDLS cases, MR spectroscopy reveals decreased N-Acetylasparate (NAA) and glutamate (Glu) concentrations and increase in Choline containing compounds (Cho) and Myo-inositol (Ins) concentrations compared to those normal databases. These findings are recognized even in asymptomatic *CSF1R* mutation carriers. MRS could be a potentially useful tool for the analysis of metabolic and pathophysiological findings of HDLS, even during the early stages of the disease.

Pathologic Features

- Cerebral atrophy is most prominent in the frontal lobes, with atrophy of the corpus callosum, brainstem, and cerebellum. Myelin loss and axonal spheroids in the cerebral white matter are recognized (see **Fig. 18**).[66]
- Degenerative changes are present in the white matter, predominantly involving the cerebral white matter, particularly in the centrum semiovale and corpus callosum, which might correspond with the diffuse high intensity in the white matter (see **Figs. 18** and **19**). Subcortical U fibers are relatively spared. Degenerative changes are also recognized in the corticospinal tract, which might correspond with the high intensity on T2-weighted image along the corticospinal tract (see **Fig. 19**).
- Abnormalities comprise a severe loss of myelinated fibers, with pigment-containing

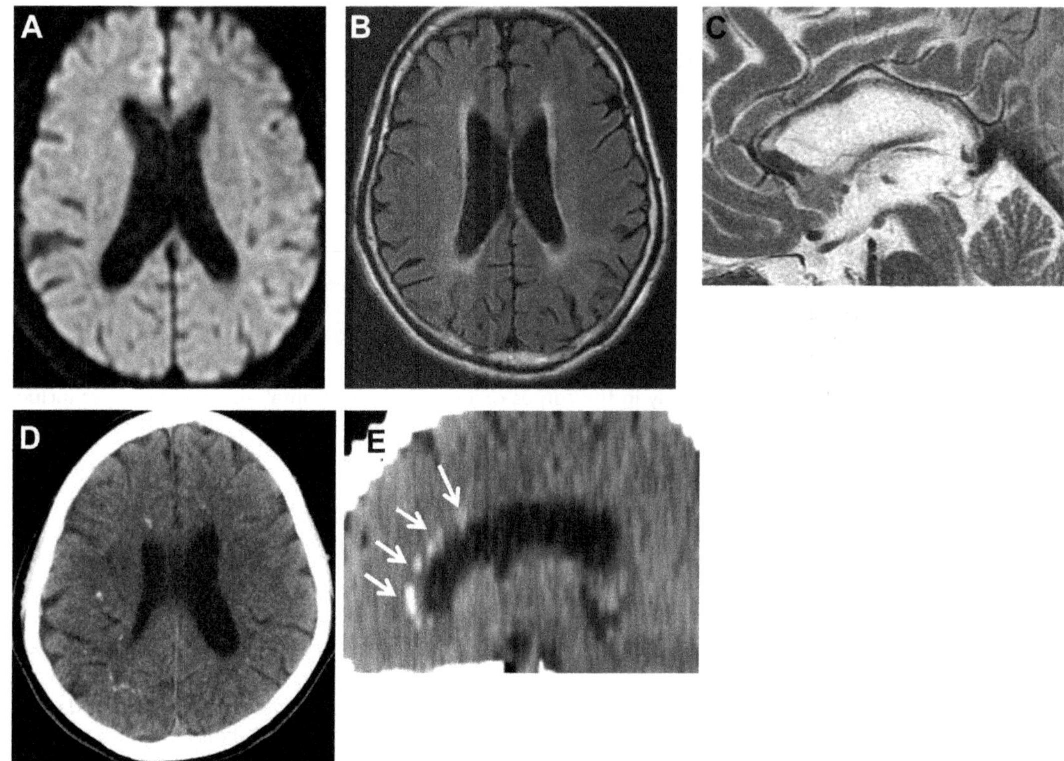

Fig. 17. A woman in her 30s with HDLS-CSF1R proved by genetic analysis. DWI (*A*) shows multiple high-intensity lesions in the deep white matter, with brain atrophy. A FLAIR axial image (*B*) shows multiple high-intensity lesions outside the lateral ventricles. A sagittal T2-weighted image (*C*) shows marked atrophy of the corpus callosum. Axial brain CT (*D*) shows multiple punctate bilateral white matter calcifications. These calcified lesions are arranged like a stepping-stone along the corpus callosum on the sagittal reconstructed CT (*E, arrows*). (Figures are adapted from reference 82 with permission.[79] *Courtesy of* Dr. Mitsuru Matsuki, Dept of Radiology, Medical School of Kinki University.)

macrophages and occasional axonal spheroids.

Proposed Diagnostic Criteria

- Konno and colleagues[69] proposed diagnostic criteria for HDLS-CSF1R/ALSP. A definite diagnosis requires proof of *CSH1R* mutation, but the presence of periventricular white matter lesions on MR imaging is useful for a probable or possible diagnosis. As mentioned earlier, the accumulation of more characteristic MR imaging and CT findings is expected to provide helpful information for reaching accurate diagnosis, with a high degree of sensitivity and specificity.

Differential Diagnosis

- AARS2 (ananyl-tRNA synthetase2)-related ovarioleukodystrophy[75–77] is an autosomal recessive adult-onset leukodystrophy with ovarian failure. All patients are female. MR imaging findings are similar to those of HDLS. Screening for mutations of AARS2 gene are recommended in patients who are CSF1R negative.
- Multiple sclerosis (especially when no signal abnormalities are observed on DWI) and neuromyelitis optica spectrum disorder are also important differentials.
- Autosomal dominant adult-onset leukodystrophy (ADLD) is another differential. Clinically, in ADLD, autonomic neuropathy is conspicuous and cognitive function is relatively maintained. Pathologically, myelin sheath disorders are conspicuous. Compared with HDLS-CSF1R/ALSP, the preservation of white matter around the ventricles differs.
- The following 3 conditions become important differentials: Binswanger disease, cerebral autosomal dominant arteriopathy with subcortical infarcts and leukoencephalopathy (CADASIL), and cerebral recessive dominant

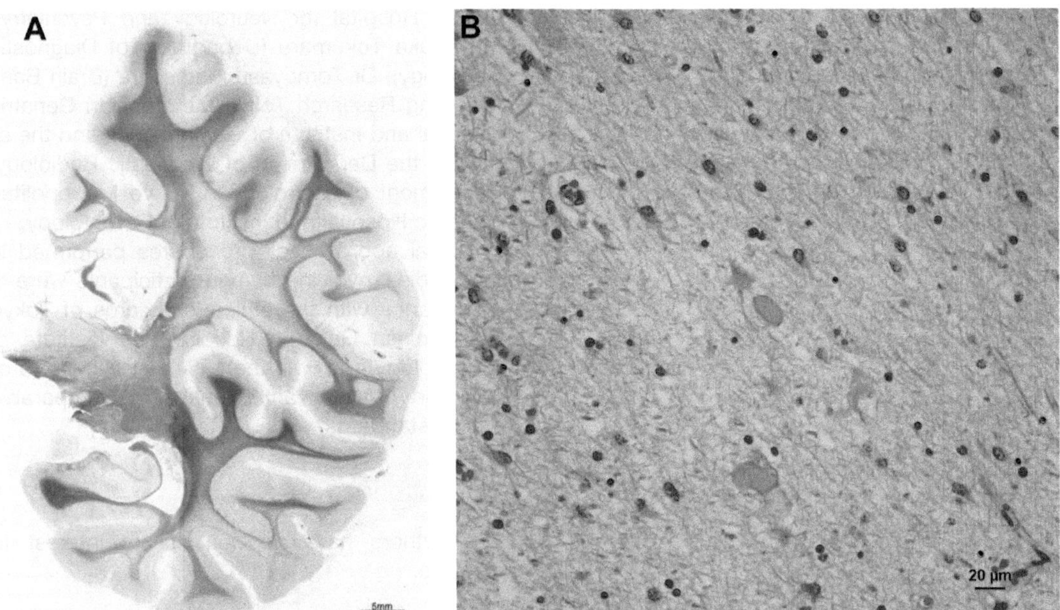

Fig. 18. Neuropathology of HDLS-CSF1R. Myelin sheath staining (coronal section) of a specimen from the cerebrum (*A*, bar = 5 mm) reveals extensive and heterogeneous degeneration in the deep white matter, with relative sparing of the subcortical white matter. H&E staining of a specimen from deep white matter (*B*, bar = 20 μm) shows abundant axonal spheroids with tissue rarefaction. (*Courtesy of* Prof. Yuishin Izumi, Department of Neurology, Tokushima University.)

arteriopathy with subcortical infarcts and leukoencephalopathy (CARASIL). In CADASIL, white matter lesions of the temporal pole and external capsule lesions are differentiation points.

Pitfalls 1

- There are a small number of cases in which persistent high signals on DWI are not observed.

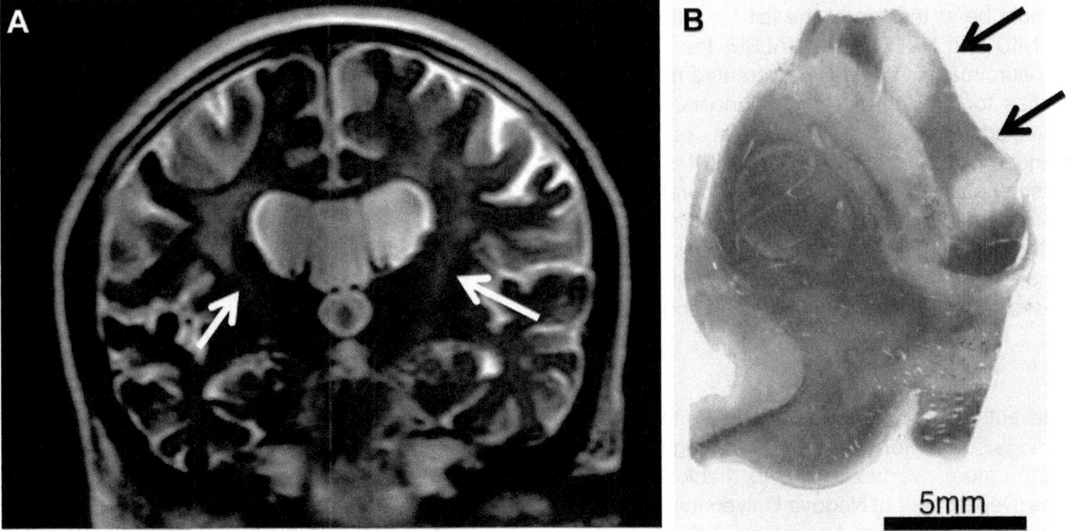

Fig. 19. HDLS. Coronal T2 weighted image (*A*) shows hyperintensity along the bilateral corticospinal tracts (*arrows*). Myelin sheath stain (*B*) in the midbrain (bar = 5 mm) reveals less stainability along the corticospinal tracts (*arrows*) with MR imaging findings. (*Courtesy of* Prof. Yuishin Izumi, Department of Neurology, Tokushima University.)

- White matter lesions have different findings, depending on the stage and condition, with punctuate, patchy, and generalized confluence.
- If DWI is performed only once during the course, especially at the early stage or as the initial examination, a misdiagnosis of acute to subacute cerebral infarcts can result.

Pitfalls 2

- A variety of names have been used for this disease, which is collectively known as ALSP, pigmentary orthochromatic leukodystrophy (POLD), and hereditary diffuse leukoencephalopathy. However, because *CSF1R* was found to be inherited in an autosomal dominant manner, it now seems to form a disease continuum. Thus, HDLS-CSF1R/ALSP integrates ALSP, which reflects the pathologic background, and HDLS-CSF1R, which reflects the genetic mutations and pathologic findings.

SUMMARY

This review provides an outline of the diseases for which persistent DWI signal abnormalities are key to their diagnosis. If signal abnormalities on DWI are in the cortex, sCJD should first be considered. If they are in the corticomedullary junction, NIID should be considered. If persistent signal abnormalities on DWI are observed around the ventricles, and CT shows calcification with a stepping-stone appearance, HDLS-CSF1R/ALSP should be at the top of the list for differentiation. In NIID and HDLS-CSF1R/ALSP, the recognition of neuroimaging findings has created major possibilities for an antemortem diagnosis, which has revealed that these diseases occur more frequently than previously thought. It is important to emphasize that accumulating accurate descriptions of neuroimaging findings and linking these with clinical, pathologic, and imaging findings help to further elucidate the nature of these diseases, including the sites of genetic abnormalities.

ACKNOWLEDGMENTS

The authors would like to thank Editage (www.editage.com) for English language editing. Furthermore, we would like to thank Dr Takashi Abe (Department of Nagoya University), Dr Yuishin Izumi (Department of Neurology, Tokushima University), Dr Mitsuru Matuki (Department of Radiology, Kinki University), Dr Ryo Kurokawa (The University of Tokyo), Ayako Shioya (Department of Pathology and Laboratory Medicine, National Center Hospital for Neurology and Psychiatry), Ms Asuka Tokumaru (Department of Diagnostic Radiology), Dr Tomoyasu Matsubara (Brain Bank for Aging Research Tokyo Metropolitan Geriatric Hospital and Institute of Gerontology), and the all staff of the Department of Diagnostic Radiology, Department of Neurology in Tokyo Metropolitan Geriatric Hospital and Institute of Gerontology.

Ethical approval: all procedures performed in the studies involving human participants were in accordance with the ethical standards of Tokyo Metropolitan Geriatric Hospital and Institute of Gerontology and with the 1964 Helsinki Declaration and its later amendments or comparable ethical standards.

DISCLOSURE

The authors have no conflicts of interest to disclose.

REFERENCES

1. Burdette J, Ricci P, Elster AD. Cerebral infarction: time course of signal intensity changes on diffusion weighted MR images. AJR Am J Roentgenol 1998; 171:791–5.
2. Fellah S, Caudal D, De Paula AM, et al. Multifocal MR imaging (diffusion, perfusion, and spectroscopy): is it possible to distinguish oligodendroglial tumor grade and 1p/19q codeletion in the pretherapeutic diagnosis? AJNR Am J Neuroradiol 2013;34: 1326–33.
3. Tung GA, Rogg JM. Diffusion-weighted imaging of cerebritis. AJR Am J Roentgenol 2003;24:110–3.
4. Schaefer PW, Huisman T, Sorensen AG, et al. Diffusion-weighted MR imaging in closed head injury: high correlation with initial Glasgow coma scale score and score on modified Rankin scale at discharge. Radiology 2004;233:58–66.
5. Vitali P, Maccagnano E, Caverzasi E, et al. Diffusion-weighted MRI hyperintensity patterns differentiate CJD from other rapid dementias. Neurology 2011; 76:1711–9.
6. Karaarslan E, Arslan A. Diffusion weighted MR imaging in non-infarct lesions of the brain. Eur J Rheumatol 2008;65:402–16.
7. Sakai M, Inoue Y, Oba H, et al. Age dependence of diffusion-weighted magnetic resonance imaging findings in maple syrup urine disease encephalopathy. J Comput Assist Tomogr 2005;229(4):524–7.
8. Ukisu R, Kushihashi T, Tanaka E, et al. Diffusion-weighted MR imaging if early-stage Creutzfeldt-Jakob disease: typical and atypical manifestations. Radiographics 2006;26(Suppl1):S191–204.
9. Sone J, Tanaka F, Koike H, et al. Skin biopsy is useful for the antemortem diagnosis of neuronal

intranuclear inclusion disease. Neurology 2011;76: 1372–6.
10. Sugiyama A, Sato N, Kimura Y, et al. MR imaging features of the cerebellum in adult-onset neuronal intranuclear inclusion disease: 8 cases. AJNR Am J Neuroradiol 2017;38:2100–4.
11. Morales H, Tomsick T. Middle cerebellar peduncles: Magnetic resonance imaging and pathophysiologic correlate. World J Radiol 2015;28:438–47.
12. Konno T, et al. Diagnostic value of brain calcifications in adult-onset leukoencephalopathy with axonal spheroids and pigmented glia. AJNR Am J Neuroradiol 2017;38:77–83.
13. Sundal C, Van Gerpen JA, Nicholson AM, et al. MRI characteristics and scoring in HDLS due to CSF1R gene mutations. Neurology 2012;79:566–74.
14. Degnan AJ, Levy LM. Inherited forms of Creutzfeldt-Jakob disease. AJNR Am J Neuroradiol 2013;34(9): 1690–1.
15. Holman RC, Belay ED, Christensen KY, et al. Human prion diseases in the United States. PLoS One 2010; 5(1):e8521.
16. Parci P, Giesa A, Capellaris S, et al. Classification of sporadic Creutzfeldt-Jakob disease based on molecular phenotypic analysis of 300 subjects. ANN Neurol 1999;46:224–33.
17. Meissner B, Kallenverg K, Sanchez-Juan T, et al. MRI lesions profiles in sporadic Creutzfeldt-Jakob disease. Neurology 2009;2:1994–2001.
18. Young GS, Geschwind MD, Fischbein NJ, et al. Diffusion weighted and fluid-attenuated inversion recovery imaging in Creutzfeldt-Jakob disease: high sensitivity and specificity for diagnosis. AJNR Am J Neuroradiol 2005;26(6):1551–62.
19. Hamaguchi T, Kitamoto T, Sato T, et al. Clinical diagnosis of MM2-type 2 sporadic Creutzfeldt-Jakob disease. Arch Neurol 2006;63:875–80.
20. Fukushima Rm, Shiga Y, Nakamura M, et al. MRI characteristics of sporadic CJD with valine homozygosity at codon 129 of the prion protein gene and PrP type 2 in Japan. J Neurol Neurosurg Psychiatry 2004;75:485–7.
21. Meissner B, Westner I, Kallenberg K, et al. Sporadic Creutzfeldt-Jakob disease: clinical and diagnostic characteristics of the rare VV1 type. Neurology 2005;65:1544–50.
22. Alvarez FJ, Bisbe J, Bisbe V, et al. Magnetic resonance imaging findings in pre-clinical Creutzfeldt-Jakob disease. Int J Neurosci 2005;115(8):1219–25.
23. CDC's diagnostic criteria for Creutzfeldt-Jakob disease. Centers for Disease Control and Prevention website. 2010. Available at: http://www.cdc.gov/prions/cjd/infection-control.html. Accessed November 23, 2020.
24. Tschampa HJ, Kallenberg K, Kretzschmar HA, et al. Pattern of cortical changes in sporadic Creutzfeldt-Jakob disease. AJNR Am J Neuroradiol 2007; 28(6):1114–8.
25. Shiga Y, Miyazawa K, Sato S, et al. Diffusion-weighted MRI abnormalities as an early diagnostic marker for Creutzfeldt-Jakob disease. Neurology 2004;63(3):443–9.
26. Eisenmenger L, Porter MC, Carswell CJ, et al. Evolution of diffusion-weighted magnetic resonance imaging signal abnormality in sporadic Creutzfeldt-Jakob disease, with histopathological correlation. JAMA Neurol 2016;73(1):76–84.
27. Collie DA, Summers DM, Sellar RJ, et al. Diagnosing variant Creutzfeldt-Jakob disease with the pulvinar sign: MR imaging findings in 86 neuropathological confirmed cases. AJNR Am J Neuroradiol 2003; 24(8):1560–9.
28. Hamaguchi T, Kitamoto T, Sato T, et al. Clinical diagnosis of MM2-type sporadic Creutzfeldt-Jakob disease. Neurology 2005;64(4):643–8.
29. Iwasaki Y, Kato H, Ando T, et al. Case report autopsy case of N180I genetic Creutzfeldt-Jakob disease with early disease pathology. Neuropathology 2018;38(6):638–45.
30. Sugiyama A, Beppu M, Kuwabara S. Teaching neuroimages: cerebral cortex swelling in Creutzfeldt-Jakob disease with V180I mutation. Neurology 2018;91:e185–6.
31. de Priester JA, Jansen GH, de Kruijk JR, et al. New MRI findings in Creutzfeldt-Jakob disease: high signal in the globus pallidus on T1-weighted images. Neuroradiology 1999;41(4):265–8.
32. Kallenberg K, Schulz-Schaeffer WJ, Jastrow U, et al. Creutzfeldt-Jakob disease: comparative analysis of MR imaging sequences. AJNR Am J Neuroradiol 2006;27(7):1459–62.
33. Poon MA, Stuckey S, Storey E. MRI evidence of cerebellar and hippocampal involvement in Creutzfeldt-Jakob disease. Neuroradiology 2001; 43(9):746–9.
34. Cohen OS, Hoffmann C, Lee H, et al. MRI detection of the cerebellar syndrome in Creutzfeldt-Jakob disease. Cerebellum 2009;8(3):373–81.
35. Geschwind MD, Potter CA, Suttavat M, et al. Correlating DWI MRI with pathologic and other features of -Creutzfeldt-Jakob disease. Alzheimer Dis Assoc Disord 2009;23:82–7.
36. Moseley ME, Kucharczyk, Mintrovitch J, et al. Early detection of regional cerebral ischemia in cats: comparison of diffusion-and T2 weighted MRI and spectroscopy. Magn Reson Med 1990; 14:330346.
37. Haik S, Dormont D, Faucheux BA, et al. Prion protein deposits match magnetic resonance imaging signal abnormalities in Creutzfeldt-Jakob disease. Ann Neurol 2002;51:797–9.

38. Kang EG, Jeon SJ, Choi SS, et al. Diffusion MR imaging of hypoglycemic encephalopathy. AJNR Am J Neuroradiol 2010;31:559–64.
39. Aoki T, Sato T, Hasegawa K, et al. Reversible hyperintensity lesion on diffusion-weighted MRI in hypoglycemic coma. Neurology 2004;27:392–3.
40. da Rocha AJ, Nunes RH, Maia AC Jr, et al. Recognizing autoimmune-mediated encephalitis in the differential diagnosis of limbic disorders. AJNR Am J Neuroradiol 2015;36(12):2196–205.
41. Bulakbasi N, Kocaoglu M. Central nervous system infections of herpesvirus family. Neuroimaging Clin N Am 2008;18(1):53–84.
42. Cianfoni A, Caulo M, Cerase A, et al. Seizure-induced brain lesions: a wide spectrum of variably reversible MRI abnormalities. Eur J Radiol 2013; 82(11):1964–72.
43. Kim JA, Chung JI, Yoon PH, et al. Transient MR signal changes in patients with generalized tonicoclonic seizure or status epilepticus: periictal diffusion-weighted imaging. AJNR Am J Neuroradiol 2001;22(6):1149–60.
44. Guler A, Alpaydin S, Sirin H, et al. A nonalcoholic Wernicke's encephalopathy case with atypical MRI findings: clinic versus radiology. Neuroradiol J 2015;28(5):474–7.
45. Tokumaru AM, Saito Y, Murayama S, et al. MRI diagnosis in other dementias. In: Matsuda H, Asada T, Tokumaru AM, editors. Neuroimaging diagnosis for alzheimer's disease and other dementias. Tokyo (Japan): Springer; 2017. p. 90–8.
46. Sone J, Kitagawa N, Sugawara e, et al. Neuronal intranuclear inclusion disease with leukoencephalopathy diagnosed via skin biopsy. J Neurol Neurosurg Psychiatry 2014;85:354–6.
47. Sone J, Mori K, Inagaki T, et al. Clinicopathological features of adult-onset neuronal intranuclear inclusion disease. Brain 2016;139:3170–86.
48. Takahashi-Fujigasaki J. Neuronal intranuclear hyaline inclusion disease. Neuropathology 2003;23: 351–9.
49. Takahashi-Fujigasaki J, Nakano Y, Uchino A, et al. Adult-onset neuronal intranuclear hyaline inclusion disease is not rare in older adults. Geriatr Gerontol Int 2016;16(Suppl 1):51–6.
50. Morimoto S, Hatsuta H, Komiya T, et al. Simultaneous skin-nerve-muscle biopsy and abnormal mitochondrial inclusions in intranuclear hyaline inclusion body disease. J Neurol Sci 2017;15(372):447–9.
51. Ishiura H, Shibata S, Yoshimura J, et al. Noncoding CGG repeat expansions in neuronal intranuclear inclusion disease, oculopharyngodistal myopathy and an overlapping disease. Nat Genet 2019;51:1222–32.
52. Sone J, Mitsuhashi S, Fujita A, et al. Long-read sequencing identifies GGC repeat expansions in NOTCH2NLS associated with neuronal intranuclear inclusion disease. Nat Genet 2019;51:1215–21.
53. Padilha LG, Nunes RH, Scortegana FA. Letters, MR imaging features of adult-onset neuronal intranuclear inclusion disease may be indistinguishable from Fragile X-Associated Tremor/Ataxia Syndrome. AJNR Am J Neuroradiol 2018;39: E100–1.
54. Greco CM, Hagerman RJ, Tassone F, et al. Neuronal intranuclear inclusions in a new cerebellar tremor/ ataxia syndrome among fragile X carriers. Brain 2002;125(Pt 8):1760–71.
55. Greco CM, Berman RF, Martin RM, et al. Neuropathology of fragile X-associated tremor/ataxia syndrome (FXTAS). Brain 2006;129(Pt 1):243–55.
56. Brunberg JA, Jacquemont S, Hagerman RJ, et al. Fragile X premutation carriers: characteristic MR imaging findings of adult male patients with progressive cerebellar and cognitive dysfunction. AJNR Am J Neuroradiol 2002;23:1757–66.
57. Kasuga K, Ikeuchi T, Arakawa K, et al. A patient with fragile x-associated tremor/ataxia syndrome presenting with executive cognitive deficits and cerebral white matter lesions. Case Rep Neurol 2011;3: 118–23.
58. Fu YH, Kuhl DP, Pizzuti A, et al. Variation of the CGG repeat at the fragile X site results in genetic instability: resolution of the Sherman paradox. Cell 1991;67:1047–58.
59. Hagerman RJ, Leeley M, Heinrichs W, et al. Intention tremor, parkinsonism, and generalized brain atrophy in male carriers of fragile X. Neurology 2001;57: 127–30.
60. Adams JS, Adams PE, Nguyen D, et al. Volumetric brain changes in females with fragile X-associated tremor/ataxia syndrome (FXTAS). Neurology 2007; 69:851–9.
61. Brown SSG, Stanfield AC. Fragile X premutation carriers: a systematic review of neuroimaging findings. J Neurol Sci 2015;352:19–28.
62. Hagerman R, Hagerman P. Advanced in clinical and molecular understanding of the FMR1 premutation and fragile X-associated tremor/ataxia syndrome. Lancet Neurol 2013;12:786–98.
63. Hashimoto R, Srivastava S, Tassone F, et al. Diffusion tensor imaging in male permutation carriers of the fragile X mental retardation gene. Mov Disord 2011;26:1329–36.
64. Hashimoto R, Javan AK, Tassone F, et al. A voxel-based morphometry study of grey matter loss in fragile X-associated tremor/ataxia syndrome. Brain 2011;134:863–78.
65. Shioya A, Ishii K, Saito Y. Fragile X-associated tremor/ataxia syndrome. Clin Neurosci 2015;33: 130–1.
66. Freeman SH, Hyman Bt, Sims KB, et al. Adult onset leukodystrophy with neuroaxonal spheroids: Clinical, neuroimaging and neuropathologic observations. Brain Pathol 2009;19:39–47.

67. Kinosita M, Yoshida K, Oyanagi K, et al. Hereditary diffuse leukoencephalopathy with axonal spheroids caused by R782H mutation in CSF1R: Case report. J Neurol Sci 2012;318:115–8.
68. Kim EJ, Shin JH, Kim JH, et al. Adult-onset leukoencephalopathy with axonal spheroids and pigmented glia linked CSF1Rmutation: Report of four Korean cases. J Neurol Sci 2015;349:232–8.
69. Konno T, Yoshida K, Mizuta I, et al. Diagnostic Criteria for Adult-onset Leukoencephalopathy with Axonal Spheroids and Pigmented Glia Due to *CSF1R* mutation. Eur J Neurol 2018;25:142–7.
70. Terasawa Y, Osaki Y, Kawarai T, et al. Increasing and persistent DWI changes in a patient with Hereditary Diffuse Leukoencephalopathy with Spheroids. J Neurol Sci 2013;335:213–5.
71. Konno T, Tada M, Tada M. Haploinsufficiency of CSF-1R and clinicopathologic characterization in patients with HDLS. Neurology 2014;82:139–48.
72. Abe T, Kawarai T, Fujita K, et al. MR Spectroscopy in patients with hereditary diffuse leukoencephalopathy with spheroids and asymptomatic carriers of colony-stimulating factor 1 receptor mutation. Magn Reson Med Sci 2017;16:297–303.
73. Inui T, Kawarai T, Fujita K, et al. A new CSF1R mutation presenting with an extensive white matter lesion mimicking primary progressive multiple sclerosis. J Neurol Sci 2013;334:192–5.
74. Rademakers R, Baker M, Nicholson AM, et al. Mutations in colony stimulating factor1 (CSF1R) gene cause hereditary diffuse leukoencephalopathy with spheroids. Nat Genet 2012;44:200–5.
75. Song C, Peng L, Wang S, et al. A novel compound heterozygous mutation in AARS2 gene (c.965 G > A, p.R322H; c.334 G > C, p.G112R) identified in a Chinese patient with leukodystrophy involved in brain and spinal cord. J Hum Genet 2019;64(10): 979–83.
76. Taglia I, Di Donato I, Bianchi S, et al. AARS2-related ovarioleukodystrophy: Clinical and neuroimaging features of three new cases. Acta Neurol Scand 2018;138:278–83.
77. Srivastava S, Butala A, Mashida S, et al. Expansion of the clinical spectrum associated with AARS2-related disorders. Am J Med Genet 2019;179A: 1556–64.
78. Tokumaru AM. Degenerative disease: FXTAS p. 320. In: Taoka T, editor. Essentials of diagnostic pearls of ne radiology pearls of neuroradiology. Japan Tokyo: Medicalview; 2021 (in print).
79. Tokumaru AM, Taoka T. Degenerative disease: HDLS p. 323. In: Essentials of diagnostic radiology pearls of neuroradiology. Japan Tokyo: Medicalview; 2021 (in print).

Diffusion Magnetic Resonance Imaging of Infants

Jeffrey J. Neil, MD, PhD[a,b,c], Christopher D. Smyser, MD, MSCI[a,b,c,*]

KEYWORDS

• MRI • Diffusion imaging • Neonate • Preterm • Brain development

KEY POINTS

- Diffusion imaging can be applied successfully and robustly in infants and offers information on both tissue physiology (injury) and microstructure.
- Diffusion parameters change throughout the course of early brain development, reflecting underlying changes in the microstructure of white matter and gray matter.
- In term neonates with neonatal encephalopathy, early diffusion imaging provides an accurate indication of the degree and location of brain injury.
- In preterm infants, abnormalities of white matter diffusion anisotropy reflect the widespread disruption of white matter development that accompanies preterm birth.

INTRODUCTION

Diffusion magnetic resonance imaging (MRI) provides several parameters for evaluation of brain structure and function. The most basic of these, derived from a single tensor formalism, are mean diffusivity (MD) and fractional anisotropy (FA). Although more sophisticated methods provide additional parameters, these are the most commonly applied in clinical practice and clinically oriented research studies in infants. Even these elementary parameters offer rich information on tissue characteristics, ranging from physiology (eg, MD reduction reflecting brain injury) to microstructure (eg, FA as an indicator of white matter structure/myelination and cortical plate maturity). This article considers how these parameters reflect the remarkable changes in tissue microstructure that accompany typical early brain development and their application to the detection of brain injury, focusing on the period from midgestation through early infancy.

TECHNICAL CONSIDERATIONS

There are several unique aspects of the developing brain that influence image acquisition but one in particular that affects diffusion imaging. Infant brains have higher water content than adult brains. As a result, MD values for infant brains are higher than for adult brains,[1,2] and the ideal b-value for measurement, if a single value is used, is approximately 1/MD,[3] or approximately 800 s/mm^2, compared with 1200 s/mm^2 commonly used for adult studies.

DETECTION OF BRAIN INJURY

By far the most common clinical use of diffusion MRI is for detection of acute and subacute brain

[a] Department of Neurology, Washington University School of Medicine, 660 South Euclid Avenue, Campus Box 8111, St Louis, MO 63110-1093, USA; [b] Department of Pediatrics, Washington University School of Medicine, 660 South Euclid Avenue, Campus Box 8116, St Louis, MO 63110-1093, USA; [c] Department of Radiology, Washington University School of Medicine, 660 South Euclid Avenue, Campus Box 8131, St Louis, MO 63110-1093, USA

* Corresponding author. Department of Neurology, Washington University School of Medicine, 660 South Euclid Avenue, Campus Box 8111, St Louis, MO 63110-1093.

E-mail address: smyserc@wustl.edu

Magn Reson Imaging Clin N Am 29 (2021) 185–193
https://doi.org/10.1016/j.mric.2021.01.004

injury, where it has proved invaluable.[4] Brain water MD values fall within minutes of stroke, and, for adults, diffusion images show areas of injury at onset in greater than 90% of patients.[5] The initial sensitivity of diffusion imaging for injury is different for infants (**Fig. 1**A). Time course studies of infants in whom the timing of injury is known indicate that approximately one-third of infants have initially normal diffusion imaging, and MD subsequently falls, reaching a nadir after 2 to 4 days.[6] The remaining two-thirds have a time course similar to adults, with sustained low MD from injury onset.

This variation may be explained by differences in the nature of the injury. In animal studies in which stroke is induced by arterial occlusion, MD falls within minutes. If the occlusion continues for greater than or equal to 60 minutes, MD remains low even if blood flow is restored. This typically is the case in adults with stroke, for whom thrombi typically persist for hours or days, hence the persistently low MD. If blood flow is restored quickly (eg, within approximately 30 minutes), however, MD may return to normal, with secondary decline after 2 to 4 days (**Fig. 1**B).[7,8] The scenario for neonates commonly may parallel that in which blood flow is restored quickly within approximately 30 minutes. For example, an intrauterine event, such as placental abruption or uterine rupture, may compromise the fetus, but blood flow and oxygenation may be restored relatively quickly through emergent delivery, which leads to MD transiently returning to normal.

Overall, diffusion imaging is most sensitive in infants 2 to 4 days after injury, and this should be borne in mind when interpreting MRI studies to detect possible injury. Beyond this window, MD rises to normal (ie, pseudonormalizes), and diffusion imaging is relatively insensitive for injury detection. T1-weighted and T2-weighted images, however, become sensitive to injury starting approximately 3 to 5 days after injury, so MRI remains highly useful. Nevertheless, there may be a gap at approximately 5 days after injury, during which it can be difficult to detect on MRI. Finally, if MRI studies are obtained weeks after injury, affected areas may be resorbed to the extent that signal abnormalities no longer are present, leaving residual tissue volume loss.

Given this timeline of MD changes following injury in infants, there are other considerations in determining when to obtain diffusion imaging. For example, in severely injured infants for whom redirection of care is being considered, early diffusion imaging is helpful because MD often stays low from injury onset, similar to the time course of adult stroke. Another consideration involves use of therapeutic hypothermia to treat neonatal encephalopathy,[9] which affects the time course of MD changes following injury in infants, extending the duration during which MD remains low.[10] The authors' standard clinical practice includes obtaining MRI studies on infants treated with therapeutic hypothermia on day of life 4, after rewarming and while diffusion imaging still demonstrates injury.

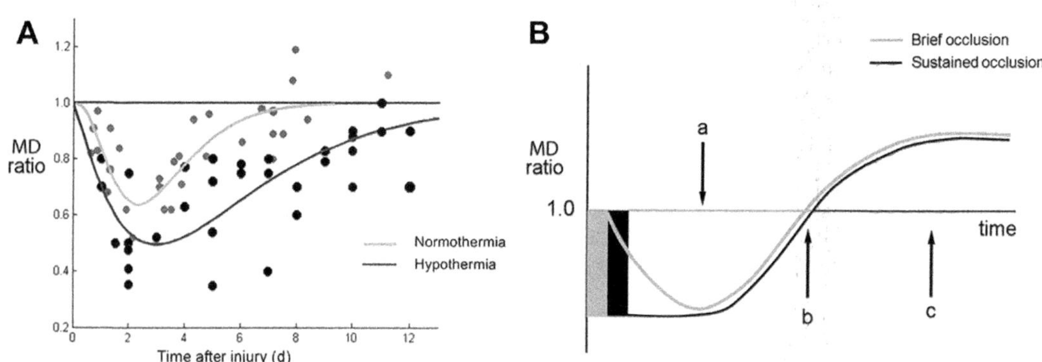

Fig. 1. The time course of change in MD following brain injury. MD is expressed as the ratio between the area of injury and the corresponding, uninjured contralateral area. MD values less than 1 represent a reduction in MD in the area of injury. (*A*) The time course of MD changes following injury in infants with and without therapeutic hypothermia treatment. Note that the time course for the reduction in MD is different between normothermic infants (*gray*) and those treated with therapeutic hypothermia (*black*). (*B*) A theoretic time course from animal studies representing brief (*gray*) and sustained (*black*) arterial occlusion. At time point a, image contrast for detecting injury is maximum. Time point b represents pseudonormalization, a time at which diffusion imaging may appear normal despite injury. At time point c, which is typically weeks after injury, MD is higher, rather than lower, in areas of injury due to tissue breakdown. (*A*) Used with permission.[10]

BRAIN DEVELOPMENT

Employing the standard terminology recommended by the American Academy of Pediatrics,[11] the time between a woman's last menstrual period before becoming pregnant and delivery of the infant is gestational age, and the time since birth is chronologic age (CA). For preterm infants, gestational age and chronologic age are summed to calculate postmenstrual age (PMA). Thus, a 4-week-old infant born at 24 weeks' gestation has a PMA of 28 weeks. A PMA of 40 weeks is labeled term-equivalent age (TEA), because human gestation normally is 40 weeks.

The youngest surviving preterm infants are born at 22 to 24 weeks' gestation, and this article focuses on the second half of gestation because that is when preterm infants can be studied. The entirety of brain development follows a remarkably choreographed sequence of events. At 24 weeks' gestation, neural migration largely is finished but cortical folding and white matter myelination are just beginning. The brain is relatively smooth, the majority of young neurons have taken their positions in the developing cortical plate, axons are extending to form neural networks, and the subplate is involuting.[12]

One unique aspect of early brain development is that MD values fall steadily during gestation. This likely is related to brain water content, because brain wet-to-dry weight falls during development.[13] As a result, barriers to diffusion move closer together and cause a reduction in MD. Also, the water content of developing white matter is higher than gray matter, and MD values for white matter are higher than gray matter (**Fig. 2**A). MD falls for both white matter and gray matter with increasing PMA, but white matter and gray matter values become closer together as the brain matures. As a result, gray–white contrast is strong on MD maps of preterm infants and gradually diminishes near TEA. Ultimately, MD maps of older children and adults show essentially no gray–white contrast, with MD values in both tissues approximately 0.9×10^{-3} mm^2/s.

FA also changes during brain development, reflecting maturational changes in tissue microstructure. Although FA usually is considered in the context of myelinated white matter, and anisotropy values taken as an indication of white matter integrity with higher values indicating healthier tissue,[14] the addition of myelin causes increases in FA during development. This is evident in the difference in FA between the anterior limb of the internal capsule (ALIC) and posterior limb of the internal capsule (PLIC). At TEA, the ALIC, which is not yet myelinated, has an FA of 0.13, whereas the PLIC, which is myelinated, has an FA of 0.21.[1] Assuming that axonal packing is similar in these structures, this difference largely is due to myelination. The ALIC, however, still has nonzero anisotropy. This is a consequence of close spacing of axons oriented in parallel, which confers a preferred direction of water displacements parallel to them even in the absence of myelin. Overall, the anisotropy values of developing white matter increase in two steps. The first, which is small, is related to maturation of not-yet-myelinated fibers and likely is caused by microstructural changes associated with premyelination.[15] This is shown in the white matter of the centrum semiovale, which shows an increase in anisotropy near TEA yet remains predominantly unmyelinated at that age (**Fig. 2**). The second

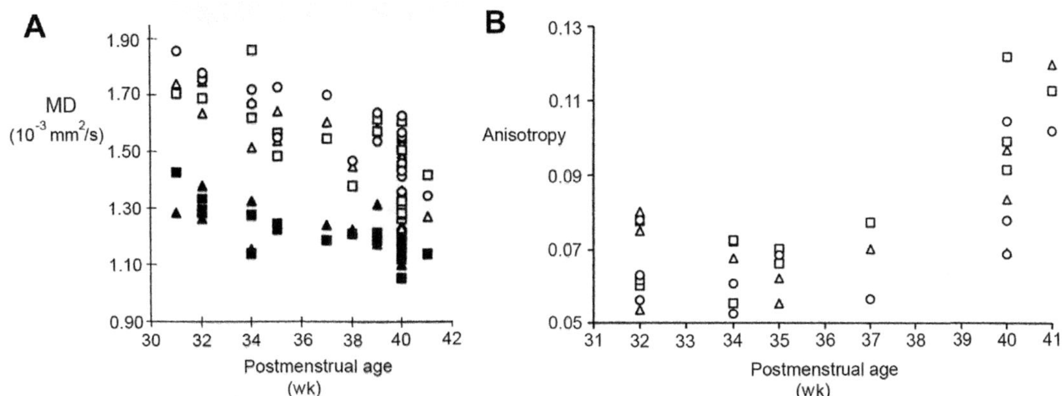

Fig. 2. (*A*) MD values versus PMA. Open symbols are from the centrum semiovale (*triangles* = anterior, *squares* = central, and *circles* = posterior) and filled symbols are cortical gray matter (*triangles* = medial and *squares* = lateral). (*B*) Diffusion anisotropy values for the centrum semiovale versus PMA. Used with permission.[1]

increase, which is larger, is associated with the addition of myelin and proceeds throughout childhood.[16]

The cortical plate also shows anisotropy changes during development. In the mature cortex, diffusion anisotropy is low, essentially zero in clinical studies. In the cortical plate, however, anisotropy values initially are high and decrease during development.[17] This is a consequence of the microstructure of the cortical plate (**Fig. 3**A).[18] Early in development, the cytoarchitecture is dominated by pyramidal cells with apical dendrites, extending to the cortical surface, and radial glial cells, which guide neuronal migration. This organization leads to a preferred direction of water displacements orthogonal to the surface of the brain and, hence, high diffusion anisotropy. As maturation proceeds, microstructural changes include the addition of basal dendrites to pyramidal cells, elaboration of dendrites from interneurons, addition and myelination of afferent axons, and involution of radial glia, which reduces anisotropy values to near zero.[17]

The anisotropy changes of the developing cortical plate reflect differential rates of development. It has been known since histology studies of the mid-nineteenth century that different areas of cortex develop at varied rates.[19] Generally speaking, primary motor and sensory areas, such as motor and visual cortex, develop earlier than association areas, such as prefrontal and parietal cortex.[20] This differential development is visible in surface representations in which cortical anisotropy is lower in faster maturing areas (**Fig. 3**B). This also can be seen in the development of Heschl's gyrus, where FA falls earlier in primary than nonprimary auditory cortex.[21] Furthermore, cortical maturation is more rapid in areas near the insula and slower moving further from the insula. This is evident in cortical anisotropy maps from fixed primate tissue.[22]

Differential rates of cortical plate development also are apparent in preterm human infant investigations. In a study of 65 preterm infants, MD and FA were measured over the entire developing cortical plate.[23] Based on the rates of change in FA from 27 through 46 weeks' PMA, the cortex was divided into 3 clusters. Areas in the cluster with the highest rates of decline also had the highest initial FA at 27 weeks' PMA and included the frontal and anterior temporal poles, superior and lateral parietal cortices, and left temporoparietal junction, regions dominated by association areas. The cluster with the lowest rate of decline in FA also had the lowest initial FA, and consisted of inferior frontal, medial occipital, and perirolandic cortices, and right temporal regions. These regions include primary motor and sensory areas, such as motor, visual, and auditory cortices. These differing rates of change during later gestation reflect the nonlinear decline of cortical FA during development. All cortical plate regions start with high FA early in development and end with low FA by TEA. As regions mature, FA drops to near zero during a period of weeks and remains there. Faster maturing primary motor and sensory areas largely complete this drop in FA by 27 weeks' PMA. These areas, therefore, had low FA on the initial MRI studies and showed small decreases

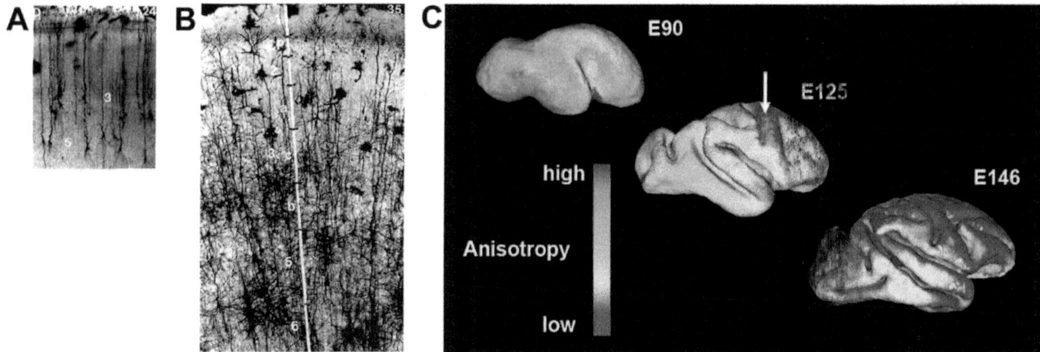

Fig. 3. (*A*, *B*) Golgi preparations of the human cortical plate. The pial surface is at the top of each panel. (*A*) Taken at 24 weeks' gestation and (*B*) taken at 35 weeks' gestation. Note the prominence of the apical dendrites from pyramidal cells at 24 weeks' gestation; their orientation confers diffusion anisotropy with a preferred direction of water displacements oriented orthogonal to the cortical surface. By 35 weeks' gestation, this microstructure has been disrupted by several structural changes, including the addition of basal dendrites to pyramidal cells and the addition of interneurons, which leads to a loss of diffusion anisotropy. Adapted with permission.[18] (*C*) Surface representations of fixed baboon brains at 90 days' through 146 days' gestation. FA of the underlying cortical plate is represented in color. Note the gradual diminution of anisotropy during development. Note also the relatively earlier reduction in FA in primary motor cortex (*arrow*), most evident at E125. Adapted with permission.[22]

in FA through to TEA. Association areas, in contrast, had not yet undergone this change. These areas started with higher FA, which fell more precipitously during later gestation. This is evident in Fig. 3C, in which the contrast in FA between early-developing and late-developing areas is strongest in mid-gestation. In a similar study of preterm infants,[24] the fastest declines in FA were observed in prefrontal cortex. These diffusion data also were evaluated using mean kurtosis, with values also declining during development but at different rates across different areas than FA. This suggests kurtosis may provide unique information regarding cortical development.

Overall, anisotropy values for the brain increase in white matter and decrease in gray matter during development, and in both instances these trajectories reflect microstructural changes associated with maturation. Although maturation often is thought of separately for white matter and gray matter, it actually occurs across neural systems, with gray matter and associated white matter maturing in tandem. Thus, anisotropy values for motor cortex and the associated corticospinal tracts both mature earlier than prefrontal cortex and its associated white matter (Fig. 4).[25]

THE ROLE OF DIFFUSION IMAGING IN PREDICTING OUTCOME IN TERM INFANTS

Brain injury in term-born infants can take numerous forms, with hypoxic-ischemic injury (HIE) a common etiology. In a simplified classification scheme, HIE is divided into two patterns: (1) basal ganglia (BG) injury, characterized by injury to the basal ganglia, thalamus, and perirolandic cortex, and (2) watershed injury, characterized by injury to the anterior and/or posterior zones between the anterior, middle, and posterior cerebral artery territories.[26,27] The BG pattern is found after acute, near-total hypoxic-ischemic insults. With more severe hypoxia-ischemia, the distribution extends to include perirolandic cortex.[27] In contrast, watershed injury is associated with less striking imaging evidence of injury and is caused by sustained, less severe hypoxia-ischemia.[27] The neurodevelopmental outcomes for these two patterns of injury differ. Outcomes for the BG pattern are poor and strongly related to imaging characteristics,[28] including an association between motor outcome and involvement of the PLIC. Watershed injury, in contrast, portends comparatively better motor and cognitive outcomes.[26] Detection of one or a combination of these two canonical forms of brain injury does not establish the diagnosis of HIE, because there are infectious[29] and metabolic[30,31] mimics.

BG and watershed patterns of injury originally were identified on T1-weighted and T2-weighted images but are readily detectable on diffusion images. As detailed previously, the sensitivity for detection depends on when after injury the images were obtained. Diffusion imaging plays an important role in the first 3 to 5 days after injury, with T1-weighted and T2-weighted imaging more helpful thereafter.[32] For prognosis, however, performance of early diffusion imaging and later T1-weighted and T2-weighted images is comparable. When MRI studies were performed at less than or equal to 6 days or greater than or equal to 7 days of life, both early and late MRIs yielded 100% sensitivity for adverse outcome, but early MRI, on which injury was detected largely using diffusion imaging, had higher specificity than late MRI (96% vs 89%, respectively).[33] Interobserver agreement also has been shown to be higher on diffusion images, perhaps because the contrast-to-noise ratio is greater.[34] One potential issue in

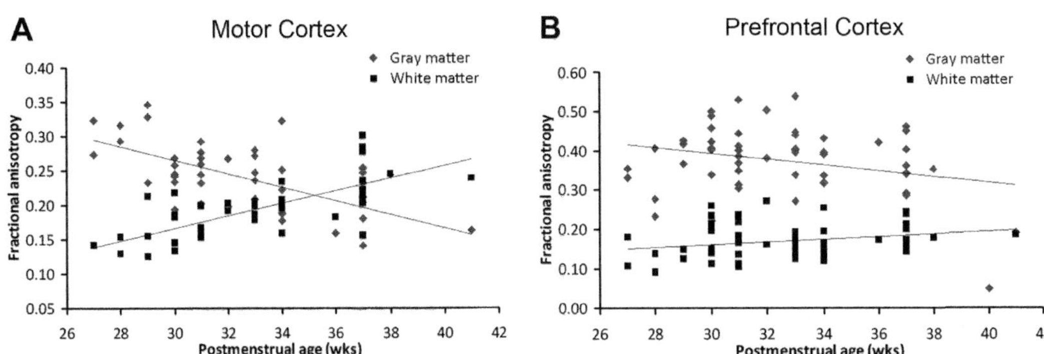

Fig. 4. Scatter plots of FA versus PMA in the white (*open squares*) and gray (*black diamonds*) matter of the (*A*) motor cortex and (*B*) prefrontal cortex. The solid lines depict results from linear regression. Note differences in the crossover point for regression lines for gray matter and white matter for the two regions, with the faster-developing motor system crossing earlier than the prefrontal system. Adapted with permission.[25]

comparing early and late scans is whether they show comparable degrees of injury in the same infant. In a study where MRI was obtained on days 4 and 10 after birth and the degree of injury was graded, 32/41 (78%) infants showed no change in grade between the first and second scans. Of the infants whose grade changed, approximately one-third improved and two-thirds worsened.[35] Overall, early diffusion imaging may hold modest advantages over later T1-weighted and T2-weighted imaging for injury detection in term infants, although which modality is employed may depend more on clinical circumstances and the desire for information earlier in the hospital course than relative performance. In many institutions, both early and late imaging are employed.

As described previously, use of therapeutic hypothermia to treat neonatal encephalopathy has an effect on the time course of MD changes following injury, and it is possible this may affect the prognostic utility of diffusion imaging. A meta-analysis showed that therapeutic hypothermia did not change the prognostic value of neonatal brain MRI. The odds ratio for adverse neurodevelopmental outcomes with severe injury on MRI was 14.0 for infants treated with therapeutic hypothermia versus 18.1 for normothermic infants ($P = .75$).[36]

THE ROLE OF DIFFUSION IMAGING IN PREDICTING OUTCOME IN PRETERM INFANTS

Brain injury in preterm infants typically manifests as white matter injury, and FA is well-suited to evaluate these findings. Both MD and FA have been employed to assess white matter injury in preterm infants and predict outcome. This injury may be focal, as in cystic periventricular leukomalacia, but more commonly is characterized by diffuse changes, or diffuse periventricular leukomalacia.[37] The nature of this injury has been defined histologically,[38] and diffusion imaging provides evidence supporting its presence via globally reduced white matter FA at TEA.[39]

White matter diffusion abnormalities have been shown to correlate with neurodevelopmental outcomes across studies. For example, high white matter[40] and cerebellar[41] MD have been associated with worse motor outcomes at age 2 years. In addition, low white matter FA, particularly in the PLIC and corpus callosum, has been associated with poor motor outcomes.[42–45] In studies of preterm children at ages 4 to 7 years, high right orbitofrontal MD has been associated with social-emotional problems,[46] and high occipital pole and cerebellar MD were associated with motor and executive function impairment.[47] In addition, low PLIC FA was associated with poor motor outcomes at age 4 years.[48]

Across studies, low white matter anisotropy was associated with impaired outcome, but this relationship is not universal. In preterm infants at age 2 years, lower right inferior temporal lobe FA, but higher left inferior temporal lobe FA, were associated with lower motor scores. In another study, lower left cingulum bundle FA was associated with better social-emotional competence.[49] The microstructural alterations underlying these apparently anomalous results have not been fully identified, although it has been hypothesized that reduced axonal branching or fewer fiber tracts crossing the tract of interest may lead to higher anisotropy in injured areas.

These studies employed region of interest (ROI) analyses, in which brain regions were drawn, often manually, to generate diffusion parameter measures. In a complementary approach, ROIs may consist of whole tracts identified using tractography. In one tractography study,[50] PLIC FA independently predicted motor delay and cerebral palsy by age 2 years, with 80% to 100% sensitivity and 66% to 69% specificity. In addition, corpus callosum MD predicted motor delay with 100% sensitivity and 65% specificity. There also are more automated approaches to evaluate diffusion data, the most popular of which is tract-based spatial statistics (TBSS).[51] With this approach, diffusion parametric maps are analyzed to identify areas where diffusion values correlate with parameters of interest, such as neurodevelopmental outcomes. Although results across these approaches generally are comparable, they do not always match and thus may not be interchangeable. Using TBSS to study preterm infants, cognitive scores at age 2 years were correlated with corpus callosum FA, and fine-motor scores were correlated with FA throughout the white matter.[52]

FA may be further divided into axial diffusivity (AD) and radial diffusivity (RD), which essentially are MD values taken perpendicular and parallel to axons. In areas where diffusion is anisotropic, AD and RD differ, with AD being greater than RD by definition. For white matter, water movement perpendicular to axons (from which RD is derived) is hindered because water molecules are moving across myelin layers or across other axons in unmyelinated white matter, resulting in lower diffusivity. In comparison, water movement parallel to white matter (from which AD is derived) is less hindered because water molecules may move within myelin layers or along axons without crossing lipid membranes. Although an oversimplification, MD can be viewed as a weighted average of AD and RD and FA as reflecting differences between AD and RD, with greater differences associated with higher FA.

Breaking diffusion into AD and RD provides insights into the etiology of reduced FA in myelinated white matter. When FA is low in myelinated white matter (ie, AD and RD are closer together), it may be because AD is lower and/or RD is higher. Lower AD suggests disruption of axons, whereas higher RD suggests injury to myelin. Although this approach is not perfect, it holds true in experimental models of axonal[53] and myelin[54] injury as well as dysmyelinating disorders.[55] As discussed previously, MD decreases during development, and FA increases as white matter is myelinated. The MD reduction is related to an overall decrease in brain water content during development, and both AD and RD decrease during white matter maturation. The relative reduction in RD is greater than AD, however, consistent with changes expected as myelin layers are added and associated with an increase in FA.

White matter FA, AD, and RD were compared with neonatal intensive care unit course and outcome in 491 preterm infants using TBSS.[56] Identified risk factors for diffuse white matter injury included lower birth GA, fetal growth restriction, increased ventilation and parenteral nutrition days, necrotizing enterocolitis, and male sex. Multivariate analysis demonstrated that fetal growth restriction and increased number of days of ventilation and parenteral nutrition were independently associated with lower FA. Infants exposed to multiple risk factors, assessed by a cumulative risk score, had lower FA and higher RD, consistent with myelin disruption (also consistent with histologic studies). FA at TEA was associated with subsequent neurodevelopmental abilities.

Relatively few studies compare cortical diffusion parameters with outcome, likely related to two factors. First, measuring diffusion parameters in the developing cortical plate is more challenging than white matter due to its thin and convoluted shape. In addition, cortical FA basically is zero at TEA, making FA relatively uninformative by this developmental stage. From 27 weeks' to 46 weeks' PMA,[23] rates of FA and MD changes in the developing cortical plate were related to GA, indicating that development was more disrupted in infants born earlier. In addition, higher developmental quotient at age 2 years was related to more rapid changes in MD, but not FA, during the preterm period. In a study of 91 preterm infants at TEA and 69 full-term controls, preterm infants demonstrated higher diffusivity in the prefrontal, parietal, motor, somatosensory, and visual cortices, suggesting delayed maturation of these areas.[57] FA was higher in preterm infants in the motor cortex only. The investigators concluded that although MD was associated with cerebral cortical dysmaturation in preterm infants, FA was not a strong marker of regional cortical maturation at TEA, a potential consequence of the issues outlined previously.

SUMMARY

Overall, diffusion imaging provides a unique and important perspective on infant brain development and injury. From a clinical perspective, it is unparalleled as a means of detecting subacute brain injury in the clinical setting. It also provides an indicator of the white matter injury that accompanies preterm birth, which, when taken in clinical context, can be helpful for predicting neurodevelopmental outcome. From a more scientific standpoint, it can be used to detect the microstructural changes associated with both white matter and cortical development, showing how this development varies regionally.

DISCLOSURE

Drs J.J. Neil and C.D. Smyser receive support through grant NIH P50 HD103525. Dr C.D. Smyser also receives support through grants R01 MH113883 and R01 MH113570.

REFERENCES

1. Neil JJ, Shiran SI, McKinstry RC, et al. Normal brain in human newborns: apparent diffusion coefficient and diffusion anisotropy measured by using diffusion tensor MR imaging. Radiology 1998;209(1):57–66.
2. Huppi PS, Maier SE, Peled S, et al. Microstructural development of human newborn cerebral white matter assessed in vivo by diffusion tensor magnetic resonance imaging. Pediatr Res 1998;44(4):584–90.
3. Conturo TE, McKinstry RC, Aronovitz JA, et al. Diffusion MRI: Precision, accuracy and flow effects. NMR Biomed 1995;8(7–8):307–32.
4. Moseley ME, Cohen Y, Mintorovitch J, et al. Early detection of regional cerebral ischemia in cats: Comparison of diffusion- and T_2-weighted MRI and spectroscopy. Magn Reson Med 1990;14(2):330–46.
5. Oppenheim C, Stanescu R, Dormont D, et al. False-negative diffusion-weighted MR findings in acute ischemic stroke. AJNR Am J Neuroradiol 2000;21(8):1434–40.
6. McKinstry RC, Miller JH, Snyder AZ, et al. A Prospective, Longitudinal Diffusion Tensor Imaging Study of Brain Injury in Newborns. Neurology 2002;59(6):824–33.

7. Dijkhuizen RM, Knollema S, van der Worp HB, et al. Dynamics of cerebral tissue injury and perfusion after temporary hypoxia-ischemia in the rat: evidence for region-specific sensitivity and delayed damage. Stroke 1998;29(3):695–704.
8. Li F, Silva MD, Liu KF, et al. Secondary decline in apparent diffusion coefficient and neurological outcomes after a short period of focal brain ischemia in rats. Ann Neurol 2000;48(2):236–44.
9. Jacobs SE, Berg M, Hunt R, et al. Cooling for newborns with hypoxic ischaemic encephalopathy. Cochrane Database Syst Rev 2013;1(1):CD003311.
10. Bednarek N, Mathur A, Inder T, et al. Impact of therapeutic hypothermia on MRI diffusion changes in neonatal encephalopathy. Neurology 2012;78(18): 1420–7.
11. Engle WA. Age terminology during the perinatal period. Pediatrics 2004;114(5):1362–4.
12. Bystron I, Blakemore C, Rakic P. Development of the human cerebral cortex: Boulder Committee revisited. Nat Rev Neurosci 2008;9(2):110–22.
13. Dodge PR, Prensky AL, Feigin RD, editors. Nutrition and the developing Nervous system. St Louis (MO): C.V. Mosby; 1975.
14. Klingberg T, Hedehus M, Temple E, et al. Microstructure of temporo-parietal white matter as a basis for reading ability: evidence from diffusion tensor magnetic resonance imaging. Neuron 2000;25(2): 493–500.
15. Wimberger DM, Roberts TP, Barkovich AJ, et al. Identification of "premyelination" by diffusion-weighted MRI. J Comput Assist Tomogr 1995; 19(1):28–33.
16. Miller JH, McKinstry RC, Philip JV, et al. Diffusion-Tensor MR Imaging of Normal Brain Maturation: A Guide to Structural Development and Myelination. AJR Am J Roentgenol 2003;180(3):851–9.
17. McKinstry RC, Mathur A, Miller JH, et al. Radial organization of developing preterm human cerebral cortex revealed by non-invasive water diffusion anisotropy MRI. Cereb Cortex 2002;12(12):1237–43.
18. Marin-Padilla M. Ontogenesis of the pyramidal cell of the mammalian neocortex and developmental cytoarchitectonics: a unifying theory. J Comp Neurol 1992;321(2):223–40.
19. Brodmann K. Vergleichende Lokalisationslehre der Grosshirnrinde in ihren Prinzipien dargestellt auf Grund des Zellenbaues. Leipzig: Verlag von Johann Ambrosius Barth; 1909.
20. Sidman RL, Rakic P. Development of the human central nervous system. In: Haymaker W, Adams RD, editors. Histology and Histopathology of the Nervous system. Springfield: C.C. Thomas; 1982. p. 3–I45.
21. Monson BB, Eaton-Rosen Z, Kapur K, et al. Differential rates of perinatal maturation of human primary and nonprimary auditory cortex. eNeuro 2018;5(1).
22. Kroenke CD, Van Essen DC, Inder TE, et al. Microstructural changes of the baboon cerebral cortex during gestational development reflected in magnetic resonance imaging diffusion anisotropy. J Neurosci 2007;27(46):12506–15.
23. Ball G, Srinivasan L, Aljabar P, et al. Development of cortical microstructure in the preterm human brain. Proc Natl Acad Sci U S A 2013;110(23):9541–6.
24. Ouyang M, Jeon T, Sotiras A, et al. Differential cortical microstructural maturation in the preterm human brain with diffusion kurtosis and tensor imaging. Proc Natl Acad Sci USA 2019;116(10): 4681–8.
25. Smyser TA, Smyser CD, Rogers CE, et al. Cortical gray and adjacent white matter demonstrate synchronous maturation in very preterm infants. Cereb Cortex 2016;26(8):3370–8.
26. Miller SP, Ramaswamy V, Michelson D, et al. Patterns of brain injury in term neonatal encephalopathy. J Pediatr 2005;146(4):453–60.
27. American College of Obstetrics and Gynecology. Executive summary: Neonatal encephalopathy and neurologic outcome, second edition. Report of the American College of Obstetricians and Gynecologists' Task Force on Neonatal Encephalopathy. Report of the American College of Obstetricians and Gynecologists' Task Force on Neonatal Encephalopathy. Obstet Gynecol 2014;123(4):896–901.
28. Martinez-Biarge M, Diez-Sebastian J, Rutherford MA, et al. Outcomes after central grey matter injury in term perinatal hypoxic-ischaemic encephalopathy. Early Hum Dev 2010;86(11):675–82.
29. Hernandez MI, Sandoval CC, Tapia JL, et al. Stroke patterns in neonatal group B streptococcal meningitis. Pediatr Neurol 2011;44(4):282–8.
30. Johnston MV, Hoon AH Jr. Possible mechanisms in infants for selective basal ganglia damage from asphyxia, kernicterus, or mitochondrial encephalopathies. J Child Neurol 2000;15(9):588–91.
31. Poretti A, Blaser SI, Lequin MH, et al. Neonatal neuroimaging findings in inborn errors of metabolism. J Magn Reson Imaging 2013;37(2):294–312.
32. Weeke LC, Groenendaal F, Mudigonda K, et al. A novel magnetic resonance imaging score predicts neurodevelopmental outcome after perinatal asphyxia and therapeutic hypothermia. J Pediatr 2018;192:33–40.
33. Charon V, Proisy M, Bretaudeau G, et al. Early MRI in neonatal hypoxic-ischaemic encephalopathy treated with hypothermia: Prognostic role at 2-year follow-up. Eur J Radiol 2016;85(8):1366–74.
34. Goergen SK, Ang H, Wong F, et al. Early MRI in term infants with perinatal hypoxic-ischaemic brain injury: interobserver agreement and MRI predictors of outcome at 2 years. Clin Radiol 2014;69(1):72–81.
35. Trivedi SB, Vesoulis ZA, Rao R, et al. A validated clinical MRI injury scoring system in neonatal

hypoxic-ischemic encephalopathy. Pediatr Radiol 2017;47(11):1491–9.
36. Sanchez Fernandez I, Morales-Quezada JL, Law S, et al. Prognostic Value of Brain Magnetic Resonance Imaging in Neonatal Hypoxic-Ischemic Encephalopathy: A Meta-analysis. J Child Neurol 2017;32(13):1065–73.
37. Volpe JJ, Inder T. Volpe's neurology of the newborn. 6th edition. Philadelphia: Elsevier; 2018.
38. Volpe JJ. Brain injury in premature infants: a complex amalgam of destructive and developmental disturbances. Lancet Neurol 2009;8(1):110–24.
39. Huppi PS, Murphy B, Maier SE, et al. Microstructural brain development after perinatal cerebral white matter injury assessed by diffusion tensor magnetic resonance imaging. Pediatrics 2001;107(3):455–60.
40. Kaukola T, Perhomaa M, Vainionpaa L, et al. Apparent diffusion coefficient on magnetic resonance imaging in pons and in corona radiata and relation with the neurophysiologic measurement and the outcome in very preterm infants. Neonatology 2010;97(1):15–21.
41. Brouwer MJ, van Kooij BJ, van Haastert IC, et al. Sequential cranial ultrasound and cerebellar diffusion weighted imaging contribute to the early prognosis of neurodevelopmental outcome in preterm infants. PLoS One 2014;9(10):e109556.
42. Rose J, Butler EE, Lamont LE, et al. Neonatal brain structure on MRI and diffusion tensor imaging, sex, and neurodevelopment in very-low-birthweight preterm children. Dev Med Child Neurol 2009;51(7):526–35.
43. Arzoumanian Y, Mirmiran M, Barnes PD, et al. Diffusion tensor brain imaging findings at term-equivalent age may predict neurologic abnormalities in low birth weight preterm infants. AJNR Am J Neuroradiol 2003;24(8):1646–53.
44. Drobyshevsky A, Bregman J, Storey P, et al. Serial diffusion tensor imaging detects white matter changes that correlate with motor outcome in premature infants. Dev Neurosci 2007;29(4–5):289–301.
45. Chau V, Synnes A, Grunau RE, et al. Abnormal brain maturation in preterm neonates associated with adverse developmental outcomes. Neurology 2013;81(24):2082–9.
46. Rogers CE, Anderson PJ, Thompson DK, et al. Regional cerebral development at term relates to school-age social-emotional development in very preterm children. J Am Acad Child Adolesc Psychiatry 2012;51(2):181–91.
47. Thompson DK, Lee KJ, Egan GF, et al. Regional white matter microstructure in very preterm infants: predictors and 7 year outcomes. Cortex 2014;52:60–74.
48. Rose J, Mirmiran M, Butler EE, et al. Neonatal microstructural development of the internal capsule on diffusion tensor imaging correlates with severity of gait and motor deficits. Dev Med Child Neurol 2007;49(10):745–50.
49. Rogers CE, Smyser T, Smyser CD, et al. Regional white matter development in very preterm infants: perinatal predictors and early developmental outcomes. Pediatr Res 2016;79(1–1):87–95.
50. De Bruine FT, Van Wezel-Meijler G, Leijser LM, et al. Tractography of white-matter tracts in very preterm infants: a 2-year follow-up study. Dev Med Child Neurol 2013;55(5):427–33.
51. Smith SM, Jenkinson M, Johansen-Berg H, et al. Tract-based spatial statistics: voxelwise analysis of multi-subject diffusion data. NeuroImage 2006;31(4):1487–505.
52. van Kooij BJ, de Vries LS, Ball G, et al. Neonatal tract-based spatial statistics findings and outcome in preterm infants. AJNR Am J Neuroradiol 2012;33(1):188–94.
53. Sun SW, Liang HF, Le TQ, et al. Differential sensitivity of in vivo and ex vivo diffusion tensor imaging to evolving optic nerve injury in mice with retinal ischemia. NeuroImage 2006;32(3):1195–204.
54. Song SK, Yoshino J, Le TQ, et al. Demyelination increases radial diffusivity in corpus callosum of mouse brain. NeuroImage 2005;26(1):132–40.
55. Song SK, Sun SW, Ramsbottom MJ, et al. Dysmyelination Revealed through MRI as Increased Radial (but Unchanged Axial) Diffusion of Water. NeuroImage 2002;17(3):1429–36.
56. Barnett ML, Tusor N, Ball G, et al. Exploring the multiple-hit hypothesis of preterm white matter damage using diffusion MRI. NeuroImage: Clin 2018;17:596–606.
57. Bouyssi-Kobar M, Brossard-Racine M, Jacobs M, et al. Regional microstructural organization of the cerebral cortex is affected by preterm birth. NeuroImage: Clin 2018;18:871–80.

Diffusion Tensor Imaging of the Spinal Cord

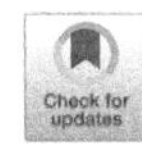

Sho-Jen Cheng, MD[a], Ping-Huei Tsai, PhD[b], Yun-Ting Lee, MS[c], Yi-Tien Li, PhD[c], Hsiao-Wen Chung, PhD[d,e,*], Cheng-Yu Chen, MD[a,c,f]

KEYWORDS

- Diffusion tensor imaging • Spinal cord • Geometric distortions • Spatial resolution
- White matter integrity

KEY POINTS

- Diffusion tensor imaging (DTI) in the spinal cord faces multiple challenges, which evoke active and continuous technical developments.
- Optimization of DTI protocols in the spinal cord currently requires a relatively lengthy scan time to maintain sufficient image quality.
- Once performed on a routine basis, the diagnostic value of DTI in addition to conventional morphologic MR imaging could be demonstrated effective for imaging of the spinal cord.

INTRODUCTION

Diffusion tensor imaging (DTI) is used widely now in routine examinations and clinical research of brain. Especially for white matter diseases or brain developments, DTI provides useful information related to microstructural integrity, hence complementary to conventional morphologic MR imaging in both diagnosis and prognosis.[1,2] Abnormalities in myelination often are reflected in reductions in fractional anisotropy (FA), a quantitative index derived from DTI data with multidirectional encoding.[3] In addition, directional changes of major white matter tracts could be visualized by tractography, a graphical tool depicting the 3-dimensional neural fiber bundles noninvasively.[4,5] Despite numerous reports documenting the success of DTI in the brain, applications of DTI in the spinal cord are comparably much less frequent, even though the pathologic alterations in the white matter of the spinal cord are no less important clinically than in the brain.

The reason for not using DTI in the spinal cord is obvious. The technical demands in MR image acquisition are higher than in the brain due to the special anatomic features, leading to inferior image quality if using scanning parameter settings for brain imaging. Adjustments of the imaging protocol are not straightforward, facing trade-offs that greatly reduce willingness applying DTI to the spinal cord, explained in detail later.

TECHNICAL CHALLENGES OF DIFFUSION TENSOR IMAGING IN THE SPINAL CORD

One major technical challenge of DTI in the spinal cord arises from the relatively small size, compared with the cerebrum. The white matter

Submitted to *Magnetic Resonance Imaging Clinics of North America*.

[a] Department of Medical Imaging, Taipei Medical University Hospital, 252 Wu-Hsing Street, Taipei 110, Taiwan; [b] Department of Medical Imaging and Radiological Sciences, Chung-Shan Medical University, No.110, Sec.1, Jianguo N. Road, Taichung 40201, Taiwan; [c] Translational Imaging Research Center, Taipei Medical University Hospital, 252 Wu-Hsing Street, Taipei 110, Taiwan; [d] Graduate Institute of Biomedical Electronics and Bioinformatics, National Taiwan University, No.1, Sec.4, Roosevelt Road, Taipei 10617, Taiwan; [e] Department of Electrical Engineering, National Taiwan University, No.1, Sec.4, Roosevelt Road, Taipei 10617, Taiwan; [f] Department of Radiology, School of Medicine, College of Medicine, Taipei Medical University, 250 Wu-Hsing Street, Taipei 110, Taiwan

* Corresponding author. Department of Electrical Engineering, National Taiwan University, No.1, Sec.4, Roosevelt Road, Taipei 10617, Taiwan.
E-mail address: chunghw@ntu.edu.tw

Magn Reson Imaging Clin N Am 29 (2021) 195–204
https://doi.org/10.1016/j.mric.2021.02.002
1064-9689/21/

tracts in the spinal cord that need to be imaged by DTI largely are confined at the level of cervical spinal cord, which is approximately 1 cm in width if viewed on an axial slice.[6] With gray matter embedded within the surrounding white matter, the limited fiber tract volume naturally leads to the requirement of high spatial resolution. Although current advances in MR imaging techniques allow clear depiction of the gray/white matter boundaries in the cervical spinal cord using routine morphologic imaging sequences, such as gradient-echo imaging, that is not the case for DTI (**Fig. 1**). Signal readout in DTI usually is achieved using single-shot spin-echo echo-planar imaging (EPI), where the entire time duration allowed for signal readout has to be confined within 2 to 3 T2* (approximately 100 ms).[7] The limitation in readout time restricts the maximum image matrix size and hence spatial resolution. Therefore, pushing the spatial resolution for spinal cord DTI is not an easy task, if using EPI as the signal readout module.[4]

A second difficulty, also related to the characteristics of EPI, is the notorious geometric distortion in the presence of main magnetic field inhomogeneity.[8] Although in the brain the magnetic field inhomogeneity often results in distorted morphology near the skull base and can be largely corrected using postprocessing algorithms, such as affine transformation,[9] in the spinal cord, the extents of distortions may vary greatly from slice to slice because of different degrees of off-resonance (see **Fig. 1**). To make things worse, the off-resonance phenomena in the spinal cord often are nonmonotonic along the body axis. The consequent jagged appearance of the spinal cord on a sagittal view not only is problematic for tractography but also may have influences on quantitative measurements of DTI parameters.[10] Good shimming before image acquisition is the ultimate key to the reduction of geometric distortion in EPI, which, however, is complicated by the irregular shape of air-tissue interface around the head and neck region.[11] Insufficient fat suppression, a necessary component in EPI sequences, is clear evidence of suboptimal shimming accompanied by geometric distortion.[12]

The third characteristic is the elongated shape of the spinal cord. The cervical spinal cord alone is approximately 15 cm long. As a result, contiguous coverage by axial images would require as many as 50 slices if using a 3-mm slice thickness. Slice interleaving with large number of slices increases the minimum repetition time to a value greater than 10 seconds, hence prolonging the scan time. Reducing the number of slices either sacrifices the coverage if the slice thickness is unchanged or leads to worsened partial volume effects if using a slice thickness greater than 3 mm. Sagittal acquisition could be a solution, but with compromise of inadequate spatial resolution along the slice direction as well as substantially enlarged EPI geometric distortions compared with axial acquisition.[13] Note that because the purpose of DTI or tractography is to probe microstructural integrity of the entire white matter tracts, the use of contiguous slices with sufficient volume coverage often is mandatory. This is unlike the depiction of single spinal cord lesions, where several image slices with gaps would suffice.

Research and development have helped continual advancements of DTI technique, such

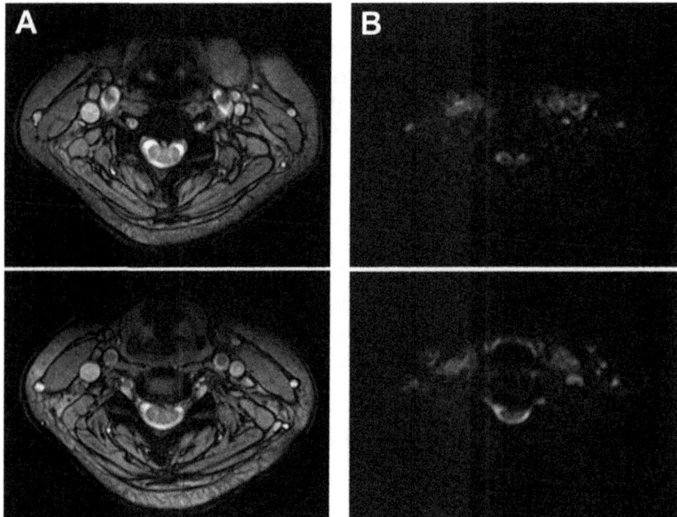

Fig. 1. Axial MR images comparing the spatial resolution that can be achieved on a routine basis for morphologic imaging versus diffusion-weighted imaging. (*A*) On two different slices (top and bottom) of the multi-echo-averaged gradient-echo images, identification of the boundaries between gray and white matter within the cervical spinal cord is possible. (*B*) Depiction of gray-white matter boundaries is hampered on the two corresponding slices (top and bottom) of the b = 0 images acquired using single-shot echo-planar imaging due to inferior spatial resolution leading to blurring.

that more alternative schemes have become commercially available for clinical practice. Some of these methods that have demonstrated potential in spinal cord DTI are addressed.

ADVANCED DIFFUSION TENSOR IMAGING ACQUISITION METHODS

One anatomic characteristic of the spinal cord that potentially could be utilized to optimize the spatial resolution is that the region of interest (ROI) is confined within a small area. With the signals from the surrounding muscle and subcutaneous fat appropriately suppressed using saturation bands, high spatial resolution theoretically could be achieved at relatively low matrix sizes without causing aliasing artifacts.[14] An obvious advantage of this approach is that it needs careful optimization of the scanning protocol only. No pulse sequence developments would be involved.[15] Alternatively, dedicated 2-dimensional spatially selective radiofrequency pulses could be used to excite the signals from a prespecified region,[16] apply the excitation and refocusing pulses at an angle such that only signals from their intersection are detected,[17] or combine both methods.[18] With detectable signals confined within a limited region, the effects resemble that of outer volume signal suppression. This technique usually is called inner volume imaging or reduced field-of-view imaging, which has been commercialized by the major manufacturers as specific packages for high-resolution diffusion-weighted MR imaging (DWI). Studies have shown that inner volume imaging helps achieve high spatial resolution DTI,[19] with applications to the spinal cord demonstrated to be effective.[20,21] For pediatric spinal cord, the use of inner volume imaging for DTI is especially critical.[22,23]

The use of inner volume imaging, however, is strictly speaking unrelated to the second problem of DTI in the spinal cord, namely the geometric distortions in EPI.[15,21] The extents of distortions in EPI are determined solely by the readout bandwidth along the phase encoding direction. As a result, reducing the time interval between successive phase encoding steps shows effectiveness. This can be accomplished by using parallel imaging with multiple receiver coils[24] or further integrated with readout segmentation.[25] The design of readout segmentation inevitably changes the EPI acquisition to multishot, with concomitant phase correction needed using navigator echo acquisition (**Fig. 2**A).[25] Encouraging results have been documented outside the brain,[26,27] which certainly include the spinal cord.[28] Other alternatives that also employ the concept of multishot acquisitions include the use of rotating blades for k-space coverage, using either EPI[29,30] or fast spin-echo[31] as the signal readout module (**Fig. 2**B). Although for fast spin-echo version the image morphology is nearly completely reserved due to the refocusing pulses,[32] in the EPI version, the reduction of distortions is due to an extraction of data that are less influenced by susceptibility-induced off-resonance.[33,34] Applications of rotating blade acquisitions to the spinal cord, however, have not yet been reported, to the best of the authors' knowledge.

The third challenge, the elongated shape of the spinal cord, potentially could be relieved by simultaneous multislice imaging.[35,36] With the advancement of phased-array receiver coils and improved reconstruction, such as controlled aliasing,[37] separation of DTI slices using parallel imaging algorithms[38] becomes increasingly reliable at high acceleration factors.[39] Maturation of simultaneous multislice imaging is expected to soon become a

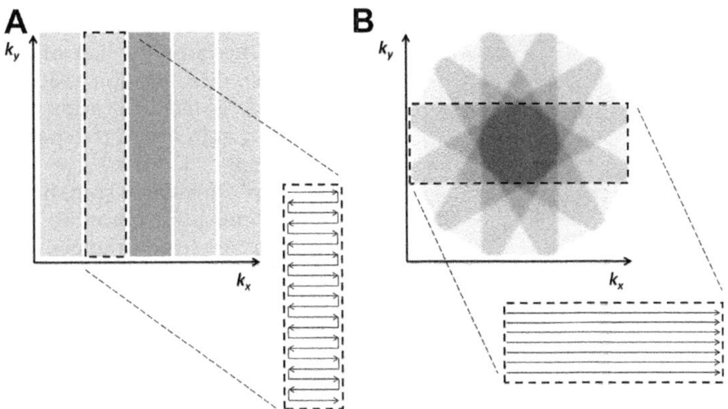

Fig. 2. Two k-space coverage schemes for multishot imaging for DTI. (*A*) The readout (k_x) direction is divided into 5 overlapping segments in this example, with each data segment acquired using EPI. The reduced time interval between successive phase-encoding steps increases the readout bandwidth along the phase-encoding direction (k_y), thereby reducing geometric distortions. (*B*) Alternatively, rotating blades could be used for multishot k-space coverage, with each data segment acquired using fast spin-echo to eliminate geometric distortions. In either of these cases, the scan time is increased by a factor of the number of data segments. The shaded areas represent the k-space overlaps, which are used for phase corrections before reconstruction.

necessary part of routine axial acquisitions of the spinal cord.

CURRENT LIMITATIONS

Even if remedies that could overcome each of the single difficulties, discussed previously, have been proposed with some success, dealing with the combinational influences of all 3 factors by no means is straightforward. Not only are the effects hard to isolate but also nearly all methods come with trade-offs causing yet other detrimental issues.

Whether or not using inner volume imaging, high spatial resolution in MR imaging is accompanied by proportional loss in the signal-to-noise ratio (SNR) due to inherent reduction in the number of protons per voxel. Multiple signal averaging is the usual way to regain SNR, which is, however, generally regarded as inefficient because SNR scales only to the square root of number of signal averaging.[40] In the authors' experience, a single DTI protocol less than 15 minutes of scan time rarely yields satisfactory quality, even at 3.0T (**Fig. 3**). To make things worse, multishot acquisitions to reduce geometric distortions further increase the scan time by a factor of the number of shots.[25] With total scan time substantially lengthened due to both of these issues, involuntary movements, including in particular the swallowing motion, ultimately may become the dominant factor determining the success of DTI acquisitions in the spinal cord. Limited success rate then precludes clinicians' willingness to place spinal cord DTI as a routine examination tool.

CLINICAL APPLICATIONS

Several clinical scenarios potentially may benefit from the addition of DWI or DTI to the routine protocol for spinal cord imaging, for instance, to reveal myelopathy that may not be clearly visible on images acquired with conventional MR sequences. Differentiation of noninfiltrative neoplasms, such as spinal ependymomas, from other infiltrative and more aggressive neoplasms like astrocytomas also is important in terms of presurgical planning, because infiltrative astrocytomas often are considered unresectable. Other conditions include the prediction of the prognosis of spinal cord injury as well as monitoring of treatment response of various conditions. These are detailed later.

Myelopathy due to External Compression Caused by Degenerative Disk Disease

Degenerative disk disease generally is regarded as the most common cause of myelopathy, especially in the cervical spinal cord. Conventional MR imaging is inadequate because discrepancy between the patient symptoms and imaging findings in myelopathy ranged from 15% to 65%. Such a discrepancy potentially could be decreased with DTI.[41] The quantitative information provided by DTI could probe the severity of myelopathy, which in turn shows strong potential to help selecting patients who may benefit from early decompression surgeries.[42] For example, compressive myelopathy most commonly demonstrates an increase in mean diffusivity (MD) and a concomitant decrease in FA (**Fig. 4**). Changes in these DTI indices likely are related to an expansion of the

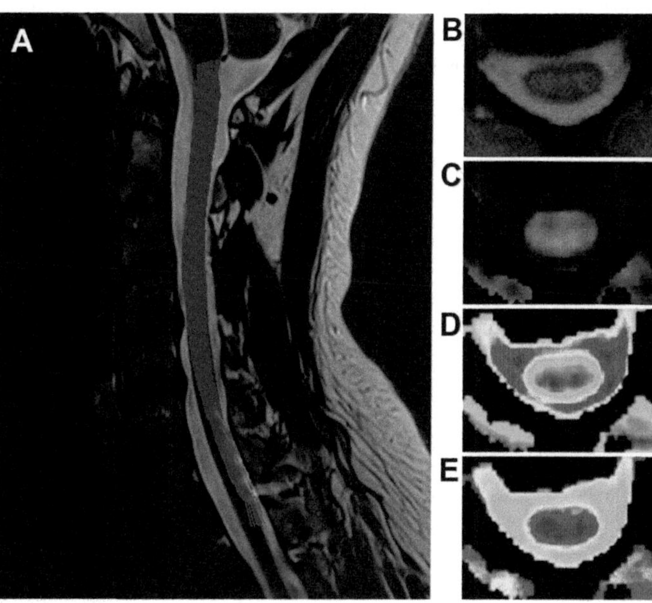

Fig. 3. Example images of the spinal cord obtained using DWI with 30 gradient directions and b values of 0 s/mm^2, 750 s/mm^2, and 1500 s/mm^2 at 3.0T, allowing derivation of mean kurtosis in addition to DTI metrics, such as FA. The large number of acquisitions per slice location (>60 in this case) is believed to provide the gain in SNR so as to afford the spatial resolution of 1 mm^3 × 1 mm^3 × 3 mm^3. This single scan, however, took 15 minutes to acquire. (*A*) Tractography results overlapped on the sagittal T2-weighted image. Also note the inconsistent location at the caudal end due to geometric distortions. A representative axial slice of the (*B*) gradient-echo T2*-weighted image, (*C*) FA, (*D*) MD, and (*E*) mean kurtosis maps.

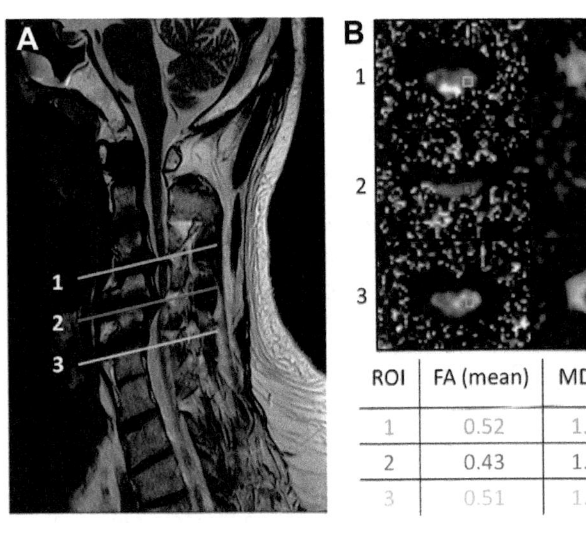

ROI	FA (mean)	MD (mm²/s)
1	0.52	1.08×10^{-3}
2	0.43	1.56×10^{-3}
3	0.51	1.09×10^{-3}

Fig. 4. A 39-year-old man suffering from persistent neck pain with radiation to the left upper limb, at the dermatome distribution of left C5 and C6, for 2 years. (*A*) Sagittal cervical MR imaging demonstrated T2 hyperintense lesion in the severely compressed spinal cord at the level of C4/5. (*B*) DTI demonstrates significant increase in MD and a concomitant decrease in FA at the compressed site, as reflected by values measured from ROIs and listed in the table for slice #2 compared with slices #1 and #3.

extracellular spaces due to a decreased number of fibers and loss of their directional organization, consequences caused by mechanical disruption of the fibers and myelin sheaths as well as physiologic deficits, such as ischemia.[42,43] In addition, FA in the spinal cord has been shown to moderately predict surgical outcomes in patients with chronic compressive myelopathy.[44] Furthermore, the diffusion metrics demonstrated superiority to T2 signal intensity in the evaluation of postoperative function assessed by the modified Japanese Orthopaedic Association score.[45] More advanced DTI techniques employing multiple b values will allow a derivation of the mean diffusional kurtosis to reflect microstructural changes of the spinal cord in patients with early chronic spondylotic myelopathy.[46]

Spinal Cord Tumors

For intramedullary spinal cord tumors, the goal of surgical treatment is to preserve the spinal cord function while achieving maximal tumor resection. Therefore, the determination of tumor resectability by means of noninvasive imaging tools before surgical operation is essential. The most frequent intramedullary tumors in adults are ependymomas, followed in order of prevalence by astrocytomas, other types of gliomas, hemangioblastomas, and metastases. Ependymomas and hemangioblastomas typically are noninfiltrative, with a distinct tumor-cord plane and thus generally are considered resectable. In contrast, most of the astrocytomas are considered unresectable due to their infiltrative nature. Several studies have demonstrated the value of DWI and DTI in predicting the resectability of intramedullary tumors. Setzer and colleagues[47] classified the patterns of DTI tractography into 3 types according to the fiber course and showed the concordance of this method with intraoperative surgical findings, namely the existence or absence of a cleavage plane. Results from Ducreux and colleagues[48,49] also suggest that DTI tractography can be used for visualization of the warped and destroyed fibers in cases of solid astrocytomas but at the same time demonstrate some limitations in pilocytic astrocytomas, which are common intramedullary neoplasms in children. In cases of extensive cervicothoracic spinal ependymoma, Granata and colleagues[50] showed that complete resection of the lesion was possible with guidance of the clear cleavage planes as detected by DTI. In these reports, DTI and tractography reveal the relationship between white matter fibers and the tumor, therefore effectively avoid damaging the fiber tracts during microsurgical procedures.

Spinal Cord Ischemia and Infarct

Acute spinal cord ischemia and/or infarct, although a relatively uncommon condition, can have devastating consequences involving severe functional neurologic loss, with permanent paralysis in up to 33% of the cases. Patients often exhibit symptoms, including acute onset of pain, paraparesis, paresthesia, and possible urinary and bowel dysfunction. Atherosclerosis, aortic dissection, and aortic surgery are the major causes of acute spinal cord ischemia. The most common location of spinal cord infarct involves the anterior two-thirds of the cord, which is supplied by the anterior spinal artery. In a majority of instances, ischemia involves the anterior horn cells within the gray matter. Sagittal MR images of anterior spinal artery infarct usually demonstrate an isolated pencil-like area of T2-hyperintensity involving the centromedullary region, whereas a limited T2-hyperintensity more prominent in the anterior gray matter as viewed from axial images leading to an owl's eye pattern.[51] These patterns allow conventional MR imaging to be valuable. Only approximately 45% of the patients, however, with acute spinal cord ischemia demonstrate signal intensity changes on T2-weighted images,[52] because spinal cord infarct lesions usually present T2 hyperintensity beyond 12 hours after onset of patient symptoms.[53] On the other hand, DWI has been reported to show signal changes as short as 3 hours after symptom onset[54]; thus, it may be helpful in early depiction of spinal cord ischemia.

The temporal evolution of diffusion abnormalities currently still is a topic under debate. Generally speaking, diffusion abnormalities found in patients with spinal cord ischemia rarely persist for longer than a week. A case of persistent diffusion abnormality at 9 days after the symptom onset, however, also has been documented.[55] The low willingness to place the technically demanding spinal cord DWI into routine protocol, as discussed previously, may be one of the reasons that comprehensive investigations on longitudinal DWI findings in spinal cord ischemia are still lacking. Consequently, specialized acquisition approaches, such as line scan diffusion imaging, could be considered as an alternative tool to conventional DWI/DTI in order to widen the assistance of DWI in diagnosing acute spinal cord infarction.[56]

Spinal Cord Trauma

The main goal of imaging patients with traumatic spinal cord injury is to avoid preventable neurologic deteriorations and to aid appropriate therapeutic management. Earlier studies reported that a substantial portion of spinal injuries have been missed and/or mismanaged in 4.6% to 10.5% of patients.[57,58] Imaging thus will play an essential role in reducing the rate of mismanagement. As long as it is safe to do so without clinical contraindications, MR imaging ideally should be performed in all cases of neural compromise after spinal trauma, even if MR examination admittedly is time consuming and relies on fully cooperative patients. Compared with CT, MR imaging risks missing a certain portion of bone injuries but has the advantage of being able to define the level of spinal cord injury clearly. In addition, the soft tissue contrast of MR imaging helps depicting causes of treatable neurologic compromise, such as spinal cord compression, by herniated disk or epidural hematoma.

In terms of added value of DTI to conventional MR imaging, several studies demonstrated the increasingly important diagnostic role of DTI owing to its ability to assess the white matter microstructural integrity via measurements of quantitative DTI indices, such as MD or FA, at the injured sites. For instance, spinal cord injury without radiographic abnormality (SCIWORA) accounts for 6% to 19% and 9% to 14% of spinal injuries in children and adults, respectively. Yet patients with SCIWORA who present with normal findings on conventional MR imaging may show hyperintense lesions on DWI.[59] DWI also is sensitive to spinal stenosis induced by trauma because it has been shown that even mild hyperextension can lead to DWI hyperintense lesions on DWI, suggesting hyperacute spinal cord injury.[60] Significantly decreased FA and tract density in the thoracic region in patients with cervical spinal cord injury has been reported by Alizadeh and colleagues,[61] further demonstrating the effectiveness of DTI and tractography in the diagnosis of spinal cord. Different opinions, however, abound. A study by Pouw and colleagues[62] suggests that T2-weighted MR imaging and DWI have comparable detection rates for traumatic spinal cord damage within 24 hours postinjury. Talbott and colleagues[63] stated that although DWI seems promising for interrogating spinal cord integrity, T2-weighted imaging is the most important sequence in acute traumatic spinal cord injury. These mysteries await well-designed prospective clinical investigations to resolve the disagreement.

Primary Myelopathies

Several morphologic MR imaging techniques (T2-weighted imaging, short TI inversion recovery, phase-sensitive inversion recovery, and so forth) have been recommended as standardized spinal cord MR imaging protocols in the clinical management of patients with multiple sclerosis, clinically isolated syndrome, and radiologically isolated syndrome.[64,65] Spinal cord DTI has been used in research related to multiple sclerosis for more than a decade in an attempt to detect occult spinal cord pathology (**Fig. 5**), even in normal-appearing spinal cord.[66] Prediction of clinical course, monitoring of disease progression, and examinations of therapeutic effects also have been explored.[66] Reductions in FA have been reported to exhibit a sensitivity of 80% to detect spinal cord abnormalities in patients with myelitis, which is superior to conventional T2-weighted imaging.[67] The study by Théaudin and colleagues[68] stated that DTI detects more extensive abnormalities than conventional T2-weighted imaging and that a less

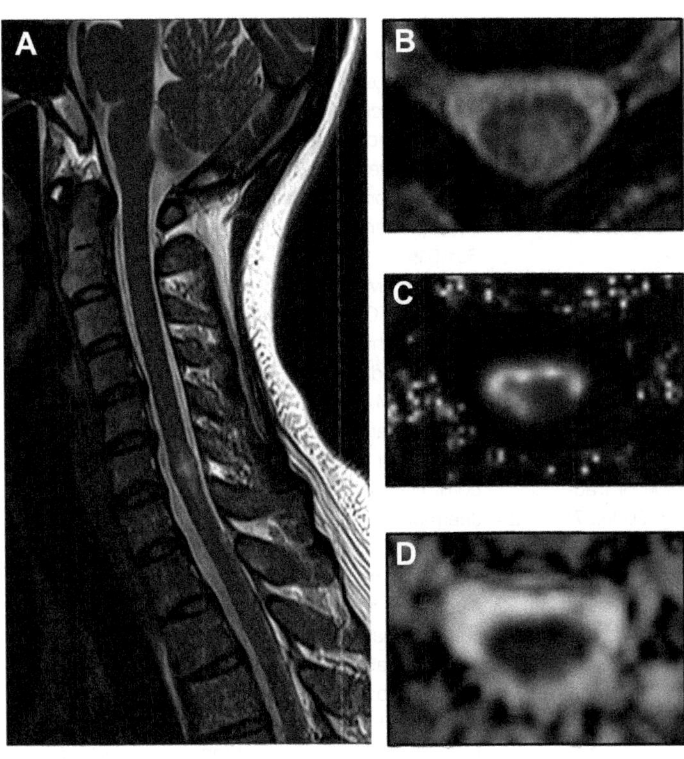

Fig. 5. A 39-year-old woman with multiple sclerosis presents with progressive numbness of bilateral lower limbs, trunk, and right upper limb. (*A*) Evidence of a demyelinating lesion at the right posterior aspect of the spinal cord shows hyperintensity on (*B*) gradient-echo T2-weighted image, (*C*) decreased FA, and (*D*) increased MD.

decrease in FA value of the inflammatory lesion seems associated with better outcome. Patients with neuromyelitis optica (NMO) also may show reduced FA and increased MD, suggesting that these DTI indices may serve as potential biomarkers to detect abnormalities, especially in early cases of NMO or NMO relapse.[69] Last but not least, research progress utilizing advanced diffusional kurtosis imaging on experimental animal model of autoimmune encephalomyelitis shows promise in the identification of spinal cord damages not only in the white matter but also in the gray matter, which correlates well with neurologic dysfunction.[70]

SUMMARY

In conclusion, DTI and tractography of the spinal cord for clinical examinations are technically challenging. Nevertheless, published literature suggests that with careful manipulation and optimization of the scanning protocols, they should be feasible if a comparably long scan time is allowed. Once performed on a routine basis, the additive diagnostic value to the conventional morphologic MR imaging could be demonstrated effectively. The authors, therefore, anticipate that DTI and tractography of the spinal cord will undergo continuous technical developments in the near future and expect to see more and more institutes to help broaden their incorporation to clinical evaluation.

ACKNOWLEDGMENTS

HWC receives support in part from the Ministry of Science and Technology under grant MOST 107-2221-E-002-038-MY3. CYC receives support in part from the Ministry of Science and Technology under grant MOST 108-2321-B-038-008.

REFERENCES

1. Mukherjee P, McKinstry RC. Diffusion tensor imaging and tractography of human brain development. Neuroimaging Clin N Am 2006;16:19–43.
2. Huston JM, Field AS. Clinical applications of diffusion tensor imaging. Magn Reson Imaging Clin N Am 2013;21:279–98.
3. Choudhri AF, Chin EM, Blitz AM, et al. Diffusion tensor imaging of cerebral white matter: technique, anatomy, and pathologic patterns. Radiol Clin North Am 2014;52:413–25.
4. Mukherjee P, Chung SW, Berman JI, et al. Diffusion tensor MR imaging and fiber tractography: technical considerations. AJNR Am J Neuroradiol 2008;29:843–52.

5. Chung HW, Chou MC, Chen CY. Principles and limitations of computational algorithms in clinical diffusion tensor MR tractography. AJNR Am J Neuroradiol 2011;32:3–13.
6. Sherman JL, Nassaux PY, Citrin CM. Measurements of the normal cervical spinal cord on MR imaging. AJNR Am J Neuroradiol 1990;11:369–72.
7. Edelman RR, Wielopolski P, Schmitt F. Echo-planar MR imaging. Radiology 1994;192:600–12.
8. Jezzard P, Clare S. Sources of distortion in functional MRI data. Hum Brain Mapp 1999;8:80–5.
9. Kybic J, Thévenaz P, Nirkko A, et al. Unwarping of unidirectionally distorted EPI images. IEEE Trans Med Imaging 2000;19:80–93.
10. Chao TC, Chou MC, Yang P, et al. Effects of interpolation methods in spatial normalization of diffusion tensor imaging data on group comparison of fractional anisotropy. Magn Reson Imaging 2009;27:681–90.
11. Chang HC, Juan CJ, Chiu HC, et al. Parotid fat contents in healthy subjects evaluated with iterative decomposition with echo asymmetry and least squares fat-water separation. Radiology 2013;267:918–23.
12. Maehara M, Ikeda K, Kurokawa H, et al. Diffusion-weighted echo-planar imaging of the head and neck using 3-T MRI: Investigation into the usefulness of liquid perfluorocarbon pads and choice of optimal fat suppression method. Magn Reson Imaging 2014;32:440–5.
13. Du YP, Joe Zhou X, Bernstein MA. Correction of concomitant magnetic field-induced image artifacts in nonaxial echo-planar imaging. Magn Reson Med 2002;48:509–15.
14. Wilm BJ, Svensson J, Henning A, et al. Reduced field-of-view MRI using outer volume suppression for spinal cord diffusion imaging. Magn Reson Med 2007;57:625–30.
15. Samson RS, Lévy S, Schneider T, et al. ZOOM or Non-ZOOM? Assessing spinal cord diffusion tensor imaging protocols for multi-centre studies. PLoS One 2016;11:e0155557.
16. Hardy CJ, Bottomley PA, O'Donnell M, et al. Optimization of two-dimensional spatially selective NMR pulses by simulated annealing. J Magn Reson 1988;77:233–50.
17. Feinberg DA, Hoenninger JC, Crooks LE, et al. Inner volume MR imaging: technical concepts and their application. Radiology 1985;156:743–7.
18. Saritas EU, Cunningham CH, Lee JH, et al. DWI of the spinal cord with reduced FOV single-shot EPI. Magn Reson Med 2008;60:468–73.
19. Finsterbusch J. High-resolution diffusion tensor imaging with inner field-of-view EPI. J Magn Reson Imaging 2009;29:987–93.
20. Hodel J, Besson P, Outteryck O, et al. Pulse-triggered DTI sequence with reduced FOV and coronal acquisition at 3T for the assessment of the cervical spinal cord in patients with myelitis. AJNR Am J Neuroradiol 2013;34:676–82.
21. Park EH, Lee YH, Jeong EK, et al. Diffusion tensor imaging focusing on lower cervical spinal cord using 2D reduced FOV interleaved multislice single-shot diffusion-weighted echo-planar imaging: comparison with conventional single-shot diffusion-weighted echo-planar imaging. Magn Reson Imaging 2015;33:401–6.
22. Alizadeh M, Intintolo A, Middleton DM, et al. Reduced FOV diffusion tensor MR imaging and fiber tractography of pediatric cervical spinal cord injury. Spinal Cord 2017;55:314–20.
23. Alizadeh M, Fisher J, Saksena S, et al. Age related diffusion and tractography changes in typically developing pediatric cervical and thoracic spinal cord. Neuroimage Clin 2018;18:784–92.
24. Jaermann T, Crelier G, Pruessmann KP, et al. SENSE-DTI at 3 T. Magn Reson Med 2004;51:230–6.
25. Porter DA, Heidemann RM. High resolution diffusion-weighted imaging using readout-segmented echo-planar imaging, parallel imaging and a two-dimensional navigator-based reacquisition. Magn Reson Med 2009;62:468–75.
26. Tokoro H, Fujinaga Y, Ohya A, et al. Usefulness of free-breathing readout-segmented echo-planar imaging (RESOLVE) for detection of malignant liver tumors: comparison with single-shot echo-planar imaging (SS-EPI). Eur J Radiol 2014;83:1728–33.
27. Friedli I, Crowe LA, de Perrot T, et al. Comparison of readout-segmented and conventional single-shot for echo-planar diffusion-weighted imaging in the assessment of kidney interstitial fibrosis. J Magn Reson Imaging 2017;46:1631–40.
28. Zhang BT, Li M, Yu LL, et al. Diffusion tensor imaging of spinal microstructure in healthy adults: improved resolution with the readout segmentation of long variable echo-trains. Neural Regen Res 2017;12:2067–70.
29. Wang FN, Huang TY, Lin FH, et al. PROPELLER EPI: an MRI technique suitable for diffusion tensor imaging at high field strength with reduced geometric distortions. Magn Reson Med 2005;54:1232–40.
30. Skare S, Newbould RD, Clayton DB, et al. Propeller EPI in the other direction. Magn Reson Med 2006;55:1298–307.
31. Pipe JG, Farthing VG, Forbes KP. Multishot diffusion-weighted FSE using PROPELLER MRI. Magn Reson Med 2002;47:42–52.
32. Forbes KP, Pipe JG, Karis JP, et al. Improved image quality and detection of acute cerebral infarction with PROPELLER diffusion-weighted MR imaging. Radiology 2002;225:551–5.
33. Chuang TC, Huang TY, Lin FH, et al. PROPELLER-EPI with parallel imaging using a circularly symmetric phased-array RF coil at 3.0 T: application to high-

resolution diffusion tensor imaging. Magn Reson Med 2006;56:1352–8.
34. Chang HC, Chuang TC, Lin YR, et al. Correction of geometric distortion in Propeller echo planar imaging using a modified reversed gradient approach. Quant Imaging Med Surg 2013;3:73–81.
35. Larkman DJ, Hajnal JV, Herlihy AH, et al. Use of multicoil arrays for separation of signal from multiple slices simultaneously excited. J Magn Reson Imaging 2001;13:313–7.
36. Barth M, Breuer F, Koopmans PJ, et al. Simultaneous multislice (SMS) imaging techniques. Magn Reson Med 2016;75:63–81.
37. Setsompop K, Gagoski BA, Polimeni JR, et al. Blipped-controlled aliasing in parallel imaging for simultaneous multislice echo planar imaging with reduced g-factor penalty. Magn Reson Med 2012; 67:1210–24.
38. Griswold MA, Jakob PM, Heidemann RM, et al. Generalized autocalibrating partially parallel acquisitions (GRAPPA). Magn Reson Med 2002;47:1202–10.
39. Eichner C, Setsompop K, Koopmans PJ, et al. Slice accelerated diffusion-weighted imaging at ultra-high field strength. Magn Reson Med 2014;71:1518–25.
40. Owen RS, Wehrli FW. Predictability of SNR and reader preference in clinical MR imaging. Magn Reson Imaging 1990;8:737–45.
41. Kara B, Celik A, Karadereler S, et al. The role of DTI in early detection of cervical spondylotic myelopathy: a preliminary study with 3-T MRI. Neuroradiology 2011;53:609–16.
42. Banaszek A, Bladowska J, Podgórski P, et al. Role of diffusion tensor MR imaging in degenerative cervical spine disease: a review of the literature. Clin Neuroradiol 2016;26:265–76.
43. Facon D, Ozanne A, Fillard P, et al. MR diffusion tensor imaging and fiber tracking in spinal cord compression. AJNR Am J Neuroradiol 2005;26: 1587–94.
44. Maki S, Koda M, Kitamura M, et al. Diffusion tensor imaging can predict surgical outcomes of patients with cervical compression myelopathy. Eur Spine J 2017;26:2459–66.
45. Wen CY, Cui JL, Liu HS, et al. Is diffusion anisotropy a biomarker for disease severity and surgical prognosis of cervical spondylotic myelopathy? Radiology 2014;270:197–204.
46. Li D, Wang X. Application value of diffusional kurtosis imaging (DKI) in evaluating microstructural changes in the spinal cord of patients with early cervical spondylotic myelopathy. Clin Neurol Neurosurg 2017;156:71–6.
47. Setzer M, Murtagh RD, Murtagh FR, et al. Diffusion tensor imaging tractography in patients with intramedullary tumors: comparison with intraoperative findings and value for prediction of tumor resectability. J Neurosurg Spine 2010;13:371–80.
48. Ducreux D, Lepeintre JF, Fillard P, et al. MR diffusion tensor imaging and fiber tracking in 5 spinal cord astrocytomas. AJNR Am J Neuroradiol 2006;27: 214–6.
49. Ducreux D, Fillard P, Facon D, et al. Diffusion tensor magnetic resonance imaging and fiber tracking in spinal cord lesions: current and future indications. Neuroimaging Clin N Am 2007;17: 137–47.
50. Granata F, Racchiusa S, Mormina E, et al. Presurgical role of MRI tractography in a case of extensive cervicothoracic spinal ependymoma. Surg Neurol Int 2017;8:56.
51. Masson C, Pruvo JP, Meder JF, et al. Spinal cord infarction: clinical and magnetic resonance imaging findings and short term outcome. J Neurol Neurosurg Psychiatr 2004;75:1431–5.
52. Nadeltchev K, Loher TJ, Stepper F, et al. Long-term outcome of acute spinal cord ischemia syndrome. Stroke 2004;35:560–5.
53. Gass A, Back T, Behrens S, et al. MRI of spinal cord infarction. Neurology 2000;54:2195.
54. Fujikawa A, Tsuchiya K, Takeuchi S, et al. Diffusion-weighted MR imaging in acute spinal cord ischemia. Eur Radiol 2004;14:2076–8.
55. Thurnher MM, Bammer R. Diffusion-weighted MR imaging (DWI) in spinal cord ischemia. Neuroradiology 2006;48:795–801.
56. Nogueira RG, Ferreira R, Grant PE, et al. Restricted diffusion in spinal cord infarction demonstrated by magnetic resonance line scan diffusion imaging. Stroke 2012;43:532–5.
57. Gerrelts BD, Petersen EU, Mabry J, et al. Delayed diagnosis of cervical spine injuries. J Trauma 1991; 31:1622–6.
58. Poonnoose PM, Ravichandran G, McClelland MR. Missed and mismanaged injuries of the spinal cord. J Trauma 2002;53:314–20.
59. Shen H, Tang Y, Huang L, et al. Applications of diffusion-weighted MRI in thoracic spinal cord injury without radiographic abnormality. Int Orthop 2007; 31:375–83.
60. Szwedowski D, Walecki J. Spinal cord injury without radiographic abnormality (SCIWORA) – clinical and radiological aspects. Pol J Radiol 2014;79:461–4.
61. Alizadeh M, Fisher J, Saksena S, et al. Reduced field of view diffusion tensor imaging and fiber tractography of the pediatric cervical and thoracic spinal cord injury. J Neurotrauma 2018;35:452–60.
62. Pouw MH, van der Vliet AM, van Kampen A, et al. Diffusion-weighted MR imaging within 24 h post-injury after traumatic spinal cord injury: a qualitative meta-analysis between T2-weighted imaging and diffusion-weighted MR imaging in 18 patients. Spinal Cord 2012;50:426–31.
63. Talbott JF, Huie JR, Ferguson AR, et al. MR imaging for assessing injury severity and prognosis in acute

traumatic spinal cord injury. Radiol Clin North Am 2019;57:319–39.
64. Muccilli A, Seyman E, Oh J. Spinal cord MRI in multiple sclerosis. Neurol Clin 2018;36:35–57.
65. Rovira A, Auger C. Spinal cord in multiple sclerosis: magnetic resonance imaging features and differential diagnosis. Semin Ultrasound CT MR 2016;37:396–410.
66. Hesseltine SM, Law M, Babb J, et al. Diffusion tensor imaging in multiple sclerosis: assessment of regional differences in the axial plane within normal-appearing cervical spinal cord. AJNR Am J Neuroradiol 2006;27:1189–93.
67. Renoux J, Facon D, Fillard P, et al. MR diffusion tensor imaging and fiber tracking in inflammatory diseases of the spinal cord. AJNR Am J Neuroradiol 2006;27:1947–51.
68. Théaudin M, Saliou G, Ducot B, et al. Short-term evolution of spinal cord damage in multiple sclerosis: a diffusion tensor MRI study. Neuroradiology 2012;54:1171–8.
69. Qian W, Chan Q, Mak H, et al. Quantitative assessment of the cervical spinal cord damage in neuromyelitis optica using diffusion tensor imaging at 3 Tesla. J Magn Reson Imaging 2011;33:1312–20.
70. Chuhutin A, Hansen B, Wlodarczyk A, et al. Diffusion kurtosis imaging maps neural damage in the EAE model of multiple sclerosis. Neuroimage 2020;208:116406.

Diffusion-Weighted Imaging of the Head and Neck (Including Temporal Bone)

Felix Boucher, MD[a], Eric Liao, MD[b], Ashok Srinivasan, MD[c,*]

KEYWORDS

• Diffusion-weighted imaging • Head and neck • Malignancy

KEY POINTS

- Diffusion imaging techniques offer complimentary information to conventional MR sequences and assist in assessing head and neck pathology.
- Advances in hardware and familiarity with diffusion techniques have expanded the role of diffusion imaging outside of stroke imaging into broader clinical applications, now routinely obtained with most head and neck protocols.
- Diffusion techniques play a particularly important role in assessing head and neck malignancies. In certain settings, a specific neoplastic diagnosis might be suggested, whereas in others, the pretreatment ADC value may suggest the likelihood of a known malignancy to respond to therapy.
- Increasing reader familiarity with the diffusion appearance of different head and neck pathologies can aid in diagnostic confidence and further establish value of imaging in clinical care.

INTRODUCTION

Diffusion-weighted imaging (DWI) revolutionized acute cerebral ischemic infarction imaging. Because hardware performance, familiarity with the technique, and sophistication of pulse sequences have advanced, so too have applications in and outside of the brain. Diffusion techniques are now the principal sequence in the detection of most high-risk prostate cancer, used in whole-body malignancy screening, and are now an indispensable adjunct to conventional T1- and T2-weighted sequences in most MR imaging protocols.[1,2] The objective of this article is to review diffusion imaging techniques and head and neck–specific imaging protocols and demonstrate selected pathology highlighting the clinical utility of diffusion-weighted techniques in the head and neck.

DIFFUSION IMAGING TECHNIQUES

Physical Basis

With conventional anatomic MR techniques (T1, T2, and proton-density–weighted sequences), observed signal reflects tissue relaxation properties, scaled on a relatively arbitrary and qualitative image.[3] In a glass of pure water, water molecules and their hydrogen atoms are free to randomly move about the container, the rate of which largely reflects thermal energy contained within the glass. If the contents of the glass become progressively more compartmentalized, the ability for water molecules to freely move about the container is impeded. This second scenario is similar to the human body where a given anatomic area is composed of highly ordered tissues organized in a specific fashion. Specifically, cellular membranes are semipermeable barriers preventing

[a] Neuroradiology Division, Radiology, Michigan Medicine, 1500 East Medical Center Drive, B1D502, Ann Arbor 48109-5030, USA; [b] Neuroradiology Division, Radiology, Michigan Medicine, 1500 East Medical Center Drive, Taubman Center B1-132, Ann Arbor 48109-5030, USA; [c] Neuroradiology Division, Radiology, Michigan Medicine, 1500 East Medical Center Drive, B2A209, Ann Arbor 48109-5030, USA

* Corresponding author.

E-mail address: ashoks@med.umich.edu

Magn Reson Imaging Clin N Am 29 (2021) 205–232

https://doi.org/10.1016/j.mric.2021.01.005

the free diffusion of extracellular water to the intracellular compartment and vice-versa. If the specific compartments have similar tissue compositions, conventional MR techniques would make differentiating between the different overall organization impossible. Three common mechanisms influence the diffusion of protons: (1) cellular size and density, (2) asymmetric cellular organization, and (3) extracellular composition.

Signal generation in MR depends on the phase coherence of similar protons in a given voxel. Magnetic gradients cause linear dephasing along the axis of the gradient; if a gradient of the opposite direction, but equal in magnitude, is applied, rephasing will occur. In this scenario, stationary protons will retain the greatest amount of phase coherence and mobile protons will experience incomplete rephrasing, thus experience signal loss proportional to distance traveled. It is by this mechanism that diffusion imaging highlights the microscopic physical movement [Brownian motion], or rather lack-thereof, of as determined by characteristics of the local environment.[4,5] The degree to which diffusion effects are accentuated in the resultant image are dependent on several factors, which are reflected in the b-value of the image.[5,6] B-value quantifies the effect of 2 different variables on a given system—amplitude of applied gradient [G], duration of the gradient [δ]—and is described by the following formula.[5]

$$b = \gamma^2 G^2 \delta^2 (\Delta - \delta/3)$$

The last term is the gyromagnetic ratio [γ], which depends on the field strength and surrounding electromagnetic environment of the protons. Unfortunately, the acquisition of quality DWI is not as straight forward as maximizing the amplitude and duration of gradients, as these effects also contribute to diminished signal-to-noise and emphasize artifacts, particularly in the head and neck. Strategies to mitigate negative imaging effects and accentuate diffusion effects are discussed later.

Not only does the visual representation of diffusion imaging often reveal strikingly different contrast than conventional anatomic sequences, because signal loss is proportional to the amount of physical motion, diffusion techniques can also provide quantitative data and generate the apparent diffusion coefficient (ADC).

Pulse Sequences

Echo-planar diffusion-weighted imaging

Most of the DWI performed in the clinical setting now uses echo-planar imaging (EPI). EPI is a sequence where altering gradients are continuously run following an excitation pulse, allowing all of k-space to be filled during the refocusing of a single excitation/echo. The major benefit to this single-shot EPI technique is rapid image acquisition (on the order of a few milliseconds per image). Rapid acquisition is particularly important for diffusion imaging, as it eliminates artifacts related to bulk patient motion: volitional motion, blood vessel pulsation, breathing, etc. from interfering with signal related to diffusion. Because EPI relies on precise gradients to manipulate a single echo, the major downside of single-shot EPI is a high degree of susceptibility to magnetic field inhomogeneities, thus causing erroneous signal and image distortion. These susceptibility effects are easily noted on single-shot EPI sequences near the petrous temporal bone, any air-skull-brain interface, or near implanted medical hardware; often, portions of the image are uninterpretable.[7–9] Techniques have been developed to diminish susceptibility effects, for example, multishot EPI, where k-space is filled in segments using a limited number of repetitions. In comparison to single-shot EPI, multishot EPI has improved spatial resolution, signal-to-noise, and decreased susceptibility artifacts, achieved at the expense of increased imaging time.[10]

Non–echo-planar diffusion-weighted imaging

The roots of diffusion imaging start in non-EPI techniques. In the 1960s, Stejkal and Tanner devised a diffusion-weighted sequence by adding time-dependent field gradients on either side of a spin echo refocusing pulse, thereby sensitizing the resultant signal to diffusion effects.[11] This technique can be limited by slow acquisition and susceptibility to motion artifacts. In the clinical setting, most DWI is based on echo-planar imaging, as discussed earlier. However, non-EPI techniques have been used to overcome some of the limitations encountered with EPI-based sequences, especially air-bone interface susceptibility. Non-EPI diffusion sequences include single-shot turbo spin-echo and multishot turbo spin-echo with non-Cartesian k-space filling.[8,12] These techniques have a longer imaging acquisition time relative to single-shot EPI but have improved diagnostic performance in specific settings, as discussed later.

Advanced diffusion techniques

Additional techniques have been developed to better demonstrate specific diffusion properties:

Diffusion tensor imaging assesses specific anisotropic directionality of diffusion within each voxel; from this, the location and orientation of white matter tracts can be inferred.[5]

Diffusion kurtosis imaging (DKI) determines the degree to which diffusion varies from a Gaussian distribution, adding an additional level of information.[13]

These, along with additional techniques, will be discussed in further details elsewhere in this diffusion-weighted series.

IMAGING PROTOCOLS

At the authors' institutions head and neck imaging protocols typically use routine T1, T2, and diffusion-weighted sequences in the axial plane, in addition to other planes that most adventitiously demonstrate the anatomy being focused on. For T1- and T2-weighted sequences, a modified Dixon technique is frequently used, allowing the option to view both non–fat-saturated and fat-saturated images without multiple acquisitions being required. If significant portions of the brain are included within the desired field of view, it is best to add additional routine brain sequences to adequately assess any incidental parenchymal findings. For example, our cranial nerve II (Orbit) protocol includes 10 imaging series: sagittal T1, axial EP-DWI, T2 FLAIR, SWI of the whole brain, in addition to T1 & T2 Dixon coronal, T1 DIXON axial, post-contrast T1 DIXON coronal and axial, and lastly a 3D postcontrast T1 of the whole brain.

Relevant head and neck imaging protocols, from the authors' institution, are included in **Table 1**.

Table 1
Summary of imaging sequences acquired in different cranial nerve and neck MR imaging protocols at the authors' institution

	Head and Neck Protocols				
	CN II (Orbit)	**CN I, III, IV, VI**	**CN V, VII, IX–XII**	**CN VIII**	**General Neck**
Series 1	T1 sagittal	T1 3D sagittal (brain)	T1 sagittal (brain)	T1 sagittal	T1 sagittal (neck)
Series 2	DWI axial (brain)	DWI axial (brain)	DWI axial (brain and neck)	DWI axial	DWI axial (neck)
Series 3	T2 FLAIR axial (brain)	T2 FLAIR axial (brain)	T2 FLAIR axial (brain)	DWI coronal thin	T2 DIXON axial (neck)
Series 4	SWI axial (brain)	T2 axial (thin)	3D SPACE/DRIVE axial optional**	T2 axial FLAIR	T1 DIXON axial (neck)
Series 5	T2 DIXON coronal (orbits)	T2 3D SPACE/ DRIVE axial	T2 DIXON axial (thin)	SWI axial	C + T1 DIXON axial (neck)
Series 6	T1 DIXON coronal (orbits)	T1 DIXON axial (thin)	T1 DIXON axial (thin)	3D DRIVE/BFFE/ FIESTA axial	C + T1 DIXON coronal (neck)
Series 7	T1 DIXON axial (orbits)	C + T1 DIXON axial	T1 perfusion optional**	T2 axial thin	
Series 8	C + T1 DIXON axial	C + T1 DIXON coronal	C + T1 DIXON axial	T1 axial thin	
Series 9	C + T1 DIXON coronal	+T1 3D sagittal (brain)	C + T1 DIXON coronal	C + T1 axial DIXON thin	
Series 10	C + T1 3D TFE sagittal		+T1 3D sagittal (brain)	C + T1 coronal thin	
Series 11				+T1 sagittal 3D TFE	
FOV	Orbit: supraorbital ridge anteriorly through the dorsum sellae posteriorly, orbital roof through orbital floor.	Top of frontal sinus through hard palate, tip of nose anteriorly through fourth ventricle posteriorly.	Top of frontal sinus through C2/C3, frontal sinus through fourth ventricle.	Routine brain coverage on axial slices, coronal slices through the IAC.	Clivus through thoracic inlet.

Irrespective of the number of series in an individual protocol or the number of planes evaluated, all head and neck imaging protocols include DWI that covers the entire brain and the relevant portion of the head and neck in order to enhance diagnostic efficacy.

IMAGING FINDINGS/PATHOLOGY

In the following section, various head and neck pathologies are further divided into subsections with discussion of the role of diffusion imaging pertaining to each pathology, especially how diffusion imaging adds valuable information beyond conventional MR sequences.

Subsections

Orbit

Although the location of abnormalities within the orbit, best determined with conventional MR sequences, assists in developing an appropriate differential diagnosis, DWI can further improve the differential.

Idiopathic orbital inflammation

- Characterized by facilitated diffusion due to higher free water content within edematous inflammatory changes (**Fig. 1**).
- Has significantly elevated ADC values relative to malignant neoplasms such as lymphoma, which can have a similar appearance.[14–16]
- Reported utility in distinguishing from abscess, which also show low ADC values that are not expected in this entity.[14]

Orbital sarcoidosis

- Characterized by facilitated diffusion, with no true diffusion restriction associated with the noncaseating granulomas that are characteristic of this entity (**Fig. 2**).
- Elevated ADC values help to differentiate malignant causes, which can share a similar imaging appearance and clinical presentation.[14]
- Clinical presentation (ie, subacute to chronic, painless) distinguishes from idiopathic orbital inflammation; systemic findings of sarcoidosis, when present, can help to discern as well.

Orbital lymphoma

- Characterized by marked restricted diffusion due to increased cellularity, similar to lymphoma throughout the other body parts (**Fig. 3**).
- Low ADC values differentiate this entity from processes such as idiopathic orbital inflammation, sarcoid, and benign lymphoproliferative disorders[17,18] and even some malignant processes as well.

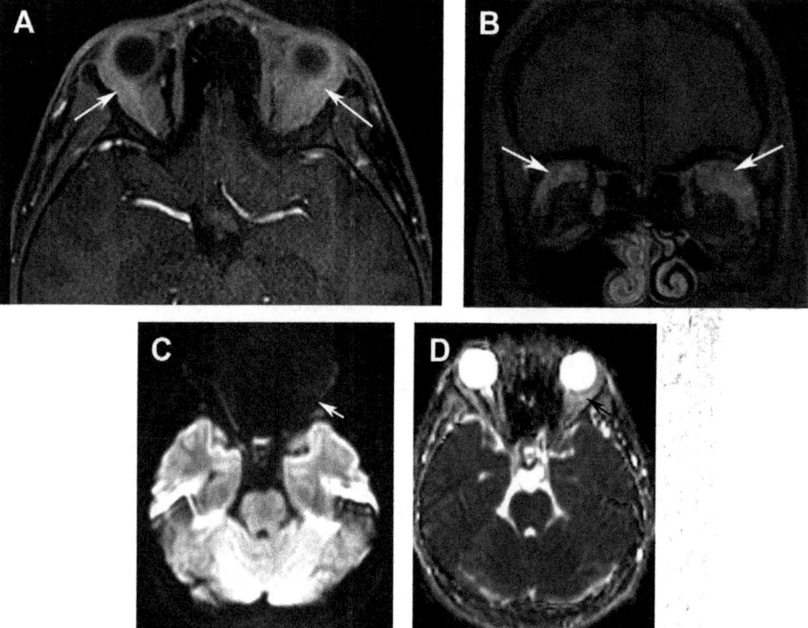

Fig. 1. A 11-year-old girl presenting with bilateral orbital swelling—idiopathic orbital inflammation (IOI). Axial (*A*) and coronal (*B*) postcontrast, axial DWI (*C*), and ADC (*D*) images demonstrate an infiltrative enhancing soft tissue involving the superior lateral aspects of the left greater than right orbits (*arrows* in *A, B*). Corresponding subtle low diffusion signal (*arrow* in *C*) signal with increased ADC values (*black arrow* in *D*) relative to the brainstem, most compatible with an inflammatory process.

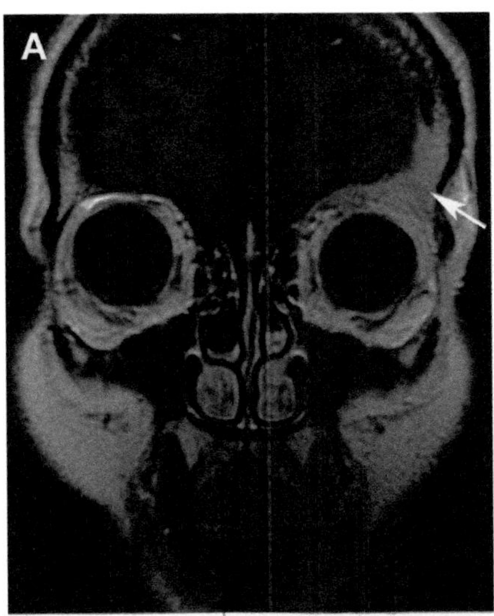

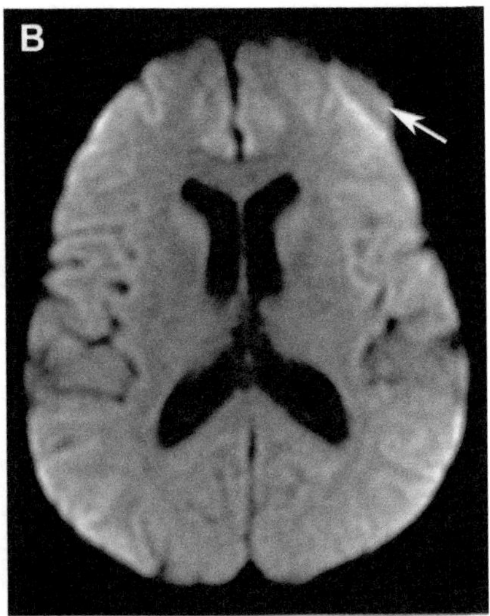

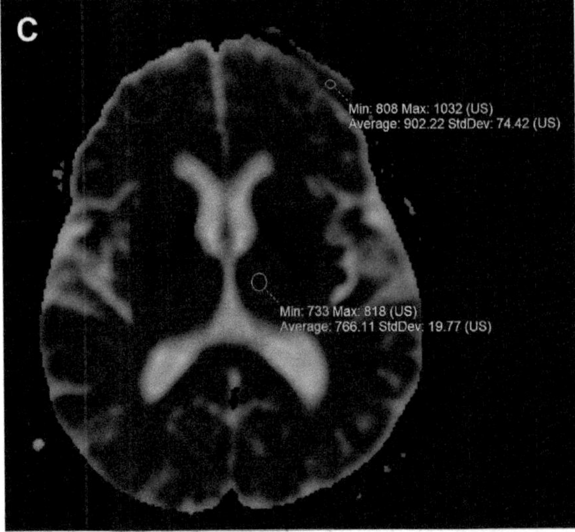

Fig. 2. A 64-year-old woman with 1-year history of dysesthesias in the left V1 distribution—sarcoidosis. Coronal postcontrast (*A*), axial DWI (*B*), and ADC (*C*) images demonstrate an aggressive enhancing soft tissue mass (*arrow* in *A*) along the superior lateral left orbit invading the calvarium and intracranial compartment. Diffusion sequences reveal hyperintense signal (*arrow* in *B*) on DWI with respect to white matter. Relatively increased ADC values, as opposed to true diffusion restriction, helping to point toward the inflammatory nature of this mass.

Venolymphatic malformation

- Unencapsulated benign hamartomatous vascular malformations can demonstrate complex cystic components, varying ages of blood products, and infiltration of local adjacent structures with multicompartmental involvement.
- Lack of cellularity results in predominantly elevated ADC values, revealing benign nature and differentiating it from malignant neoplasms (**Fig. 4**).[19] Of note, considerable overlap can be visualized between these cohorts, as susceptibility artifacts from blood products can distort the local magnetic field, and resulting inhomogeneities can result in artifactual signal on DWI (**Fig. 5**); results in this setting therefore should be interpreted with caution and in conjunction with conventional imaging sequences.[15]

Rhabdomyosarcoma

- Soft tissue sarcoma that demonstrates restricted diffusion due to increased cellularity.
- On conventional MR sequences, it can be nearly indistinguishable from vascular lesions of the orbit such as capillary hemangiomas; however, significantly lower ADC values help

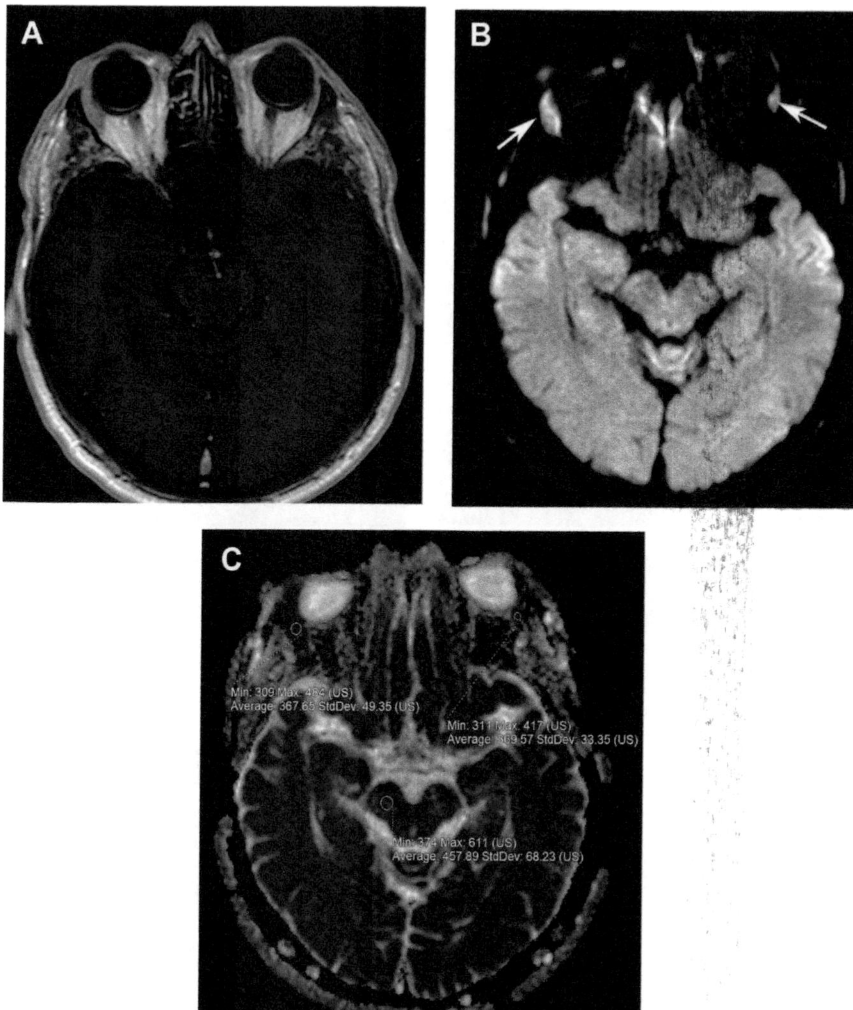

Fig. 3. A 69-year-old man with known history of lymphoma, presenting with headache and right sided eye swelling—lymphoma. Axial postcontrast (*A*), DWI (*B*), and ADC (*C*) images show bilateral lacrimal region orbital masses with postcontrast enhancement. Strikingly hyperintense DWI signal (*arrows* in *B*) and corresponding low ADC values, which reflect the densely cellular nature of lymphoma.

to characterize the true nature of these lesions (**Fig. 6**).[19,20]

Retinoblastoma

- Small round-cell tumors that demonstrate restricted diffusion due to high cellularity (**Fig. 7**A).
- Low ADC values have been shown to help differentiate residual viable neoplasm and/or locoregional metastases from posttreatment inflammatory changes (**Fig. 7**B), which can have a similar appearance on conventional sequences.[21,22]

Choroidal melanoma

- Restricted diffusion likely reflects high cellularity of melanoma, similar to melanoma elsewhere in the head and neck, and indeed throughout the body (**Fig. 8**).[23]
- Changes in ADC values seem to correlate with treatment response even earlier than conventional sequences, providing prognostic information to the clinician caring for the patient.[24]

Lacrimal gland benign mixed tumor

- Also known as pleomorphic adenomas, these are encapsulated slow-growing painless masses.
- Although benign, imaging features can demonstrate irregular lobulation, satellite lesions, and adjacent bony remodeling, with areas of cystic degeneration resulting in a heterogeneous appearance, all of which can mimic more aggressive lacrimal masses.

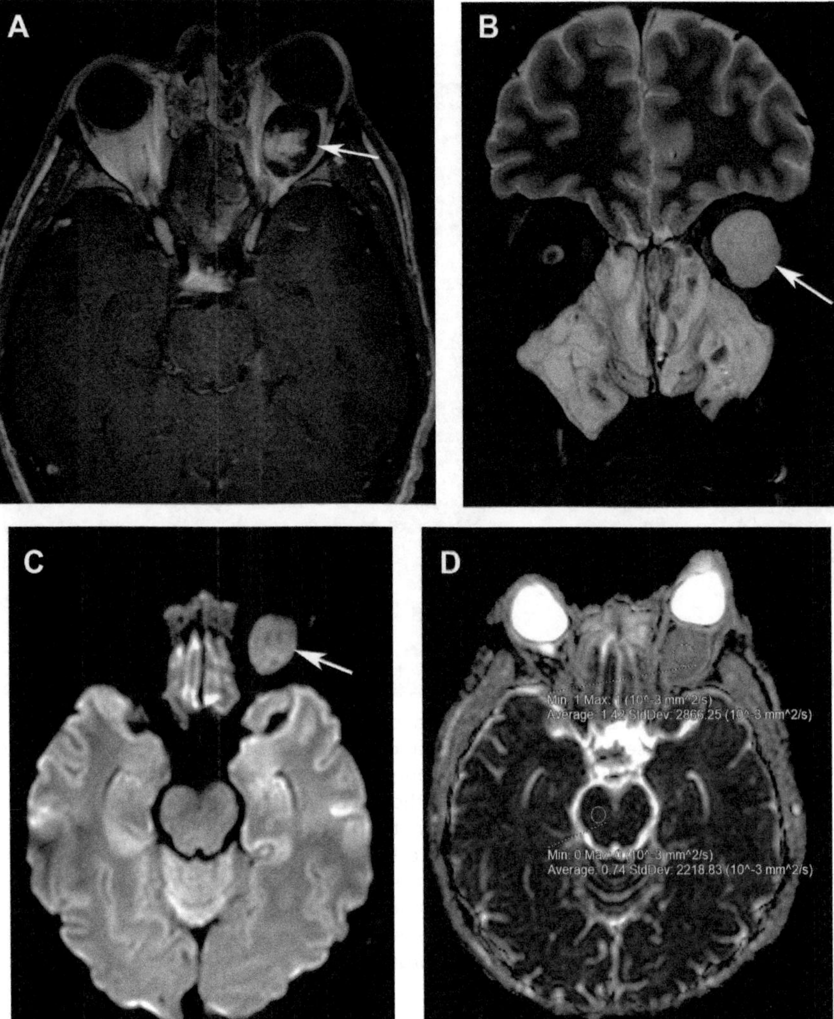

Fig. 4. A 36-year-old man with 7-year history of slowly progressive proptosis—venolymphatic malformation. Axial postcontrast (*A*), coronal T2 (*B*), axial DWI (*C*), and axial ADC map (*D*) images show a well-circumscribed T2 hyperintense mass (*arrow* in *B*) with progressive avid enhancement (*arrow* in *A*) and hyperintense DWI (*arrow* in *C*) signal. ADC values are nearly twice that of brain parenchyma, pointing away from a cellular tumor, favoring benign causes including vascular malformations like this one. Also evident is extensive sinonasal polyposis.

- Have significantly increased ADC values relative to malignant neoplasms of the lacrimal gland (such as adenoid cystic carcinoma, mucoepidermoid carcinoma, adenocarcinoma, squamous cell carcinoma, and undifferentiated carcinomas).[25]
- Decreased ADC values also associated with malignant transformation into carcinoma ex pleomorphic adenoma and are therefore a clue when assessing serial examinations in patients with known lacrimal benign mixed tumor (Fig. 9).

Maxillofacial

Pathology affecting the maxillofacial region may originate from the mucosa lining the paranasal sinuses, bones, or minor salivary glands.

Inverted papilloma

- Also known as Schneiderian papilloma, classically with a convoluted cerebriform pattern on conventional MR imaging sequences. Similar to other sinonasal polypoid diseases, it is characterized by facilitated diffusion (Fig. 10A).
- Risk of malignant transformation, most commonly into squamous cell carcinoma. On transformation, changes in architecture of the papilloma result in statistically decreased ADC values when compared with the benign lesion (Fig. 10B).[26]

Langerhans cell histiocytosis

- A monoclonal proliferation of Langerhans cells with high cellularity resulting in diffusion restriction.

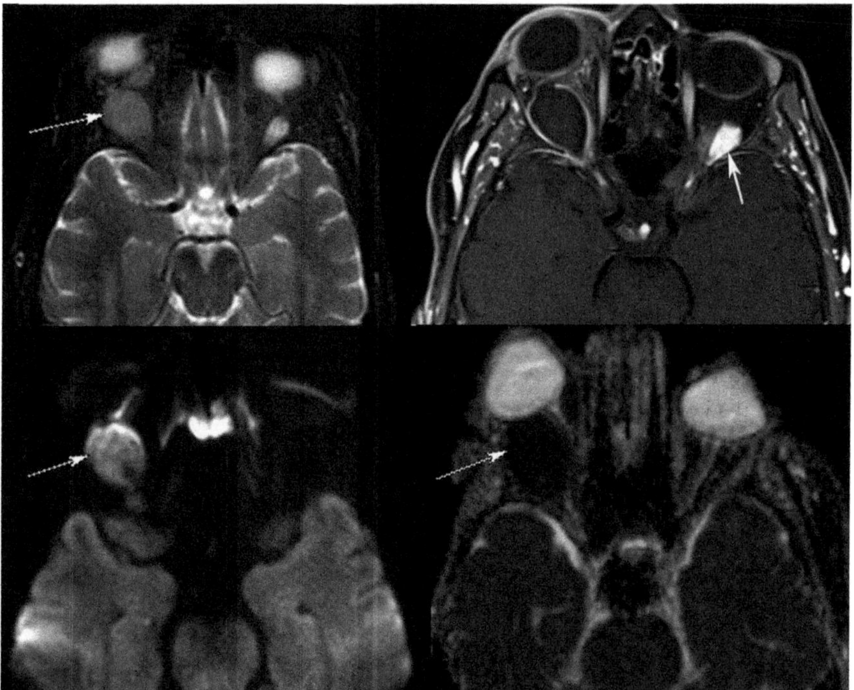

Fig. 5. A 67-year-old woman with 2-day history of headache, 1-day decreased vision in right eye—thrombosed varix. Care should be taken in cases of vascular malformations that have been complicated by hemorrhage, post-treatment changes, or thrombosis. Susceptibility distortions in the magnetic field can result in artifactual signal on DWI, such as in the case of this thrombosed varix. Although bland thrombus often has increased ADC values, care should be taken as increased viscosity or paramagnetic effects from deoxyhemoglobin or methemoglobin may decrease ADC values. In this patient with bilateral orbital varices, the right orbital lesion has intermediate intrinsic T2-weighted signal (*dashed arrow, top left*), peripheral enhancement, hyperintense DWI signal (*dashed arrow, bottom left*), and strikingly hypointense ADC signal (*dashed arrow, bottom right*). A smaller left orbital lesion is occult on diffusion sequences and has similar T2-weighted signal as the right orbital lesion and avid post-contrast enhancement (*white solid arrow, top right*), consistent with a patent varix.

- Conventional MR imaging appearance of Langerhans cell histiocytosis, most often demonstrating hypointense to isointense signal on T1, hyperintense T2/STIR signal, and avid postcontrast enhancement, can mimic an aggressive neoplastic process.
- May be a potential pitfall in interpretation, as both conventional and DWI appearance can mimic a malignant process (**Fig. 11**).[27]

Aneurysmal bone cyst

- Benign, expansile lytic lesions that on conventional imaging appearance classically demonstrates a well-circumscribed multiseptated mass with internal fluid-fluid levels.
- Characterized by facilitated diffusion (**Fig. 12**A).
- Most of these lesions primarily arise from bone, although can secondarily arise from an underlying bony lesion.
- As such, differentiating primary benign aneurysmal bone cysts (ABCs) from secondary lesions as well as malignant neoplasms such as telangiectatic osteosarcomas or giant cell tumors, which can mimic both the expansile nature and internal architecture of ABCs, is an important distinction (**Fig. 12**B).
- Statistically elevated ADC values associated with ABCs when compared with the ADC values associated with malignant tumors; even small areas of diffusion restriction within these lesions can point toward a secondary ABC with underlying pathology.[28]

Juvenile nasopharyngeal angiofibroma

- Benign tumors of vascular origin that nonetheless demonstrate locally aggressive features, confounding diagnosis on conventional MR imaging.
- Characterized by facilitated diffusion, with markedly elevated ADC values relative to similar-appearing malignancies on the differential (**Fig. 13**).[29,30]

Esthesioneuroblastoma

- Also known as olfactory neuroblastomas, these are neoplasms of neural crest origin arising from the superior olfactory recess.

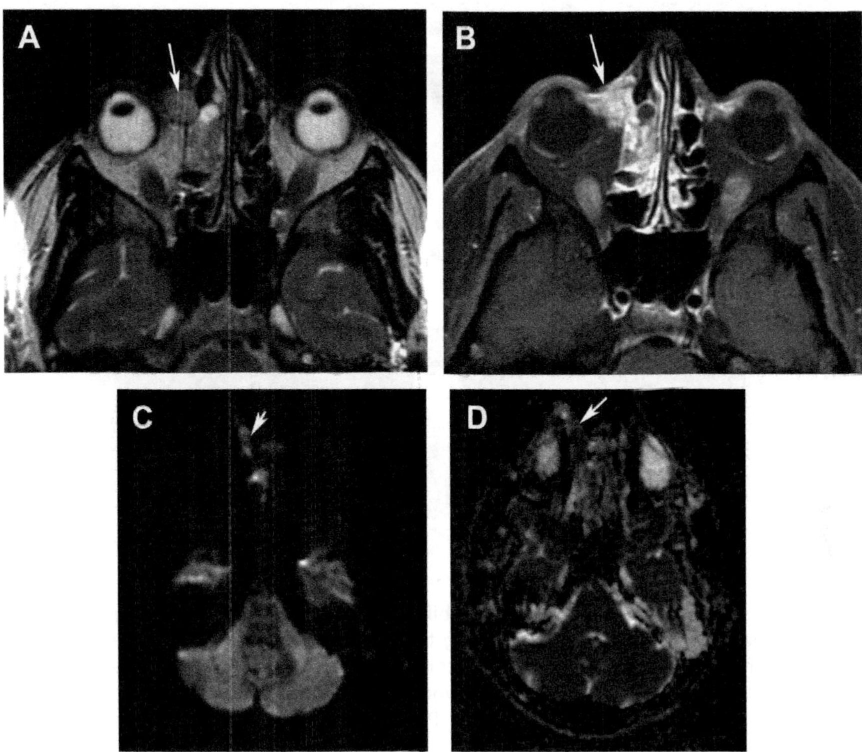

Fig. 6. A 54-year-old woman with right epiphora and facial swelling—rhabdomyosarcoma. Axial T2 (*A*), postcontrast (*B*), DWI (*C*), and ADC (*D*). Mass along the medial inferior aspect of the right orbit seems relatively well circumscribed on T2 imaging (*arrow* in *A*); however, avid infiltrative enhancement (*arrow* in *B*) with corresponding DWI hyperintensity (*short arrow* in *C*) and low ADC signal (*arrow* in *D*) indicate a more ominous process, in this case a pathology-proven rhabdomyosarcoma.

- On conventional sequences, this diagnosis can be suggested by location, locally aggressive margins, and intracranial peritumoral cysts, although other aggressive malignancies of the head and neck can have a similar appearance (**Fig. 14**).
- Reports suggest diffusion imaging can differentiate this lesion from both benign and other malignant causes,[31] with statistically increased ADC values (proposed cutoff >1.1 x 10^{-3} mm^2/s) characterizing esthesioneuroblastoma with high specificity when compared with other malignancies and esthesioneuroblastoma demonstrating lower ADC values than those associated with benign lesions.
- Application of diffusion kurtosis imaging, particularly in combination with additional advanced MR techniques such as perfusion, is reported to offer increased sensitivity and specificity when delineating these tumors from other malignancies, with significantly higher kurtosis on DKI when compared with squamous cell carcinomas.[32]

Nasopharyngeal carcinoma

- Highly cellular tumor, with expected diffusion restriction (**Fig. 15**A).
- DWI is shown to provide both diagnostic and prognostic values.
  - In endemic areas, both conventional DWI and advanced diffusion techniques such as intravoxel incoherent motion (IVIM) DWI have been used to differentiate early stage NPC from benign lymphoid hyperplasia, as well as from additional malignant causes such as lymphoma (**Fig. 15**B).[33–35]
  - Used to improve detection of lymph node metastases.[36]
  - Able to track treatment effects in both the primary site and nodal metastases and increase sensitivity for tumor recurrence.[37] Good treatment response results in interval increase of ADC within the treated area, and tumor recurrence causes an interval decrease in ADC in the area of interest after ADC values have normalized.
  - Conventional and advanced techniques, including RESOLVE DWI and DKI, have

A

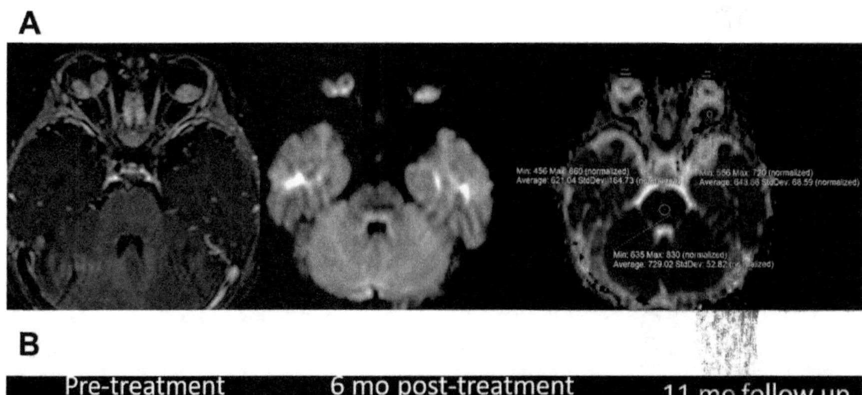

B

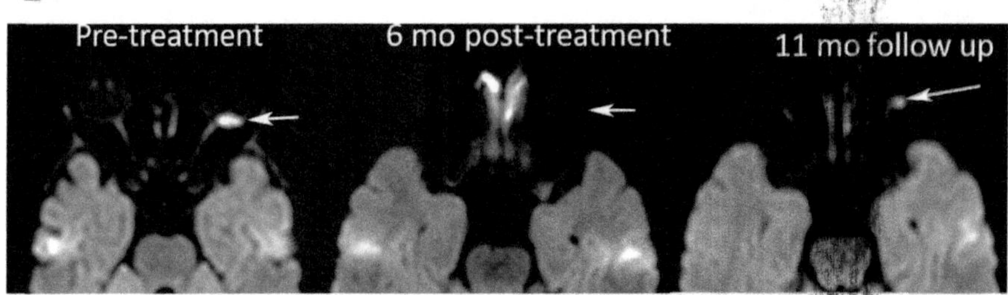

Fig. 7. (*A*) A 9-month-old girl with absent red reflex bilaterally—retinoblastoma. Axial postcontrast, DWI, and ADC map images. Enhancing soft tissue masses along the posterior globes in a pediatric patient, concerning for retinoblastoma. Diffusion imaging demonstrates corresponding increased DWI signal and low ADC values, reflective of high cellularity. (*B*). Five-month-old woman originally presenting with wandering left eye, nystagmus, and poor eye contact—retinoblastoma. Pretreatment, 6-month posttreatment, and 11-month follow-up DWI images. In a pediatric patient with unilateral retinoblastoma, index images show an ocular mass with restricted diffusion compatible with retinoblastoma. Interval examination demonstrates complete resolution of restricted diffusion approximately 6 months later. However, subsequent imaging 11 months posttreatment reveals new left ocular restricted diffusion compatible with recurrence.

been suggested to provide prognostic value in NPC cases, predicting response to chemotherapy treatment, although varying results have been reported in the literature, and additional validation studies are required.[38,39]

- Several studies, including those by Yan and colleagues[38] and Zhang and colleagues,[40] suggested pretreatment ADC values greater than 0.72 or 0.747 x 10^{-3} mm^2/s, respectively, demonstrated significantly longer overall survival, as well as local relapse-free survival, when compared with those whose pretreatment tumors had ADC values lower than the aforementioned cutoff.
- Other studies that failed to find a significant difference in pretreatment ADC values, however, found low absolute early posttreatment minimum ADC values, a lower percent change in ADC values, and increased mean of the kurtosis coefficient, K_{means}, predictive of a failure to respond to treatment.[41,42]

Temporal bone

Temporal bone contents include nerves, mucosa, ossicular chain, and small blood vessels.

Cholesteatoma

- Strikingly apparent on DWI, thought to reflect trapped water associated with microstructure of increased keratin.
- Technical considerations:
  - Conventional single-shot EPI sequences suffer from susceptibility artifacts and geometric distortion particularly at the air-bone and air-soft tissue interfaces where cholesteatomas reside, as well as inherent image resolution limitations, hindering evaluation for lesions smaller than 5 mm.[9]
  - Non-EPI sequences, such as single-shot turbo spin-echo sequences, have been recommended, given their decreased sensitivity to susceptibility mismatches and geometric distortion and higher resolution matrix (although at the cost of lower signal-to-noise ratio and longer imaging times) (**Fig. 16**A).
  - Additional refinements, such as HASTE (a half Fourier single-shot TSE sequence), PROPELLER (a multishot TSE sequence, in which k-space is acquired in a rotating manner), RESOLVE (an EPI sequence with reduced echo spacing), and TGSE BLADE (a Propeller type sequence with hybrid

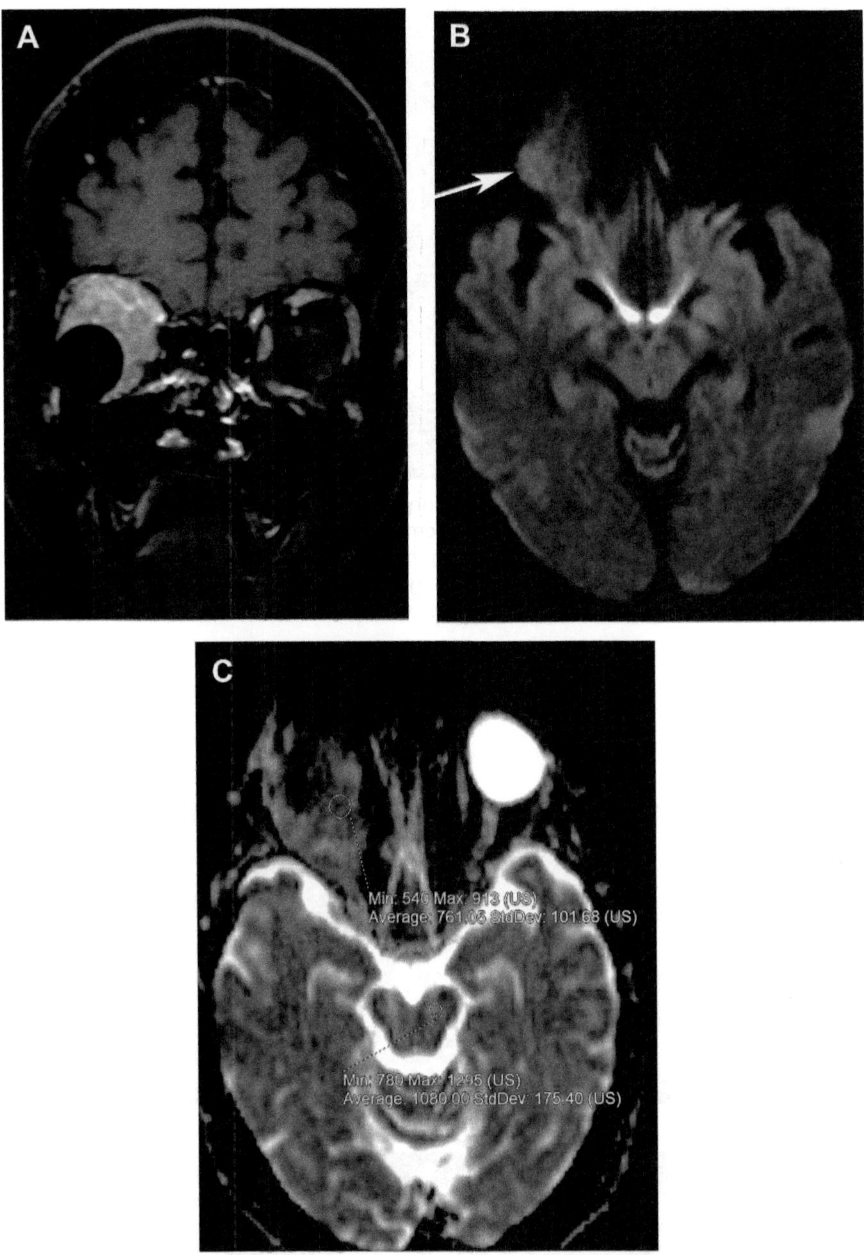

Fig. 8. A 68-year-old woman with history of choroidal melanoma status post enucleation, presenting with 1-week history of sudden onset ptosis—recurrent choroidal melanoma. Coronal postcontrast (*A*), DWI (*B*), and ADC map (*C*) images. Infiltrative enhancing soft tissue mass displacing the right orbital prosthesis is seen with associated diffusion restriction (*arrow*) and low ADC, pointing to the cellular nature of melanoma in this case of recurrent disease.

gradient-echo spin-echo readouts) sequences, have all been proposed in efforts to further improve image quality and diagnostic accuracy, with progressive reduction in artifacts and increased ability to visualize smaller and smaller lesions.[43–45]

- The exquisite sensitivity provided by DWI has been reported to obviate postcontrast sequences in routine follow-up imaging for cholesteatomas (**Fig. 16**B).[46] Diffusion imaging in this setting has also helped surgeons reduce the need for second-look surgeries.

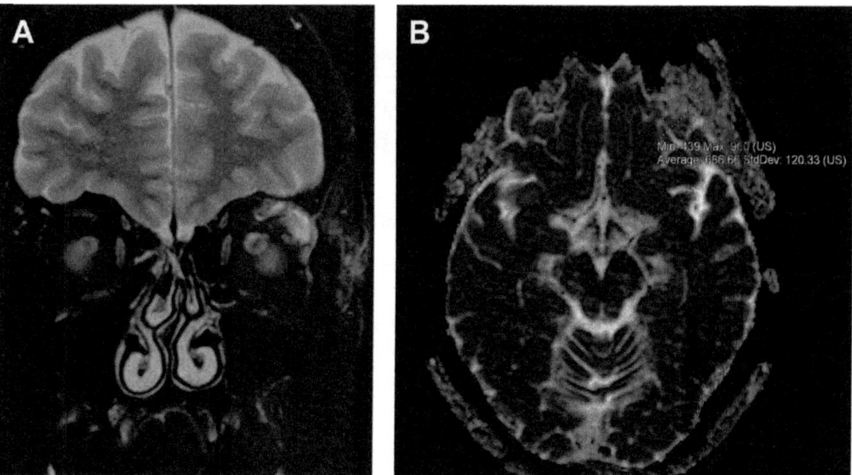

Fig. 9. A 58-year-old man presenting with 6-month history of progressive orbital swelling and proptosis—carcinoma ex pleomorphic adenoma. Coronal T2 image (*A*) demonstrates enhancing (not shown) infiltrative T2 signal centered in the region of the lacrimal gland, extending into the lateral body orbit and periorbital soft tissues. ADC map (*B*) demonstrates decreased ADC values involving infiltrative periorbital enhancing soft tissue, concerning for malignant transformation to a carcinoma ex pleomorphic adenoma, as subsequently demonstrated on pathology.

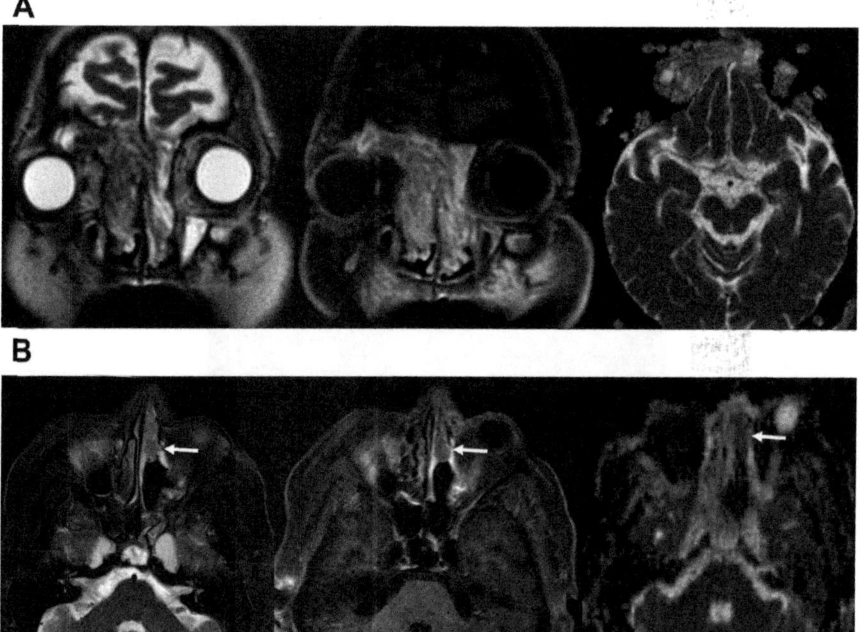

Fig. 10. (*A*) A 64-year-old man with nasal obstructive symptoms—inverted papilloma. Expansile mass occupying the right greater than left paranasal sinuses and nasal cavity demonstrates "convoluted cerebriform" pattern on T2 and postcontrast imaging. As with other benign sinonasal polyps, this mass demonstrated facilitated diffusion with relatively increased ADC values present. (*B*) A 63-year-old woman with previously resected inverted papilloma, clinically asymptomatic enlarging nasal mass—inverted papilloma with squamous transformation. Imaging in a different patient with previously resected inverted papilloma demonstrates development of a heterogeneous T2 hyperintense soft tissue lesion (*arrow, left image*) with mild enhancement (*middle arrow*) occupying the left nasal cavity. Diffusion imaging revealed low ADC values (*right arrow*) concerning for recurrence with transformation into squamous cell carcinoma, as was shown later on pathology.

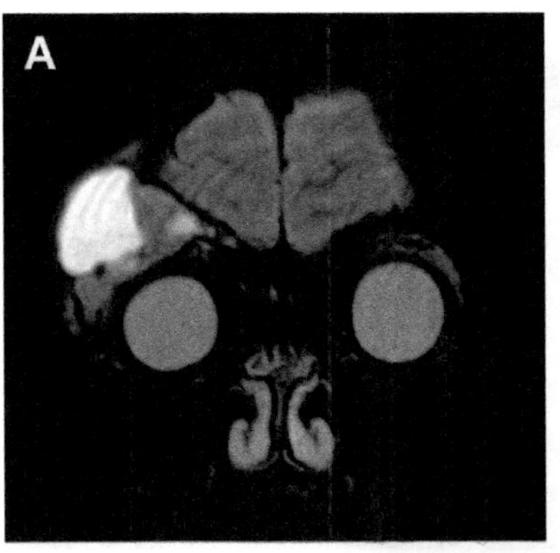

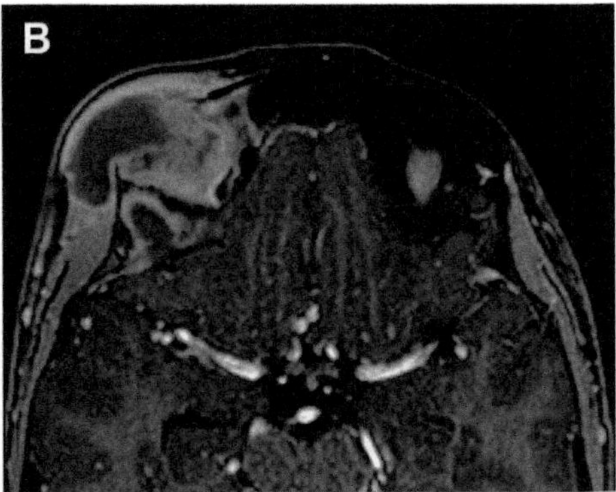

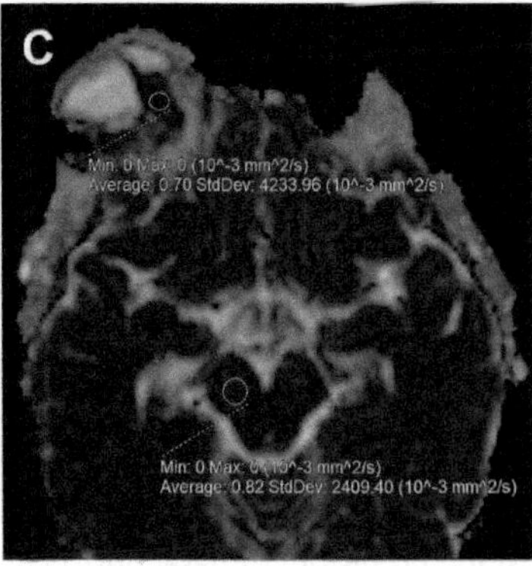

Fig. 11. A 12-year-old boy presenting with sudden onset enlarging right orbital mass following minor trauma - Langerhans cell histiocytosis. Conventional MR imaging (coronal T2 fat sat [*A*], axial post-contrast fat sat [*B*]) sequences demonstrate a solid and cystic mass involving the right superior lateral bony orbit, with eccentric enhancing soft tissue component, and extension into the intracranial compartment. The soft tissue component demonstrates relatively decreased ADC values on diffusion weight imaging (*C*), which indicate the cellular nature of Langerhans cell histiocytosis. Given the locally aggressive features and cellularity of histiocytosis, this entity can be difficult to differentiate from other malignancies, which can have a similar appearance.

Cholesterol granuloma

- Benign expansile cystic lesions, reflecting inflammatory response to cholesterol deposits from repeat bleeding, and thus characterized by facilitated diffusion (**Fig. 17**).
- Classic conventional imaging demonstrates marked hyperintense T1 and T2 signal without associated enhancement, helping to differentiate these lesions from additional petrous apex lesions including asymmetric marrow signal, effusions, or cholesteatomas.
- In more complex cases, the absence of restricted diffusion can help to differentiate these lesions from cholesteatomas or malignant processes as well.[47]

Petrous apicitis

- Infection involving the petrous apex classically presents with Gradenigo syndrome (otorrhea, abducens nerve palsy, and facial pain), secondary to involvement of Dorello canal and Meckel cave.
- In earlier cases where the only manifestation on computed tomography (CT) might be a fluid collection in the petrous apex, MR imaging is more sensitive for signs of infection, with conventional fat-saturated T2 and postcontrast imaging able to demonstrate marrow edema and abnormal enhancement.
- The addition of DWI helps to elucidate the progression of the infectious process as well, able to depict small areas of abscess formation that are otherwise difficult to identify on conventional sequences, and thus helping to guide clinical management (**Fig. 18**).[48]

Major salivary glands

Located in separate head and neck regions, the salivary glands are grouped together here by their common function and relatively common pathologies. As a special anatomic consideration, the parotid gland is the last major salivary gland to be encapsulated by investing fascia; as such, it contains intraparotid lymph nodes that drain the scalp, cheek, and external ear.

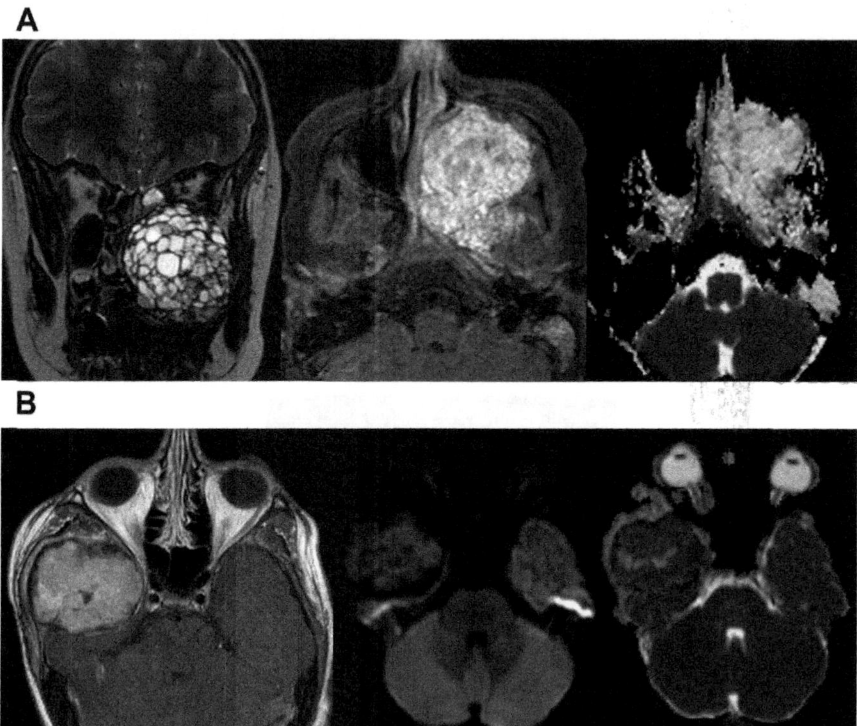

Fig. 12. (*A*) An 8-year-old girl with longstanding history of nasal obstruction and 4-month history of enlarging left cheek mass—aneurysmal bone cyst. Enhancing multiloculated expansile fluid signal mass centered in the region of the left sinonasal cavity. Markedly elevated ADC values associated with this lesion reassure of the benign nature of this aneurysmal bone cyst, which is in contrast to causes such as giant cell tumors, as demonstrated in the next figure. (*B*) A 13-year-old man presenting with right-sided facial swelling—giant-cell tumor. This heterogeneously enhancing expansile mass centered along the right sphenoid wing demonstrates increased diffusion signal and relatively decreased ADC values, as opposed to the elevated ADC values seen in aneurysmal bone cyst. This was a giant-cell tumor.

Sjogren syndrome

- A chronic autoimmune disease affecting the salivary and lacrimal glands, in which acinar destruction by lymphocytes results in progressive salivary gland dysfunction and progressive fatty replacement of the involved glands.
- Changes in the pathophysiology of the glandular tissue as the disease evolves seem to result in variance in imaging appearance of the glands throughout this process.
  - At early stages, Sjogren syndrome without obvious morphologic abnormalities can be indistinguishable from an uninvolved gland on conventional MR imaging. However, studies have suggested that the early pathologic changes of Sjogren result in elevated ADC values relative to normal age-matched controls, apparent even when no appreciable difference can be visualized on conventional MR imaging (**Fig. 19**).[49]
  - Conversely, late-stage Sjogren demonstrates statistically decreased ADC values relative to early stage Sjogren and nonafflicted individuals.
- These imaging differences are increasingly apparent on application of further refinements to traditional DWI, such as intravoxel incoherent motion[50] and whole-volume ADC histogram analysis.[51]

Sialadenitis

- The most common pathology affecting the salivary glands, this entity encompasses a broad spectrum of causes, including infectious, obstructive, autoimmune, granulomatous, and treatment-related causes, with imaging appearance dependent on the instigating process.
- DWI proves useful in specific situations:
  - In cases of acute bacterial sialadenitis, complications such as early or small abscess formation can be detected at a

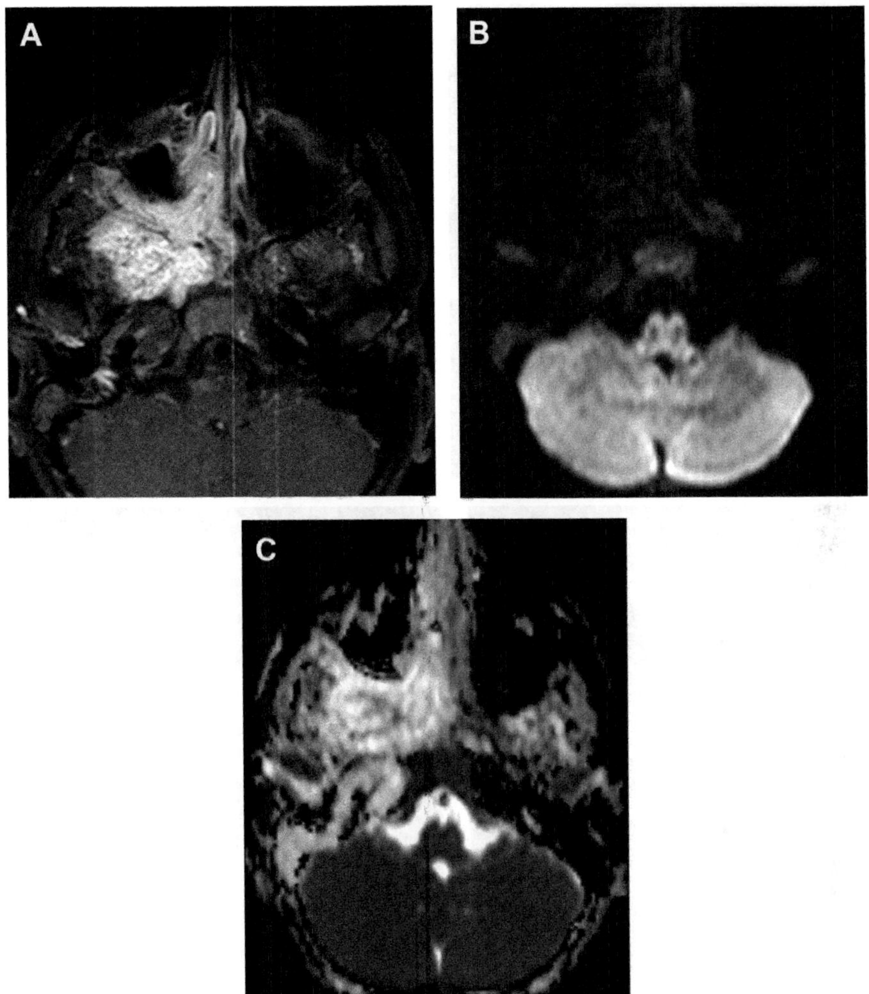

Fig. 13. A 10-year-old boy presenting with progressive headaches and severe epistaxis following an episode of trauma—juvenile nasopharyngeal angiofibroma (JNA). This locally aggressive, avidly enhancing soft tissue mass centered in the region of the sphenopalatine foramen (*A*) demonstrates lack of increased signal on diffusion-weighted images (*B*) and increased ADC values (*C*), suggesting a benign entity such as JNA as opposed to a more cellular malignant process.

greater sensitivity using DWI than conventional imaging (**Fig. 20**).

- In cases of subacute necrotizing sialadenitis, a locally aggressive, however self-limited, inflammatory process that can mimic an aggressive malignancy on conventional imaging, the lack of diffusion restriction can help suggest this less concerning cause.[52]

Benign mixed tumor/pleomorphic adenoma

- Encapsulated well-circumscribed masses containing both epithelial and mesenchymal tissues. Lack of increased cellularity indicates that these lesions are characterized by facilitated diffusion (**Fig. 21**).
- Although imaging appearance on conventional MR imaging sequences can resemble both other benign and malignant parotid masses, ADC values associated with pleomorphic adenomas are statistically elevated relative to Warthin tumors as well as parotid malignancies. These elevated values are thought to reflect areas of accumulated fluid in the adenomatous and glandular components within the pleomorphic adenoma.[53]

Xerostomia

- Salivary gland dysfunction is a known risk of radiation therapy in the head and neck when radiation fields encompass the major salivary glands, and xerostomia remains one of the

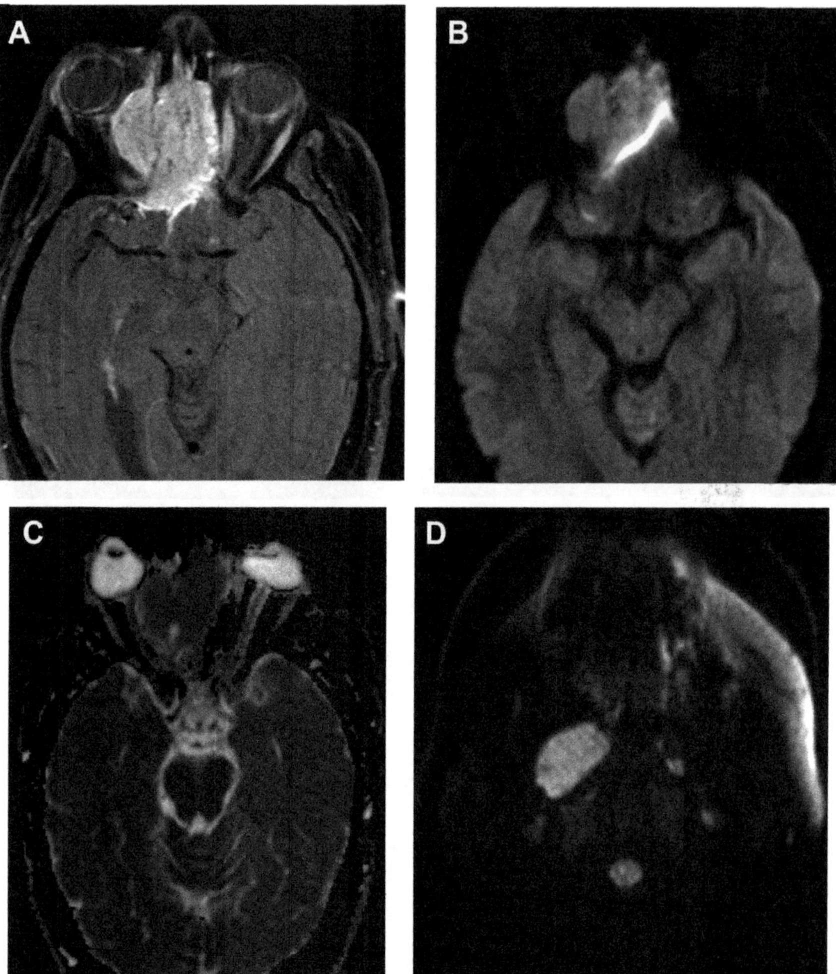

Fig. 14. A 41-year-old woman presenting with 3-week history of severe frontal headaches, blurry vision—esthesioneuroblastoma. As opposed to the JNA described earlier, this locally aggressive avidly enhancing mass centered in the region of the olfactory recess (*A*) shows increased diffusion signal (*B*) and corresponding low ADC values (*C*), compatible with the densely cellular nature of this malignancy. The enlarged metastatic retropharyngeal node demonstrates similar diffusion characteristics (*D*).

most frequent complications of radiation therapy despite mitigation strategies such as intensity modulation.

- There is heterogeneity in the reported changes of ADC values within the literature, which likely reflects variance in technique and b-value selection.
  - Propensity of recent literature suggests an increase in ADC values in the immediate postradiation therapy period.[54]
- Despite this heterogeneity, there is general agreement that these early changes in ADC values seem to provide functional and long-term prognostic value.
  - Correlates with clinically reported functional grading of xerostomia
  - Associated with the degree of residual xerostomia 6 to 12 months following treatment, with a higher grade of xerostomia associated with relatively increased ADC values and percent change following gustatory stimulation 1 to 2 weeks after initiation of treatment.[55,56]

Tumors

- With the possible exception of lymphoma, which demonstrates significantly decreased ADC values relative to other malignancies, the diverse histologic and radiologic appearances of malignant tumors of the salivary gland precludes accurate differentiation.

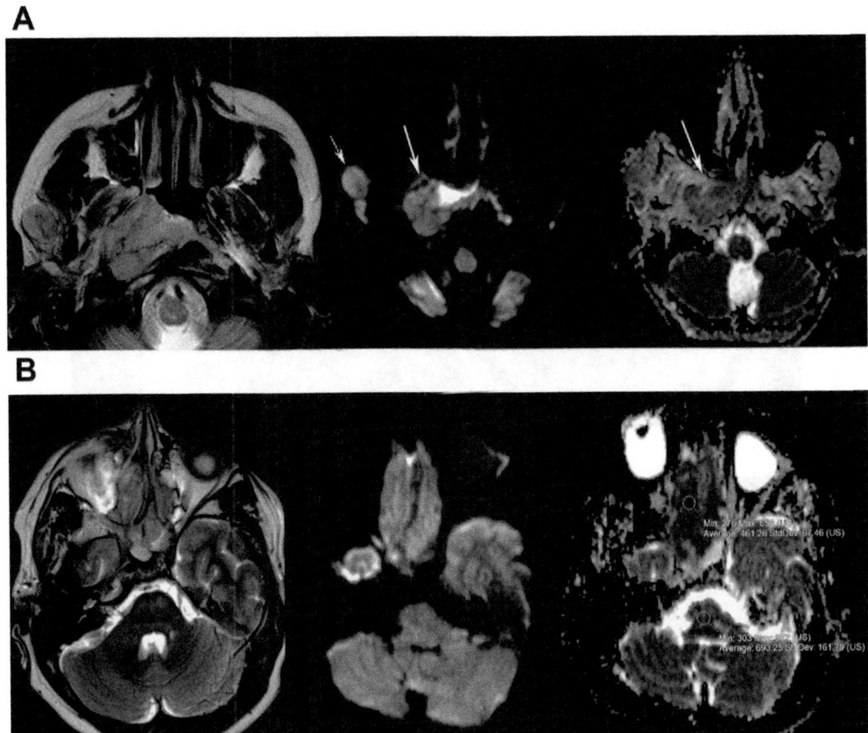

Fig. 15. (*A*) A 21-year-old woman with 5-month history of right-sided headaches—nasopharyngeal carcinoma: aggressive-appearing soft tissue mass along the posterior nasopharynx, which demonstrates DWI hyperintensity (*solid arrow, middle image*) and low ADC signal (*solid arrow, right image*) compatible with increased cellularity. A metastatic right periparotid node is evident as well (short dashed arrow). (B) A 59-year-old woman presenting with progressive sinus headaches and pressure—nasopharyngeal lymphoma: a comparison case of nasal lymphoma reveals marked decreased ADC values, to an even greater degree than is seen in nasopharyngeal carcinoma, as reported in the literature.

- DWI nonetheless offers valuable information once the primary tumor type has been identified.
  - Similar to elsewhere in the head and neck region, residual and recurrent tumors display decreased ADC values reminiscent of the pretreatment appearance of the primary mass, thought to be reflective of the hypercellularity maintained by viable tumor, and in contrast to the facilitated diffusion present in areas of posttreatment changes and radiation necrosis.

Pharynx/larynx

Squamous cell carcinoma

- Clinical presentation and imaging appearance can vary depending on HPV status (especially in the oropharynx), site of primary, and locoregional extent.
- The larynx in particular offers unique challenges to MR imaging, given its complex structure, propensity for motion, and air-tissue interfaces.
  - Despite these technical difficulties, DWI has been shown to accurately differentiate precancerous lesions from carcinomas including squamous cell carcinoma.[57]
- More broadly, DWI has been used for an expanding role in the diagnosis, staging, prognosis, and follow-up of squamous cell carcinoma throughout the head and neck mucosal space.
  - Despite early concerns about the interobserver reproducibility of measured ADC values between readers and scanners,[58] DWI has been proved to be a robust and valuable clinical tool.
  - Utilization of advanced techniques such as IVIM and ADC histogram analyses has been reported to allow for the differentiation of HPV+ and HPV− squamous cell carcinoma, with lower mean ADC, increased positive skewness, and increased excess kurtosis associated with HPV+ carcinomas.[59,60]

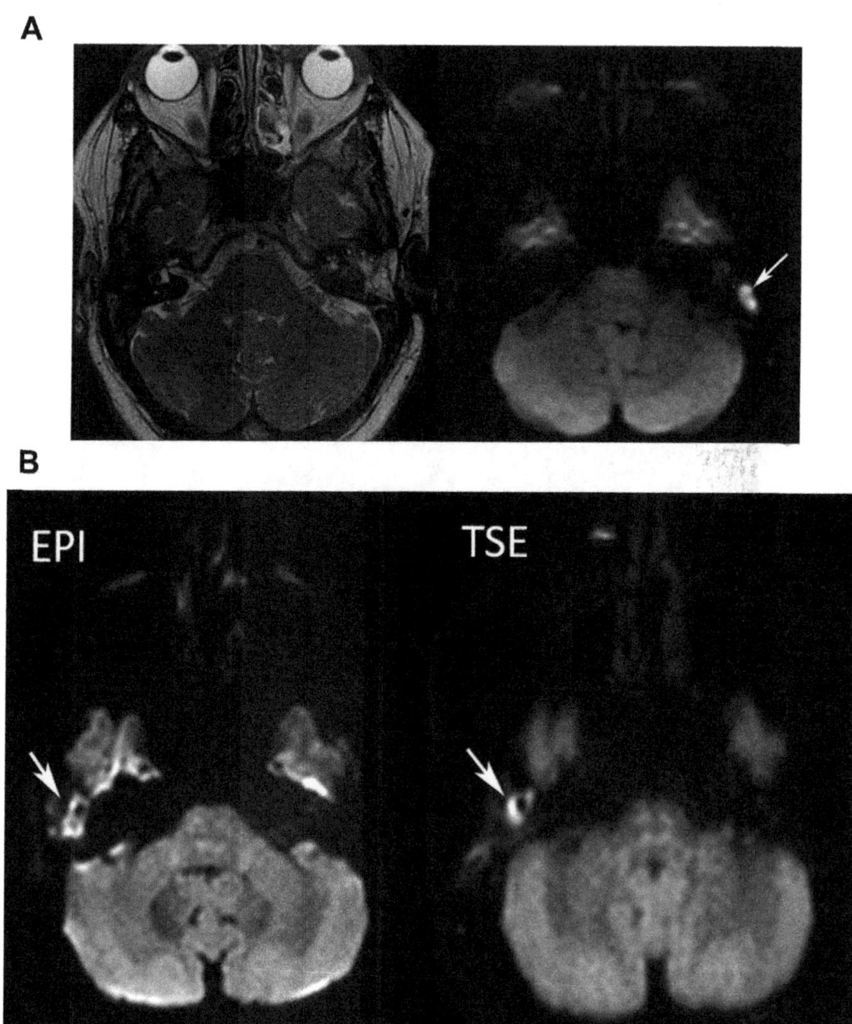

Fig. 16. (*A*) A 58-year-old woman with history of chronic left suppurative otitis media status postmultiple revisions, left aural fullness, and chronic otalgia—cholesteatoma. Evaluation for recurrent cholesteatoma on conventional MR imaging can be difficult in previously treated patients, as seen in this example, where there is nonspecific heterogenous T2 signal seen in the left middle ear cavity. However, the area of recurrent cholesteatoma is strikingly apparent on diffusion imaging (*arrow*). (*B*) A 39-year-old man with history of metastatic adenoma of right middle ear status post resection, presenting with recurrent otorrhea—cholesteatoma: a companion case demonstrates the utility of TSE versus EPI and multiplanar diffusion imaging in evaluation of cholesteatoma. As noted, susceptibility artifacts and geometric distortion can complicate traditional EPI diffusion sequences, as in this case, where linear high signal on the axial EPI diffusion sequence is reminiscent of the artifactual high signal seen at normal air-bone interfaces (*left arrow*). The abnormal diffusion signal is more easily appreciated on coronal diffusion imaging (not shown), appearing less artifactual and more mass-like. TSE diffusion sequences are less susceptible to susceptibility mismatches and distortion. In this same case, a rounded focus of abnormal diffusion compatible with recurrent cholesteatoma is revealed on the axial and coronal TSE diffusion-weighted sequences (*right arrow*). TSE, turbo spin-echo.

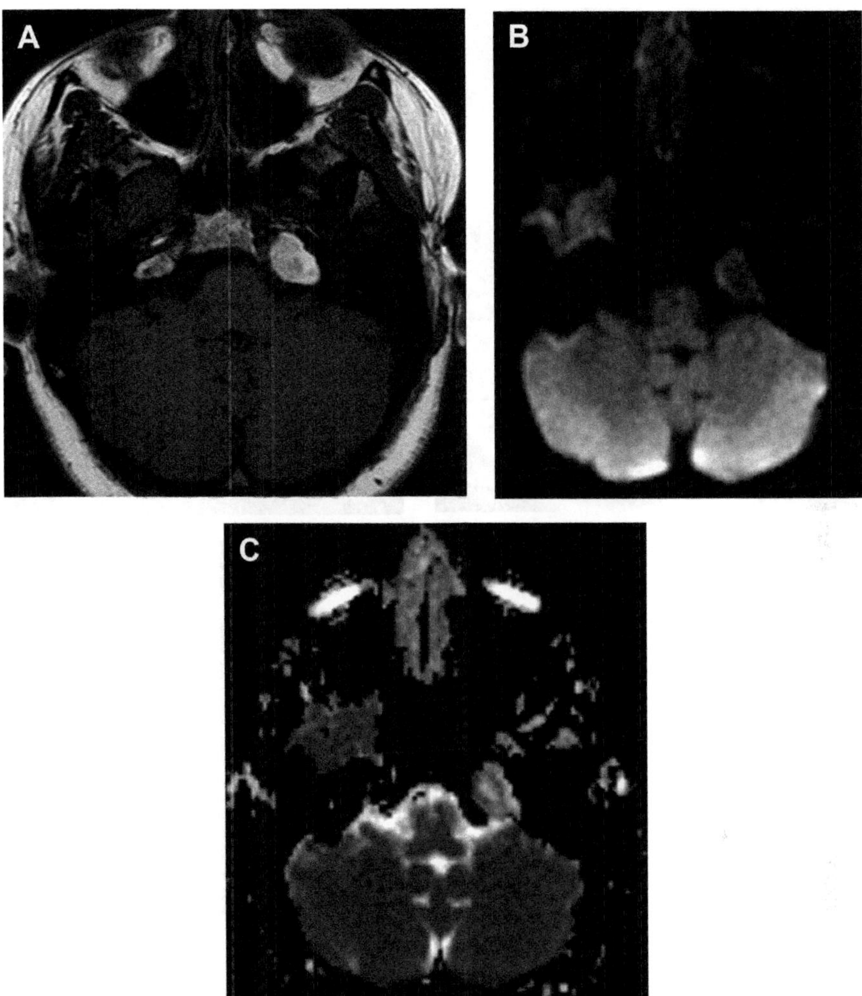

Fig. 17. A 27-year-old woman with intermittent imbalance and headaches—cholesterol granuloma. T1 hyperintense lesion centered in the left petrous apex (*A*), suggesting a cholesterol granuloma. Diffusion imaging (*B, C*) demonstrates increased ADC values, further corroborating the suggested diagnosis.

- Multiple studies have demonstrated the utility of DWI in differentiating benign and pathologic lymphadenopathy associated with primary squamous cell carcinoma. Although results are not entirely consistent in the literatures, a recent meta-analysis reported that, overall, lymph nodes with ADC values lower than suggested thresholds ranging from 0.749 to 1.39 x 10^{-3} mm^2/s demonstrated neoplastic involvement with statistical significance (**Fig. 22**).[61] Using more advanced diffusion techniques also reveals significant differences in benign and malignant nodes; as reported by Park and colleagues,[62] texture analysis of malignant nodes in multishot EPI-DWI demonstrated significantly increased complexity, energy, and roundness when compared with benign nodes.
- Diffusion changes seem to correlate with clinical prognosis:
  - Detection of residual or recurrent tumors,[63,64] with pathologic recurrence detected by residual restricted diffusion on follow-up examinations with sensitivity equivalent and complementary to the sensitivity of F-18 fluorodeoxy glucose PET/CT.[65,66] Differentiation seemed improved when combined with morphologic criteria.[67]
  - Intermediate and slow diffusion rates (D_2 and D_3) derived from triexponential fitting was reported to correlate with tumor growth rate, thought to reflect difference

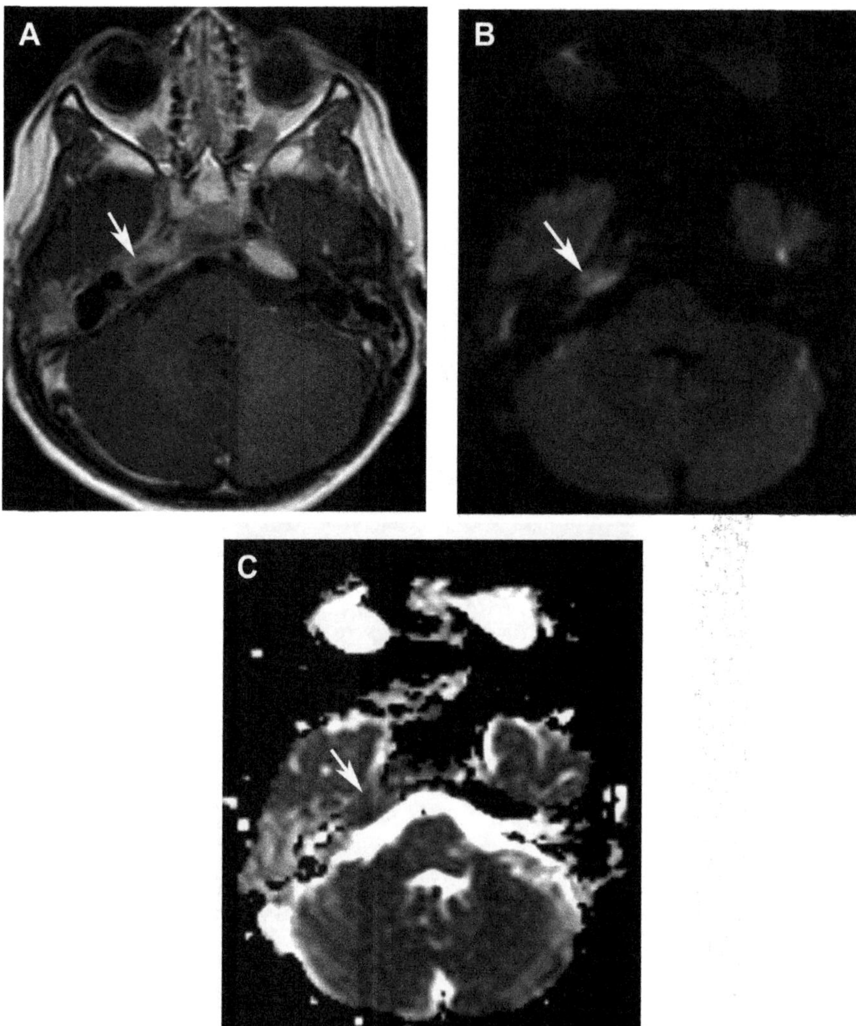

Fig. 18. A 6-year-old girl with several month history of intermittent fevers, noted to have abducens nerve palsy - petrous apicitis. Axial post-contrast (*A*), DWI (*B*), ADC (*C*). Diffuse opacification of the right middle ear cavity and the petrous apex on T2 imaging (not shown) in the patient who presented with Gradenigo syndrome. There is corresponding postcontrast enhancement (*arrow* in *A*), compatible with otomastoiditis and petrous apicitis. There is a linear area of hypoenhancement along the posterior medial aspect of the petrous apex, which demonstrates increased signal on diffusion (*arrow* in *B*) and low ADC signal (*arrow* in *C*), consistent with intraosseous abscess.

in microstructure related to high cell turnover,[68] with D_2 speculated to reflect diffusivity in the extracellular extravascular space and D_3 encompassing the cellular space as well.

- Provides predictive value regarding early treatment response and long-term recurrence/residual tumor following treatment.
  - Brenet and colleagues[69] suggested that initial ADC values less than 0.7 x 10^{-3} mm^2/s on pretreatment MR imaging are associated with residual tumor on follow-up, and increase in ADC values by less than 0.7 x 10^{-3} mm^2/s at 3 months postinitiation of treatment was associated with increased risk of recurrence.
  - Similarly, Nakajo and colleagues[70] reported ADC values greater than 0.88 x 10^{-3} mm^2/s on pretreatment MR imaging had significantly improved 2-year disease-free survival. Vandecaveye and colleagues[71] reported changes in ADC values from the pretreatment

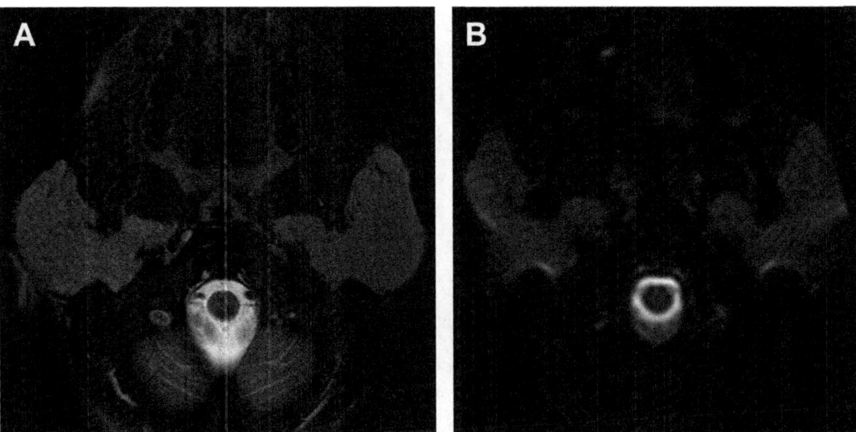

Fig. 19. A 38-year-old woman with several year history of salivary gland swelling and enlargement, severe sicca - Sjogren syndrome. In this patient with known Sjogren syndrome, there is diffuse enlargement of the bilateral parotid glands without atrophy, compatible with early stage involvement (*A*). ADC maps reveal relatively increased ADC values (*B*), compatible with degree of clinical involvement. No low ADC values to suggest lymphomatous involvement are identified.

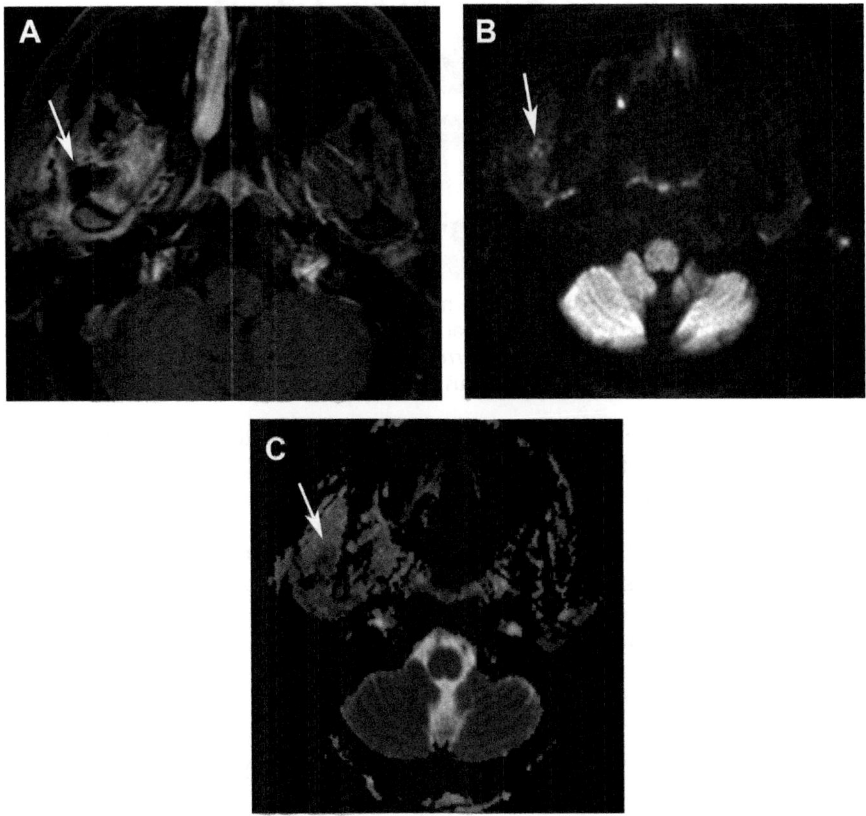

Fig. 20. A 24-year-old woman with 2-month history right facial swelling and pain—sialadenitis. Axial postcontrast (*A*), DWI (*B*), and ADC (*C*). In this patient with history of parotiditis complicated by abscess after placement of a drainage catheter, diffuse edematous inflammatory and posttreatment changes limit evaluation. Postcontrast imaging reveals a small focus of hypoenhancement (*arrow* in *A*) which also demonstrates increased diffusion signal (*arrow* in *B*) and low ADC signal (*arrow* in *C*), compatible with residual abscess.

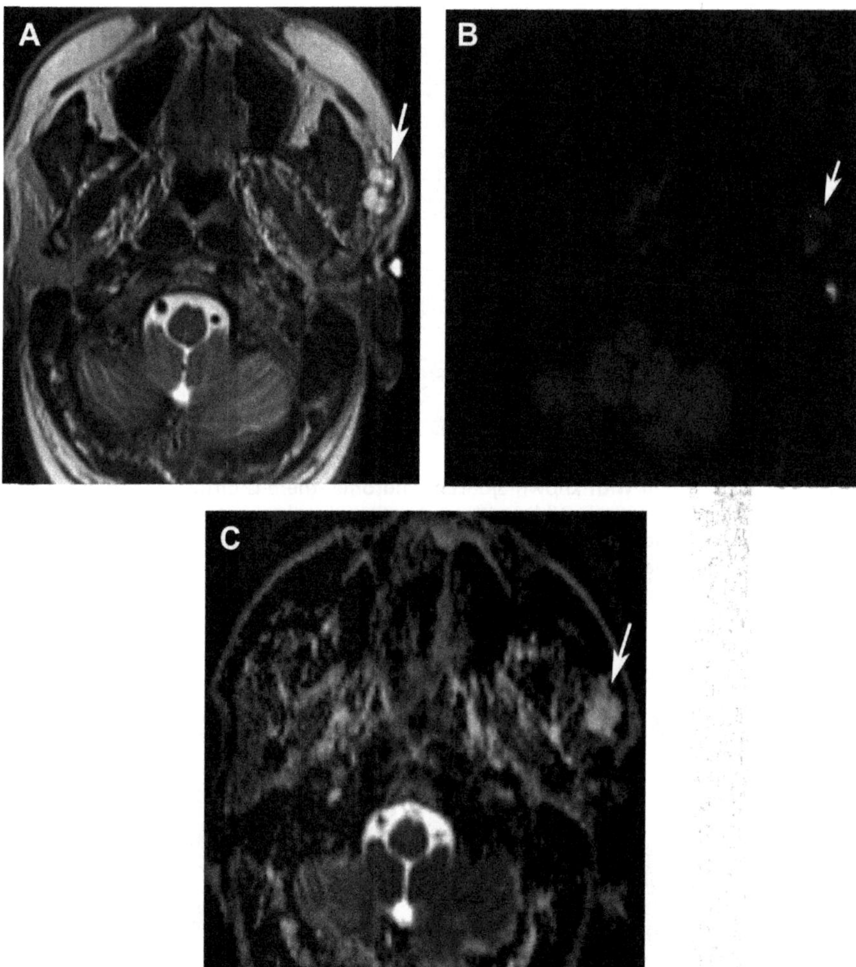

Fig. 21. A 38-year-old man presenting with palpable mass over left masseter—pleomorphic adenoma. Axial T2 (*A*), DWI (*B*), ADC (*C*). Lobulated hyperintense T2 signal (*arrow* in *A*) involving the left parotid gland, which demonstrates facilitated diffusion and high ADC values (*arrows* in *B*, *C*) characteristic of benign mixed tumors, reflective of the accumulated fluid within the adenomatous and glandular components of these masses.

scan to early posttreatment imaging (2–3 weeks following initiation of treatment) correlates with long-term prognosis as well, with nonresponding masses demonstrating significantly smaller changes in ADC values after treatment.

- Martens and colleagues[65] used histogram analysis on pretreatment MR imaging and found maximal ADC values and standard deviation of ADC values within primary tumors were significantly elevated in cases of treatment failure.

Chondrosarcoma

- Low-grade chondrosarcomas demonstrate characteristically elevated ADC values, thought to be secondary to facilitated diffusion within the chondroid tumoral component (Fig. 23).
- Development of a low ADC component has been reported to correlate with an area of dedifferentiation,[72] with associated increased risk of recurrence, metastasis, and poorer survival.

Thyroid

Graves' disease

- Differentiation between Graves disease and painless thyroiditis, a variant of Hashimoto thyroiditis, can be difficult, as early stage painless thyroiditis can present with a transient hyperthyroidism that can mimic the findings of Graves disease.
  - In these cases, DWI can play a role, with ADC values in Graves disease being

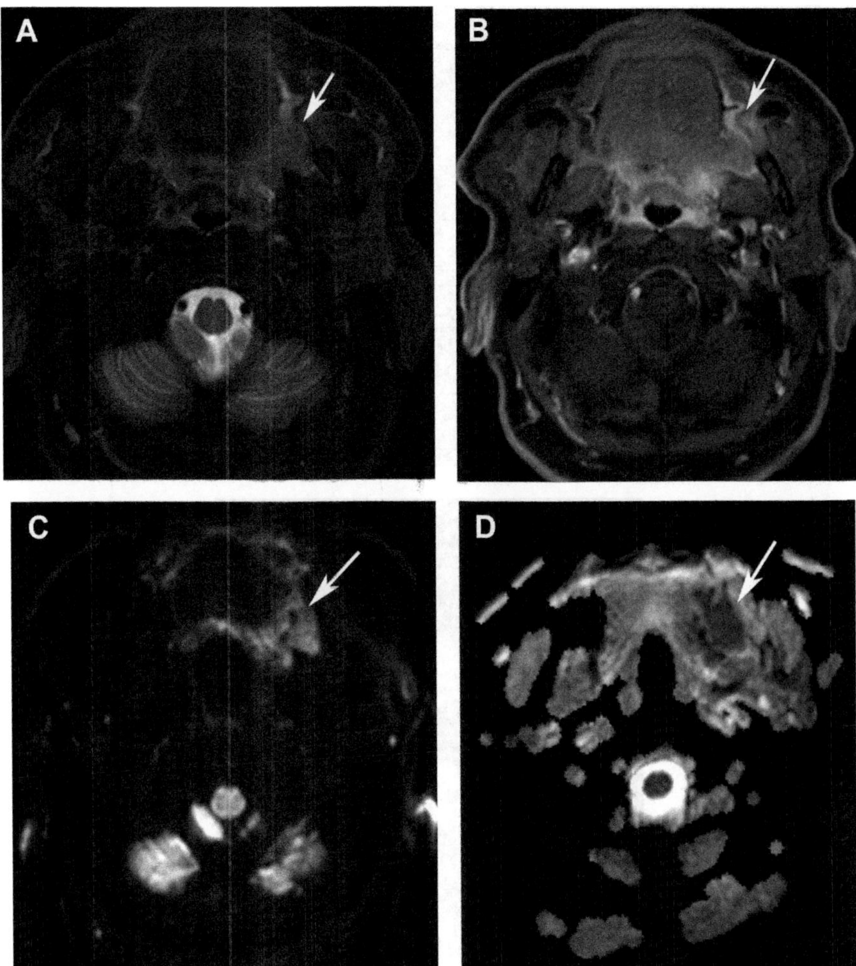

Fig. 22. A 78-year-old man with history of left soft palate/retromolar trigone squamous cell carcinoma after chemotherapy and radiation therapy, presenting with feeling of left ulcer, tongue swelling, new left otalgia—recurrent squamous cell carcinoma. Axial T2 (*A*), post-contrast (*B*), DWI (*C*), ADC (*D*). Circumscribed hyperintense T2 (*arrow* in *A*) enhancing (*arrow* in *B*) signal in the region of the left retromolar trigone in this patient with history of left soft palate squamous cell carcinoma after chemoradiation. Corresponding diffusion signal (*arrow* in *C*) and low ADC signal (*arrow* in *D*) are compatible with pathologically proven recurrent squamous cell carcinoma.

significantly elevated when compared with the ADC values found in painless thyroiditis (optimal cutoff suggested at 1.837 x 10^{-3} mm^2/s).[73]

- It has been suggested that MR imaging might play a role in monitoring patients during treatment of Graves as well, as ADC values in patients with active Graves disease are significantly lower than patients in remission (suggested cutoff 0.82 x 10^{-3} mm^2/s).[74]

Thyroid nodules

- Fine-needle aspiration results can be indeterminate or of uncertain significance, and benign and malignant nodules can demonstrate overlapping pathology on needle aspiration.
- Multiple studies have demonstrated value in DWI as a noninvasive method of differentiating benign from malignant nodules with relatively high sensitivity and specificity.
  - ADC values of malignant thyroid nodules measured significantly lower when compared with the ADC values associated with benign nodules (**Figs. 24** and **25**).[75–78]
  - Intravoxel incoherent motion DWI has been shown to improve reproducibility of ADC measurements in heterogeneous thyroid nodules.[79]

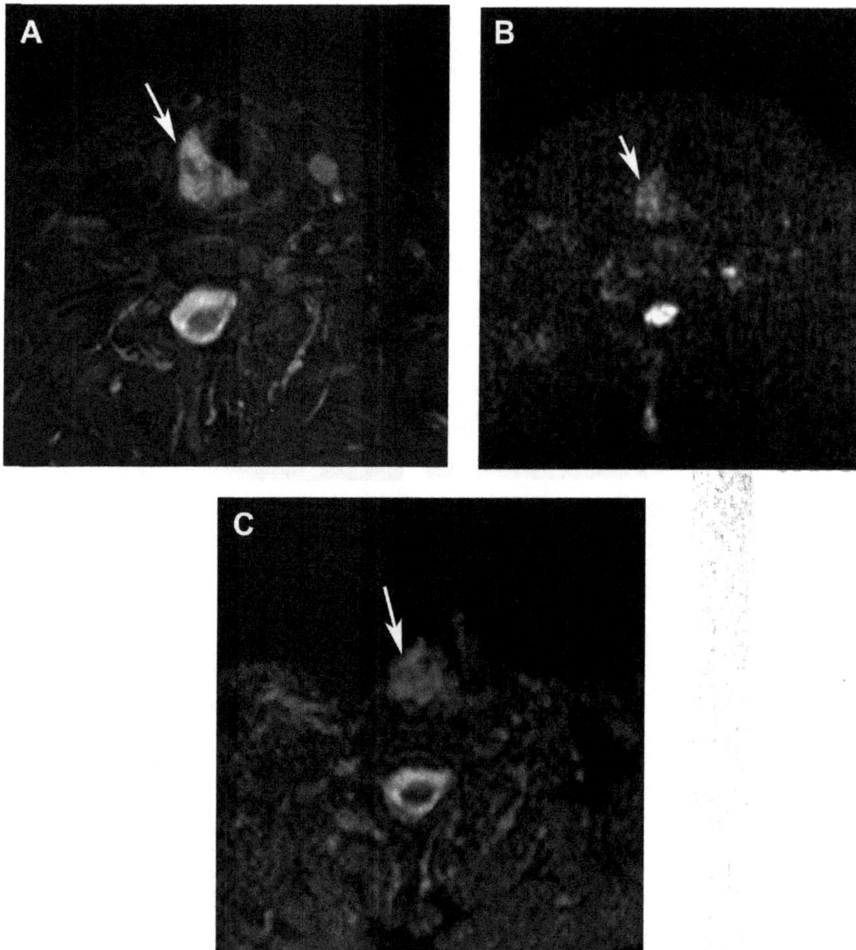

Fig. 23. A 78-year-old man with 1-year history of dystonia—chondrosarcoma. Axial T2 (*A*), DWI (*B*), ADC (*C*). Expansile heterogeneously enhancing (postcontrast sequences not shown) mass centered along the right cricoid cartilage, which shows hyperintense T2 signal (*arrow* in *A*) and facilitated diffusion (*arrow* in *B* and *C*), compatible with a chondroid lesion such as chondrosarcoma.

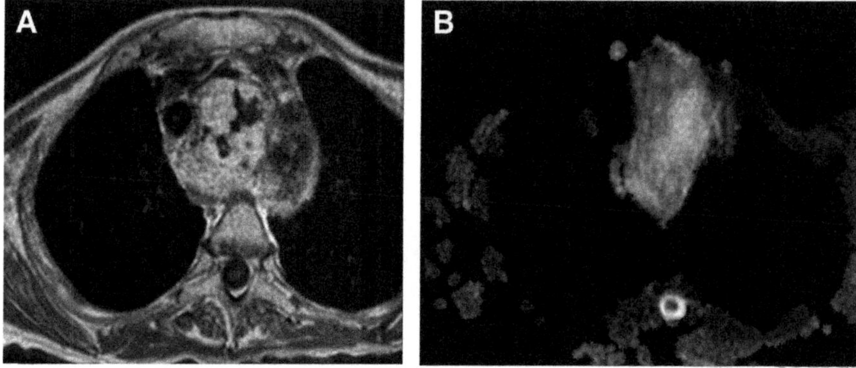

Fig. 24. An 89-year-old woman with history of Graves disease, thyroid ophthalmopathy - Graves disease. Axial post-contrast (*A*) and ADC (*B*). Extensive substernal extension of the thyroid, which demonstrates heterogeneous enhancement following administration of intravenous contrast. Diffuse high ADC values throughout this region were however reassuring for a lack of underlying malignant neoplastic process, and this large substernal extension was stable on follow-up serial imaging.

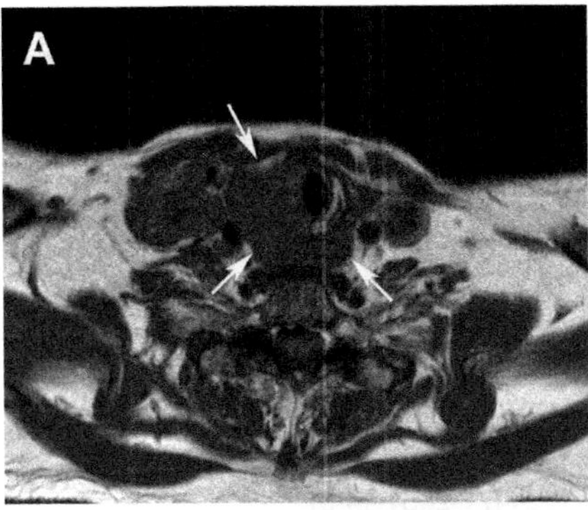

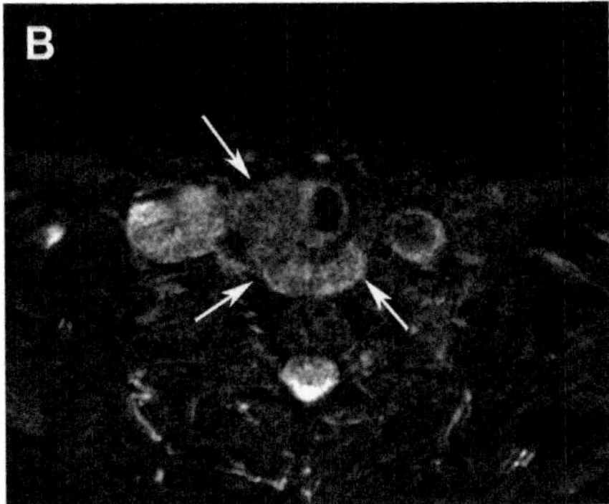

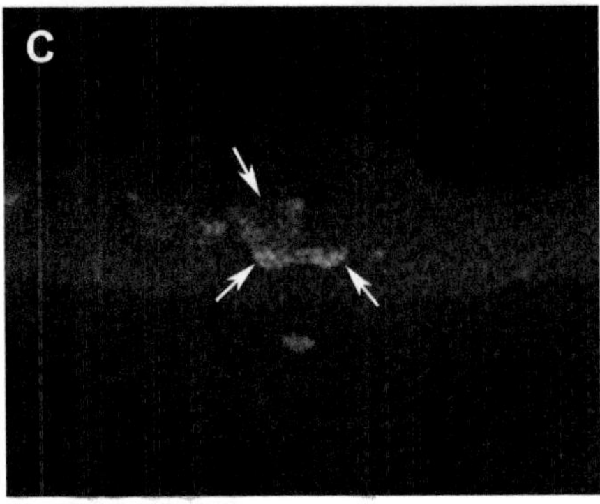

Fig. 25. An 83-year-old man with 5-week history of dysphagia, voice changes—thyroid cancer. Axial T1 (*A*), T2 (*B*), DWI (*C*). Aggressive infiltrative hypointense T1 (*arrows* in *A*), heterogeneous T2 (*arrows* in *B*) signal involving the right aspect of the thyroid, effacing the right larynx and the right aspect of the esophagus. Associated diffusion restriction (*arrows* in *C*) compatible with abnormal increased cellularity in this case of Hurthle cell carcinoma.

- High b-value RESOLVE diffusion imaging has been reported to delineate not only papillary thyroid carcinoma but also microcarcinomas less than 10 mm, from benign nodules.[80]

SUMMARY

Technological advancements and increasing familiarity with diffusion imaging have expanded the role of DWI outside of the brain, now including meaningful application in head and neck imaging. Advancements will only continue to provide more valuable information, better informing our clinical colleagues with treatment decisions. Diffusion information may suggest whether a process is benign or malignant, suggest a specific diagnosis, or indicate the probable response to treatment.

CLINICS CARE POINTS

- While there is some overlap in mean ADC values between benign and malignant lesions, ADC values less than 1.3×10^{-3} mm^2/s predict malignancy for head and neck lesions.[81]
- Lymphoma often has the lowest mean ADC values for malignant lesions.[82]
- While each modality may have a role in cancer follow up imaging, DWI has shown to have fewer false positive results at the primary site and for persistent adenopathies when compared with FDG-PET, CT, and conventional MR sequences.[71]

DISCLOSURE

The authors have nothing to disclose.

REFERENCES

1. Vilanova JC, Catala V, Algaba F, et al. Atlas of multiparametric prostate MRI : with PI-RADS approach and anatomic-MRI-pathological correlation. Cham (Switzerland): Springer; 2018. p. xi, 156.
2. Koh DM, Blackledge M, Padhani A, et al. Whole-body diffusion-weighted MRI: tips, tricks, and pitfalls. AJR Am J Roentgenol 2012;199:252–62.
3. Chenevert TL, Meyer CR, Moffat BA, et al. Diffusion MRI: a new strategy for assessment of cancer therapeutic efficacy. Mol Imaging 2002;1:336–43.
4. Schaefer PW, Grant PE, Gonzalez RG. Diffusion-weighted MR imaging of the brain. Radiology 2000;217:331–45.

5. Hagmann P, Jonasson L, Maeder P, et al. Understanding diffusion MR imaging techniques: from scalar diffusion-weighted imaging to diffusion tensor imaging and beyond. Radiographics 2006;26 Suppl 1:S205–23.
6. Higaki T, Nakamura Y, Tatsugami F, et al. Introduction to the Technical Aspects of Computed Diffusion-weighted Imaging for Radiologists. Radiographics 2018;38:1131–44.
7. De Foer B, Vercruysse JP, Spaepen M, et al. Diffusion-weighted magnetic resonance imaging of the temporal bone. Neuroradiology 2010;52:785–807.
8. Lingam RK, Nash R, Majithia A, et al. Non-echoplanar diffusion weighted imaging in the detection of post-operative middle ear cholesteatoma: navigating beyond the pitfalls to find the pearl. Insights Imaging 2016;7:669–78.
9. Mas-Estelles F, Mateos-Fernandez M, Carrascosa-Bisquert B, et al. Contemporary non-echo-planar diffusion-weighted imaging of middle ear cholesteatomas. Radiographics 2012;32:1197–213.
10. Skare S, Newbould RD, Clayton DB, et al. Clinical multishot DW-EPI through parallel imaging with considerations of susceptibility, motion, and noise. Magn Reson Med 2007;57:881–90.
11. Stejskal EO, Tanner JE. Spin diffusion measurements: Spin echoes in the presence of a time-dependent field gradient. The Journal of Chemical Physics 1965;42(1):288–92. https://doi.org/10.1063/1.1695690.
12. Yiping L, Hui L, Kun Z, et al. Diffusion-weighted imaging of the sellar region: a comparison study of BLADE and single-shot echo planar imaging sequences. Eur J Radiol 2014;83:1239–44.
13. Steven AJ, Zhuo J, Melhem ER. Diffusion kurtosis imaging: an emerging technique for evaluating the microstructural environment of the brain. AJR Am J Roentgenol 2014;202:W26–33.
14. Ferreira TA, Saraiva P, Genders SW, et al. CT and MR imaging of orbital inflammation. Neuroradiology 2018;60:1253–66.
15. Sepahdari AR, Politi LS, Aakalu VK, et al. Diffusion-weighted imaging of orbital masses: multi-institutional data support a 2-ADC threshold model to categorize lesions as benign, malignant, or indeterminate. AJNR Am J Neuroradiol 2014;35:170–5.
16. Mombaerts I, Bilyk JR, Rose G, et al. Consensus on Diagnostic Criteria of Idiopathic Orbital Inflammation Using a Modified Delphi Approach. JAMA Ophthalmol 2017;135:769–76.
17. Haradome K, Haradome H, Usui Y, et al. Orbital lymphoproliferative disorders (OLPDs): value of MR imaging for differentiating orbital lymphoma from benign OPLDs. AJNR Am J Neuroradiol 2014;35:1976–82.
18. Ren J, Yuan Y, Wu Y, et al. Differentiation of orbital lymphoma and idiopathic orbital inflammatory pseudotumor: combined diagnostic value of conventional MRI and histogram analysis of ADC maps. BMC Med Imaging 2018;18:6.
19. Lope LA, Hutcheson KA, Khademian ZP. Magnetic resonance imaging in the analysis of pediatric orbital tumors: utility of diffusion-weighted imaging. J AAPOS 2010;14:257–62.
20. Hassold N, Warmuth-Metz M, Winkler B, et al. Hit the mark with diffusion-weighted imaging: metastases of rhabdomyosarcoma to the extraocular eye muscles. BMC Pediatr 2014;14:57. https://doi.org/10.1186/1471-2431-14-57.
21. Chen S, Ji X, Lie M, et al. The value of MRI in evaluating the efficacy and complications with the treatment of intra-arterial chemotherapy for retinoblastoma. Oncotarget 2017;8:38413–25.
22. Habib YS, Youssif AA, Alkiki HA, et al. High Resolution MR imaging guidelines in retinoblastoma: prospective study correlated with histopathological results. Egyption J Radiol Nucl Med 2020;51–62.
23. Erb-Eigner K, Willerding G, Taupitz M, et al. Diffusion-weighted imaging of ocular melanoma. Invest Radiol 2013;48:702–7.
24. Foti PV, Longo A, Reibaldi M, et al. Uveal melanoma: quantitative evaluation of diffusion-weighted MR imaging in the response assessment after proton-beam therapy, long-term follow-up. Radiol Med 2017;122:131–9.
25. Purohit BS, Vargas M, Ailianou A, et al. Orbital tumours and tumour-like lesions: exploring the armamentarium of multiparametric imaging. Insights Imaging 2016;7:43–68.
26. Yan CH, Tong CC, Pent M, et al. Imaging predictors for malignant transformation of inverted papilloma. Laryngoscope 2019;129:777–82.
27. Ginat DT, Mangla R, Yeaney G, et al. Diffusion-weighted imaging for differentiating benign from malignant skull lesions and correlation with cell density. AJR Am J Roentgenol 2012;198:W597–601.
28. Pekcevik Y, Kahya MO, Kaya A. Diffusion-weighted Magnetic Resonance Imaging in the Diagnosis of Bone Tumors: Preliminary Results. J Clin Imaging Sci 2013;3:63.
29. Alimli AG, Ucar M, Oztunali C, et al. Juvenile Nasopharyngeal Angiofibroma: Magnetic Resonance Imaging Findings. J Belg Soc Radiol 2016;100:63.
30. Das A, Bhalla A, Sharma R, et al. Can Diffusion Weighted Imaging Aid in Differentiating Benign from Malignant Sinonasal Masses?: A Useful Adjunct. Pol J Radiol 2017;82:345–55.
31. Miracle AC, El-Sayed IH, Glastonbury CM, et al. Diffusion weighted imaging of esthesioneuroblastoma: Differentiation from other sinonasal masses. Head Neck 2019;41:1161–4.
32. Xiao Z, Tang Z, Qiang J, et al. Differentiation of olfactory neuroblastomas from nasal squamous cell carcinomas using MR diffusion kurtosis imaging and

dynamic contrast-enhanced MRI. J Magn Reson Imaging 2018;47:354–61.
33. Ai QY, King A, Chan J, et al. Distinguishing early-stage nasopharyngeal carcinoma from benign hyperplasia using intravoxel incoherent motion diffusion-weighted MRI. Eur Radiol 2019;29:5627–34.
34. Song C, Cheng P, Cheng J, et al. Differential diagnosis of nasopharyngeal carcinoma and nasopharyngeal lymphoma based on DCE-MRI and RESOLVE-DWI. Eur Radiol 2020;30:110–8.
35. Zhang SX, Jia QJ, Zhang ZP, et al. Intravoxel incoherent motion MRI: emerging applications for nasopharyngeal carcinoma at the primary site. Eur Radiol 2014;24(8):1998–2004.
36. Jin GQ, Yang J, Liu LD, et al. The diagnostic value of 1.5-T diffusion-weighted MR imaging in detecting 5 to 10 mm metastatic cervical lymph nodes of nasopharyngeal carcinoma. Medicine (Baltimore) 2016; 95(32):e4286. https://doi.org/10.1097/MD.0000000000004286.
37. Wang C, Liu L, Lai S, et al. Diagnostic value of diffusion-weighted magnetic resonance imaging for local and skull base recurrence of nasopharyngeal carcinoma after radiotherapy. Medicine (Baltimore) 2018; 97(34):e11929.
38. Yan DF, Zhang WB, Ke SB, et al. The prognostic value of pretreatment tumor apparent diffusion coefficient values in nasopharyngeal carcinoma. BMC Cancer 2017;17:678.
39. Zheng D, Lai G, Chen Y, et al. Integrating dynamic contrast-enhanced magnetic resonance imaging and diffusion kurtosis imaging for neoadjuvant chemotherapy assessment of nasopharyngeal carcinoma. J Magn Reson Imaging 2018;48:1208–16.
40. Zhang Y, Liue X, Zhang Y, et al. Prognostic value of the primary lesion apparent diffusion coefficient (ADC) in nasopharyngeal carcinoma: a retrospective study of 541 cases. Sci Rep 2015;5:12242.
41. Hong J, Yao Y, Zhang TT, et al. Value of magnetic resonance diffusion-weighted imaging for the prediction of radiosensitivity in nasopharyngeal carcinoma. Otolaryngol Head Neck Surg 2013;149:707–13.
42. Huang WY, Li MM, Lin SM, et al. Vivo Imaging Markers for Prediction of Radiotherapy Response in Patients with Nasopharyngeal Carcinoma: RESOLVE DWI versus DKI. Sci Rep 2018;8:15861.
43. Henninger B, Kremser C. Diffusion weighted imaging for the detection and evaluation of cholesteatoma. World J Radiol 2017;9:217–22.
44. Khemani S, Lingam RK, Kalan A, et al. The value of non-echo planar HASTE diffusion-weighted MR imaging in the detection, localisation and prediction of extent of postoperative cholesteatoma. Clin Otolaryngol 2011;36:306–12.
45. Sheng Y, Hong R, Sha Y, et al. Performance of TGSE BLADE DWI compared with RESOLVE DWI in the diagnosis of cholesteatoma. BMC Med Imaging 2020;20:40.
46. Kavanagh RG, Liddy S, Carroll AG, et al. Rapid diffusion-weighted MRI for the investigation of recurrent temporal bone cholesteatoma. Neuroradiol J 2020;33:210–5.
47. Kuruma T, Tanigawa T, Uchida Y, et al. Large Cholesterol Granuloma of the Middle Ear Eroding into the Middle Cranial Fossa. Case Rep Otolaryngol 2017; 2017:4793786.
48. Ibrahim M, Shah G, Parmar H. Diffusion-weighted MRI identifies petrous apex abscess in Gradenigo syndrome. J Neuroophthalmol 2010;30:34–6.
49. Ding C, Xing X, Guo Q, et al. Diffusion-weighted MRI findings in Sjogren's syndrome: a preliminary study. Acta Radiol 2016;57:691–700.
50. Chu C, Zhou N, Zhang H, et al. Correlation between intravoxel incoherent motion MR parameters and MR nodular grade of parotid glands in patients with Sjogren's syndrome: A pilot study. Eur J Radiol 2017;86:241–7.
51. Chu C, Feng Q, Zhang H, et al. Whole-Volume ADC Histogram Analysis in Parotid Glands to Identify Patients with Sjogren's Syndrome. Sci Rep 2019;9:9614.
52. Abdel Razek AAK, Mukherji S. Imaging of sialadenitis. Neuroradiol J 2017;30:205–15.
53. Zhang Z, Song C, Zhang Y, et al. Apparent diffusion coefficient (ADC) histogram analysis: differentiation of benign from malignant parotid gland tumors using readout-segmented diffusion-weighted imaging. Dentomaxillofac Radiol 2019;48:20190100.
54. Munhoz L, Ramos EADA, Im DC, et al. Application of diffusion-weighted magnetic resonance imaging in the diagnosis of salivary gland diseases: a systematic review. Oral Surg Oral Med Oral Pathol Oral Radiol 2019;128(3):280–310.
55. Zhang Q, Wei YM, Qi YG, et al. Early Changes in Apparent Diffusion Coefficient for Salivary Glands during Radiotherapy for Nasopharyngeal Carcinoma Associated with Xerostomia. Korean J Radiol 2018;19:328–33.
56. Zhang Y, Ou D, Gu Y, et al. Evaluation of Salivary Gland Function Using Diffusion-Weighted Magnetic Resonance Imaging for Follow-Up of Radiation-Induced Xerostomia. Korean J Radiol 2018;19:758–66.
57. Shang DS, Ruan LX, Zhou SH, et al. Differentiating laryngeal carcinomas from precursor lesions by diffusion-weighted magnetic resonance imaging at 3.0 T: a preliminary study. PLoS One 2013;8:e68622.
58. Kolff-Gart AS, Pouwels PJ, Noij DP, et al. Diffusion-weighted imaging of the head and neck in healthy subjects: reproducibility of ADC values in different

MRI systems and repeat sessions. AJNR Am J Neuroradiol 2015;36:384–90.

59. de Perrot T, Lenoir V, Ayllon MD, et al. Apparent Diffusion Coefficient Histograms of Human Papillomavirus-Positive and Human Papillomavirus-Negative Head and Neck Squamous Cell Carcinoma: Assessment of Tumor Heterogeneity and Comparison with Histopathology. AJNR Am J Neuroradiol 2017;38:2153–60.
60. Vidiri A, Marz S, Gangem E, et al. Intravoxel incoherent motion diffusion-weighted imaging for oropharyngeal squamous cell carcinoma: Correlation with human papillomavirus Status. Eur J Radiol 2019;119:108640.
61. Payabvash S, Brackett A, Forghani R, et al. Differentiation of lymphomatous, metastatic, and non-malignant lymphadenopathy in the neck with quantitative diffusion-weighted imaging: systematic review and meta-analysis. Neuroradiology 2019;61:897–910.
62. Park JH, Bae YJ, Choi BS, et al. Texture Analysis of Multi-Shot Echo-planar Diffusion-Weighted Imaging in Head and Neck Squamous Cell Carcinoma: The Diagnostic Value for Nodal Metastasis. J Clin Med 2019;8:1767.
63. Driessen JP, Van Kempen PMW, VanderHeijden GJ, et al. Diffusion-weighted imaging in head and neck squamous cell carcinomas: a systematic review. Head Neck 2015;37:440–8.
64. Fujima N, Yoshida D, Sakashita T, et al. Residual tumour detection in post-treatment granulation tissue by using advanced diffusion models in head and neck squamous cell carcinoma patients. Eur J Radiol 2017;90:14–9.
65. Martens RM, Noij DP, Koopman T, et al. Predictive value of quantitative diffusion-weighted imaging and 18-F-FDG-PET in head and neck squamous cell carcinoma treated by (chemo)radiotherapy. Eur J Radiol 2019;113:39–50.
66. Schroeder C, Lee JH, Tetzner U, et al. Comparison of diffusion-weighted MR imaging and (18)F Fluorodeoxyglucose PET/CT in detection of residual or recurrent tumors and delineation of their local spread after (chemo) radiotherapy for head and neck squamous cell carcinoma. Eur J Radiol 2020;130:109157.
67. Ailianou A, Mundada P, De-Perrot T, et al. MRI with DWI for the Detection of Posttreatment Head and Neck Squamous Cell Carcinoma: Why Morphologic MRI Criteria Matter. AJNR Am J Neuroradiol 2018;39:748–55.
68. Fujima N, Sakashita T, Homma A, et al. Non-invasive prediction of the tumor growth rate using advanced diffusion models in head and neck squamous cell carcinoma patients. Oncotarget 2017;8:33631–43.
69. Brenet E, Barbe C, Hoeffel C, et al. Predictive Value of Early Post-Treatment Diffusion-Weighted MRI for Recurrence or Tumor Progression of Head and Neck Squamous Cell Carcinoma Treated with Chemo-Radiotherapy. Cancers (Basel) 2020;12:1234.
70. Nakajo M, Nakajo M, Kajiya Y, et al. FDG PET/CT and diffusion-weighted imaging of head and neck squamous cell carcinoma: comparison of prognostic significance between primary tumor standardized uptake value and apparent diffusion coefficient. Clin Nucl Med 2012;37:475–80.
71. Vandecaveye V, Dirix P, DeKeyzer F, et al. Diffusion-weighted magnetic resonance imaging early after chemoradiotherapy to monitor treatment response in head-and-neck squamous cell carcinoma. Int J Radiat Oncol Biol Phys 2012;82:1098–107.
72. Purohit BS, Dulguerov P, Burkhardt K, et al. Dedifferentiated laryngeal chondrosarcoma: combined morphologic and functional imaging with positron-emission tomography/magnetic resonance imaging. Laryngoscope 2014;124:E274–7.
73. Meng Z, Zhang G, Sun H, et al. Differentiation between Graves' disease and painless thyroiditis by diffusion-weighted imaging, thyroid iodine uptake, thyroid scintigraphy and serum parameters. Exp Ther Med 2015;9:2165–72.
74. Abdel Razek AA, Sadek AG, Gaballa G. Diffusion-weighed MR of the thyroid gland in Graves' disease: assessment of disease activity and prediction of outcome. Acad Radiol 2010;17:779–83.
75. Bozgeyik Z, Coskun S, Dagli AF, et al. Diffusion-weighted MR imaging of thyroid nodules. Neuroradiology 2009;51:193–8.
76. Noda Y, Kanematsu M, Goshima S, et al. MRI of the thyroid for differential diagnosis of benign thyroid nodules and papillary carcinomas. AJR Am J Roentgenol 2015;204:W332–5.
77. Vandecaveye V, Dirix P, DeKeyzer F, et al. Diagnostic efficacy of multiple MRI parameters in differentiating benign vs. malignant thyroid nodules. BMC Med Imaging 2018;18:50.
78. Chen L, Xu J, Bao J, et al. Diffusion-weighted MRI in differentiating malignant from benign thyroid nodules: a meta-analysis. BMJ Open 2016;6:e008413.
79. Song M, Yue Y, Jin Y, et al. Intravoxel incoherent motion and ADC measurements for differentiating benign from malignant thyroid nodules: utilizing the most repeatable region of interest delineation at 3.0 T. Cancer Imaging 2020;20:9.
80. Wang Q, Guo Y, Zhang J, et al. Utility of high b-value (2000 sec/mm2) DWI with RESOLVE in differentiating papillary thyroid carcinomas and papillary thyroid microcarcinomas from benign thyroid nodules. PLoS One 2018;13:e0200270.
81. Srinivasan A, Dvorak R, Perni K, et al. Differentiation of benign and malignant pathology in the head and neck using 3T apparent diffusion coefficient values: early experience. AJNR Am J Neuroradiol 2008;29(1):40–4.
82. Koontz NA, Wiggins RH 3rd. Differentiation of Benign and Malignant head and NECK lesions with diffusion tensor imaging and DWI. AJR Am J Roentgenol 2017;208(5):1110–5.

Measuring Perfusion

Intravoxel Incoherent Motion MR Imaging

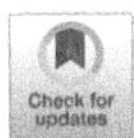

Christian Federau, MD, MSc[a,b,*]

KEYWORDS

• IVIM • Intravoxel incoherent motion • Perfusion • Diffusion • Review

KEY POINTS

- Intravoxel incoherent motion (IVIM) perfusion MR imaging is a method that extracts microvascular perfusion information from a standard diffusion-weighted sequence.
- The perfusion information obtained with IVIM is local and quantitative, which contrasts with other perfusion methods such as dynamic susceptibility MR imaging or arterial spin labeling, which are inflow dependent.
- The IVIM perfusion method does not require intravenous contrast media injection and can therefore be applied without arm in all groups of patients, such as newborns or patients with renal failure.

Perfusion imaging plays an important role in the diagnosis, monitoring, and therapy decision-making of many important neurologic diseases such as stroke and tumors. In clinical brain examinations using MR imaging, perfusion is usually acquired using dynamic susceptibility contrast (DSC), which requires the intravenous injection of gadolinium chelate. A rare, but catastrophic, complication associated with the intravenous injection of gadolinium-based contrast agents is the development of nephrogenic systemic fibrosis in patients with renal disease. The long-term potential risks of repeated injection of gadolinium-based contrast agents are unknown, especially because Gadolinium deposition has been observed in the brain.[1] Intravoxel incoherent motion (IVIM) perfusion MR imaging offers an elegant alternative way to acquire perfusion information. The IVIM method measures microcirculatory blood-flow properties directly, without the need of an intravenous contrast injection. The method exploits the fact that the signal acquired using a diffusion-weighted MR imaging (DWI) sequence is influenced not only by the incoherent motion of water due the thermal energy but also by the incoherent motion of water due to blood flow circulation in the microvasculature. The effects that arise from both compartments (the thermal diffusion compartment and the microvascular compartment) can be separated using a biexponential signal equation model (each exponential corresponding to one of the compartments), as proposed by in the late 1980s by Le Bihan and colleagues.[2] The growing interest in IVIM perfusion methods in the past decade, which can largely be attributed to recent hardware and software developments, has accumulated a series of reports demonstrating both the validity and clinical applicability of these methods. This review summarizes the idea behind IVIM perfusion imaging and its clinical application to diagnostic neuroradiology.

THE IDEA BEHIND INTRAVOXEL INCOHERENT MOTION PERFUSION IMAGING: NOT EVERY INCOHERENT MOTION IS RELATED TO THERMAL ENERGY

DWI uses magnetic field gradients to diphase the spins of a given volume as a function of the distribution of their displacements during the so-called

[a] University and ETH Zürich, Institute for Biomedical Engineering, Gloriastrasse 35, Zürich 8092, Switzerland; [b] Ai Medical AG, Goldhaldenstr 22a, Zollikon 8702, Switzerland
* Corresponding author. University and ETH Zürich, Institute for Biomedical Engineering, Gloriastrasse 35, Zürich 8092, Switzerland.
E-mail address: federau@biomed.ee.ethz.ch

Magn Reson Imaging Clin N Am 29 (2021) 233–242
https://doi.org/10.1016/j.mric.2021.01.003

diffusion time, inducing a drop in echo signal. The larger the distribution of the spin's displacements, the larger the drop in echo signal. In a chemical solute, a distribution of displacement arises from thermal energy in the form of Brownian motion, leading to (self-)diffusion, and this can in turn be measured with DWI. In a biological tissue, Brownian motion of water is somewhat restricted through the presence of biological macromolecules, such as carbohydrates, lipids, proteins, and nucleic acids. Therefore, the quantity measured with DWI in a biological tissue is reduced in comparison to what would be measured at the same temperature for freely moving water molecules and was therefore named apparent diffusion coefficient (ADC), in order to distinguish it from the physical quantity diffusion. Further, in a living biological tissue, there is another source of distribution of displacement, namely blood motion in the microvasculature. The energy of this motion arises from mechanical propulsion in the heart. The effects on the drop in diffusion-weighted signal arising from the blood motion and thermal motion can be separated (up to a given point), because the effects arising from the motion in the blood compartment are more pronounced than the ones arising from the thermal compartment. On the other hand, the size of the blood compartment is much smaller compared with the thermal compartment. The quantity arising from the blood compartment and measured by this method has been coined "pseudodiffusion," to distinguish it from the thermal diffusion.

In the standard diffusion-weighted sequence used in the clinical practice, magnetic field gradients used for diffusion encoding are typically Stejskal-Tanner pulsed gradients[3] or a modification thereof (eg, bipolar gradients). The "imaging gradients," on the other hand, are used to localize the position of the signal. They also produce some spin dephasing, which is usually neglected for a diffusion-weighted or an IVIM measurement.

The term "*incoherent motion*" refers to the displacements that lead to a distribution of position of the water molecules in a given direction and after a given amount of time, whereas the term "*coherent motion*" refers to the displacements that lead to an identical translation in a given direction of all particles. In other words, incoherent motion leads to a measured drop in signal amplitude in a DW sequence, whereas coherent motion leads to an unchanged signal amplitude. The terms "diffusion-weighted imaging" and "intravoxel incoherent motion imaging" refer to the same physical principle, and both methods also use the exact same sequence. The existence of these 2 terms is a source of confusion, but the distinction arose for historical reasons. The term "diffusion-weighted imaging" is mostly used when referring to the use of a single exponential model (or more complicated model, but excluding perfusion effects) for measuring the ADC, whereas the term "intravoxel incoherent motion imaging" is used to refer to the measurement of perfusion effects with a diffusion-weighted sequence, using a biexponential or any other more advanced models.

The effect of the diffusion-weighting gradients of a given sequence on the measured signal can be summarized in the so-called *b-value*. When applying a typical standard diffusion-weighted sequence on a simple chemical solute, such as pure water, the slope of the signal decay is, on a logarithmic scale, linearly dependent on the diffusion coefficient and the aforementioned b-value. This provides a simple method to measure the diffusion coefficient. In a biological tissue that consists of many molecular components, of both heterogeneous size and complexity, and in which many active processes, such as membrane transport, biomolecular synthesis, and perfusion, take place, the signal drop is as a function of the b-value, on a logarithmic scale, remarkably linear (for b-values greater than 200 s/mm^2). For this reason, the apparent diffusion coefficient can be modeled by using a single exponential model, often requiring only two b-values to evaluate it. For b-values less than 200 s/mm^2, the signal curve digresses from a single exponential decay because of perfusion effects. Although more complicated models can and have been proposed, usually these perfusion effects are modeled using a second exponential decay function.

Usually multiple b-values (>10) are acquired between 0 and 1000 s/mm^2, including several b-values (usually half of them) acquired between 0 and 200 s/mm^2, and IVIM parameters are derived by fitting a biexponential signal equation model (**Fig. 1**). This is usually done using a two-step method, by first fitting a single exponential for the signal at b-values greater than 200 s/mm^2 and then the second exponential using the signal at all b-values.[4] Although some studies show that a simplified acquisition with less b-values is feasible,[5–8] this is not without the drawback of reducing signal to noise. The most common method to estimate the IVIM parameters is by using the Levenberg-Marquardt algorithm,[9,10] but several alternative methods have been proposed.[11–14]

The correct interpretation of IVIM perfusion maps requires a good understanding of the underlying method. There are 3 IVIM perfusion parameters, the perfusion fraction f, the pseudodiffusion coefficient D*, and the blood flow–related parameter fD*. The perfusion parameter f should be understood as the "incoherently flowing" blood

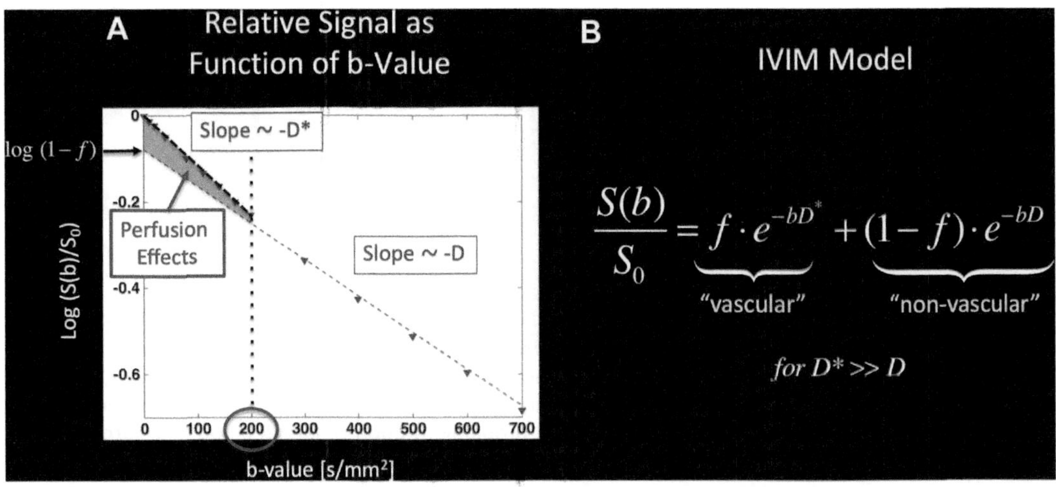

Fig. 1. (*A*) Relative signal as function of b-value, in logarithmic scale. A b-value threshold greater than 200 s/mm^2 the signal is linearly decreasing with a slope of −D due to "apparent thermal diffusion." Below this threshold, a deviation from this linear decay is visible (surface in red) due to perfusion effects. The negative slope of the decay less than the threshold of 200 s/mm^2 is related to the pseudodiffusion coefficient D* (it is not exactly D* because thermal diffusion effects are still present as well). The perfusion fraction, which is related to microvascular blood volume, can be derived from the intercept. (*B*) The IVIM biexponential signal equation model. The first exponential corresponds to the "vascular" compartment and the second exponential to the "nonvascular" compartment or "apparent thermal diffusion" compartment. The assumption that D* is much larger than D is very reasonable from a biological stand point, given the biological function of perfusion and the fact that the blood flow is produced under large energy consumption. This assumption is also necessary to be able to separate mathematically both compartments.

microvascular blood volume. The pseudodiffusion coefficient D* holds information on blood speed, but in "units of diffusion," that is, m^2/s (usually given in mm^2/s) and not m/s as a "ballistic speed." The blood flow–related parameter fD* has been suggested to be related to blood flow, that is, to the quantity of blood flowing through a unit tissue per unit time.

Several important artifacts should be kept in mind while interpreting IVIM perfusion maps in the brain. For example, cerebrospinal fluid (CSF) pulsations, such as in the sulci and at the foramen of Monroe, can also lead to intravoxel dephasing effects, but of course those voxels are extraparenchymatous and should not lead to misinterpretations. Partial volume effects in voxels including both CSF and brain parenchyma could also lead to artefactually increased IVIM perfusion parameters because of the difference in ADC between the CSF and the brain parenchyma compartments.

APPLICATIONS OF IN-VIVO INTRAVOXEL INCOHERENT MOTION PERFUSION NEUROIMAGING

Experimental evidence demonstrating the feasibility of in-vivo perfusion imaging with IVIM MR imaging have been mounting, including phantoms and ex-vivo studies, studies correlating IVIM perfusion parameters with histologic findings, as well as with physiologically and pharmaceutically induced perfusion state changes, and with standard perfusion parameters using other methods (see[15] for a review). In the brain in particular, an increase in IVIM perfusion parameters was observed under hypercapnia,[4,16] which is well known to increase brain perfusion. In addition, a dependence on the cardiac cycle of those parameters was demonstrated.[17] For clinical application, the IVIM perfusion method has several interesting properties. The IVIM method does not require injection of contrast agent. Further, this method is in essence local (both excitation and read-out are done in the same plane) and in essence quantitative. Finally, because it is essentially different than other perfusion methods, it might provide additional and complementary perfusion information, which are not available otherwise.

Stroke

Perfusion imaging, either by computer tomography (CT) or MR imaging with DSC, plays an essential role in diagnosis and therapeutic decision-making in acute stroke.[18] In stroke, the IVIM perfusion fraction f is decreased in the infarcted tissue as depicted on DWI (ie, infarct

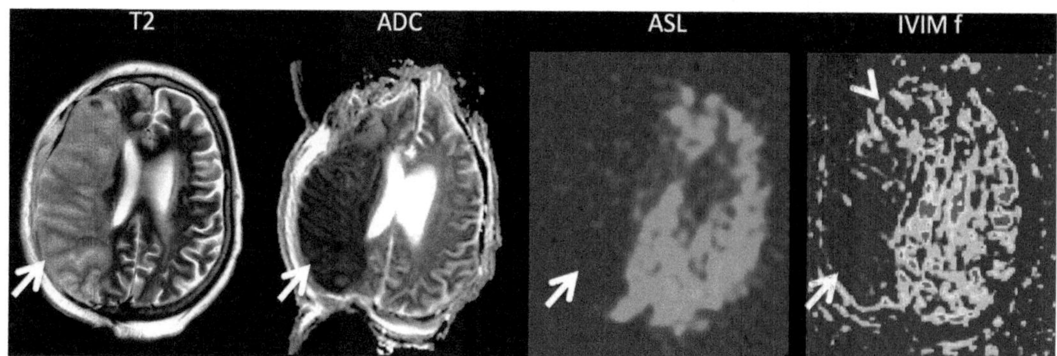

Fig. 2. An example of a large right-sided middle cerebral artery infarct, clearly visible on T2 and ADC (*arrow*), with clear hypoperfusion on both arterial spin labeling and the IVIM perfusion fraction f (*arrow*). Note that the frontal region shows some residual IVIM perfusion, probably through collateral blood flow (*arrowhead*).

core) compared with the contralateral hemisphere[19–21] (**Fig. 2**). In hyperacute stroke, one recent study found that the IVIM perfusion fraction was significantly reduced in the infarct core but globally retained in the penumbra (which was defined as Tmax >6 seconds on DSC), suggesting that IVIM perfusion imaging could be used to assess the local microvascular perfusion maintained in the penumbra through the collateral blood flow.[22] Therefore, IVIM perfusion imaging could be used as a tool to assess the quality of the collateral in the context of hyperacute stroke.

In addition, this study found that if a confluent zone of perfusion reduction was seen on the IVIM f map within the DSC penumbra volume, this zone systematically underwent infarction on follow-up imaging in all patients, independent of treatment. The finding of a confluent zone of perfusion reduction on the IVIM f map within the DSC penumbra also correlated with a larger infarct growth after hyperacute imaging, as well as with a larger final infarct size. The number of patients with such a zone was small ($n = 9$), and these findings needs to be confirmed by larger studies, but

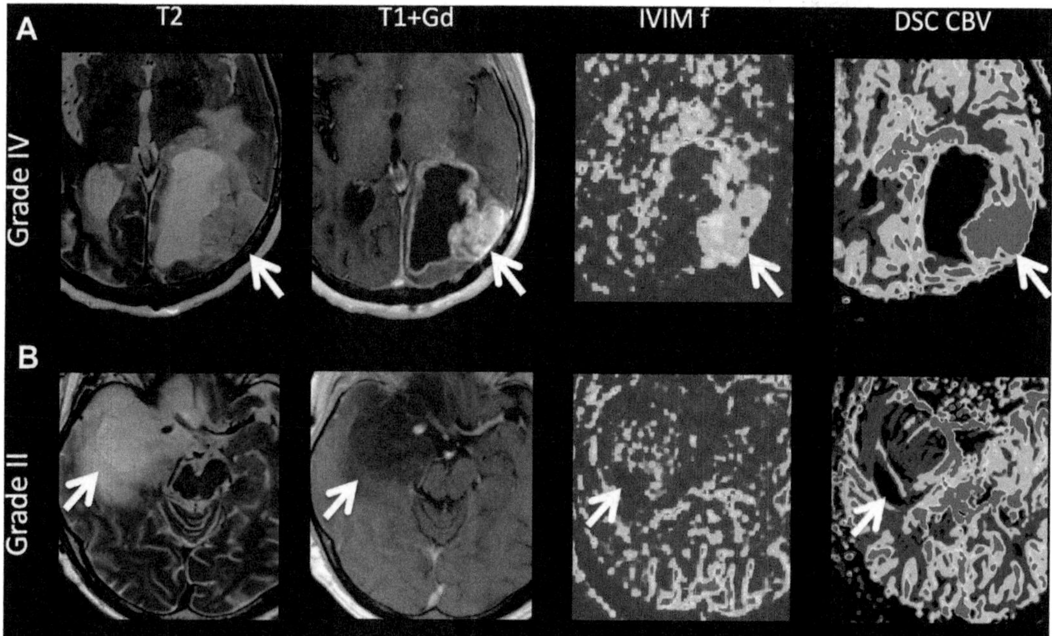

Fig. 3. Perfusion imaging can be useful for differentiating low- and high-grades gliomas. (*A*) High-grade gliomas typically show an increase in perfusion, as in this case clearly visible on both the IVIM perfusion fraction and the cerebral blood volume on DSC (*arrow*). (*B*) Low-grade gliomas do not show hyperperfusion (*arrow*), as in the case in the bottom row, which was classified on pathology as low grade despite its large size.

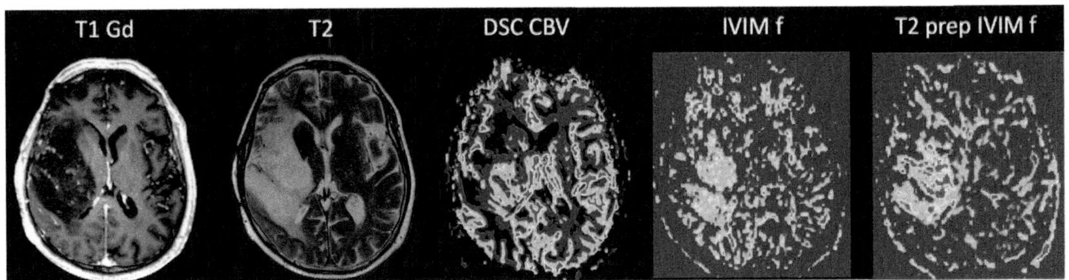

Fig. 4. The contrast between pathologic and normal perfusion fractions can be improved using T2 prep IVIM, as can be seen in this case of glioblastoma. The T2 prep prepulse suppresses CSF signal while retaining (some) blood signal.

they nevertheless suggested that the presence such a zone could be a marker of nonsalvageable tissue despite treatment with thrombectomy, in addition to the stroke core defined by DWI. Its presence might therefore speak against a therapeutic intervention in borderline cases.

Tumors

Gliomas are the most common primary tumor of the central nervous system. Neoangiogenesis is an important differentiating criterion in the diagnosis of high-grade glioma compared with low-grade, both on histopathology and imaging. A significant increase in the IVIM perfusion fraction f in high-grade glioma compared with low-grade has been reported in several independent studies (**Fig. 3**).[23–30]

In an attempt to increase contrast between pathologic tumorous tissue and normal brain, the addition of a T2-prepared prepulse to the IVIM sequence has been proposed, in order to suppress the confounding IVIM signal from CSF

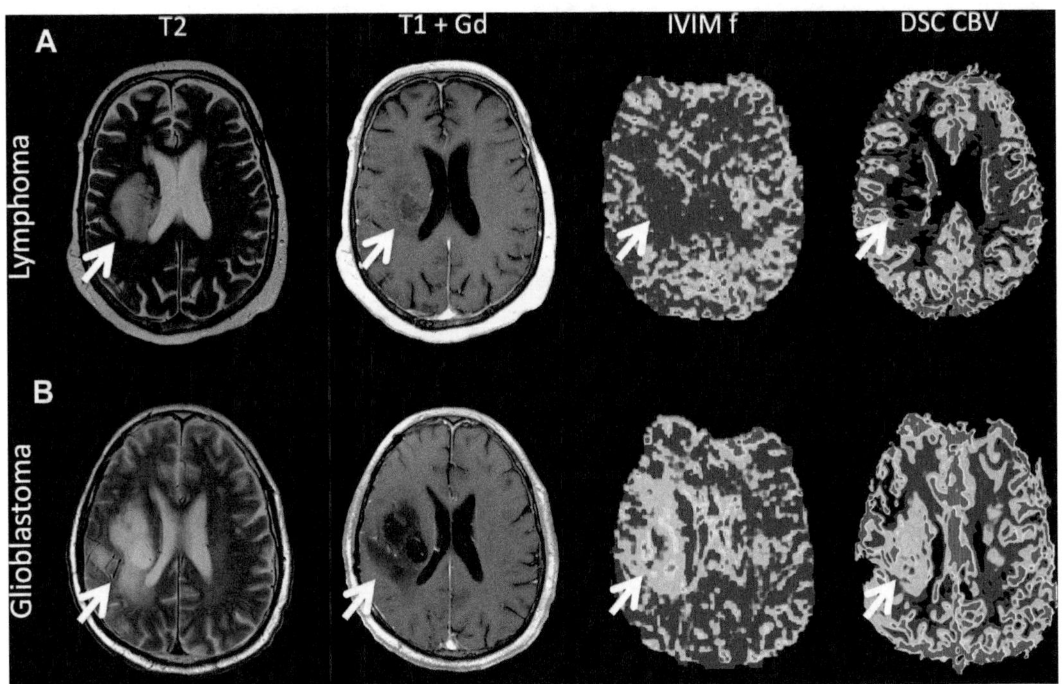

Fig. 5. Lymphoma and glioblastoma can usually be differentiated from one another, as they typically show a different contrast enhancement patterns: lymphoma typically shows homogenous enhancement pattern, whereas glioblastomas tend to have a peripheral enhancement with central necrosis. However, in some atypical cases, they can look very similar on both T2 and T1 postcontrast studies, as in this example. In such a case, perfusion imaging can be very useful, because lymphoma typically shows a reduced perfusion (as can be seen on both IVIM f and DSC cerebral blood volume [CBV] in [*A*] [*arrows*]), whereas glioblastoma shows an increased perfusion due to neoangiogenesis (*arrows*), as in the example in (*B*).

pulsation (**Fig. 4**).[31] The benefits of using a T2 prepared prepulse compared with a 180° inversion recovery magnetization preparation is that the former permits to recover more signal from the blood pool than the latter.[31]

Furthermore, IVIM perfusion imaging can be used to differentiate high-grade glioma from lymphoma, which is very useful in doubtful cases (**Fig. 5**) or in cases where a contrast-agent injection is contraindicated. Indeed, the IVIM perfusion fraction has been shown to decrease in CNS lymphoma when compared with normal brain parenchyma.[32,33] Finally, there is evidence that the IVIM perfusion fraction is prognostic for survival in patients with glioma,[34–36] and in particular, when only considering the subgroup of patients with histopathologically proven glioblastoma,[34,35] although these 2 studies were done in 2 relatively small cohorts of patients (n = 15 in both studies). This suggests that the perfusion fraction may serve as a complementary biomarker for histopathology. Further, an increase in IVIM perfusion fraction could be an early marker of tumor progression (**Fig. 6**). Interestingly, IVIM have recently been recommended as a marker of isocitrate dehydrogenase 1 (IDH1) mutational status.[7,29] In addition, IVIM D* has been suggested to act as a marker for monitoring tumor vascular normalization in glioblastoma after dual inhibition of vascular endothelial growth factor and the glycolytic activator PFKFB3.[37] Finally, IVIM perfusion abnormalities have been demonstrated in other neoplasms, such as meningioma[38–40] (**Fig. 7**) and pituitary adenoma.[41]

Cerebral Death

The diagnosis of cerebral death is in most countries based on clinical evaluation of symptoms such as coma, apnea, and absence of brainstem reflexes.[42] Brain perfusion imaging plays an important role in the preliminary assessment of brain death in critically ill patients, in which the clinical evaluation cannot be performed because they are intubated and are under general anesthesia, and the demonstration of lack of cerebral circulation is often required as an ancillary test before the declaration of brain death.[43] An interesting property of IVIM perfusion imaging might be particularly useful in the evaluation of cerebral death: because both excitation and read-out are performed in-plane, its measurement is totally

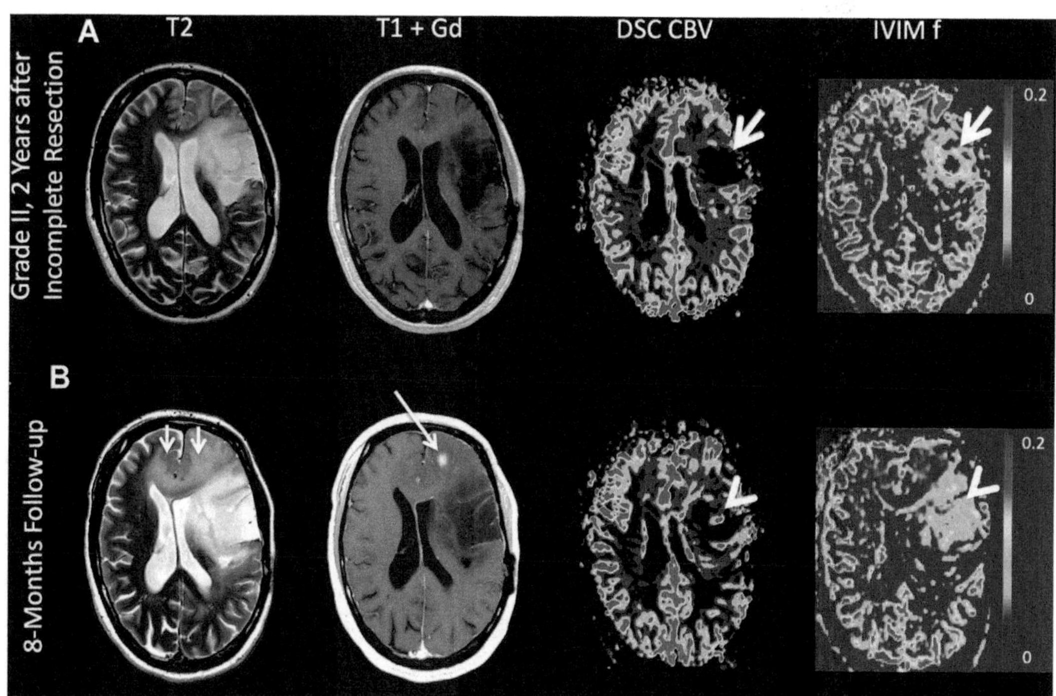

Fig. 6. (*A*) In this patient imaged 2 years after resection of an oligoastrocytoma grade II otherwise unchanged in size, the IVIM perfusion fraction seems to be increased, whereas DSC CBV seems decreased (*arrows*). Increased perfusion in low-grade glioma is known to be of bad prognosis, the so-called angiogenic switch. (*B*) On the follow-up study 8 months later, the tumor showed a significant increase in extension on the T2-weighted images, a new site of contrast uptake (*arrows*), and an increase in IVIM perfusion fraction (*arrowheads*). This case suggests that IVIM perfusion imaging can bring additional information to the currently broadly used DSC perfusion in glioma follow-up imaging.

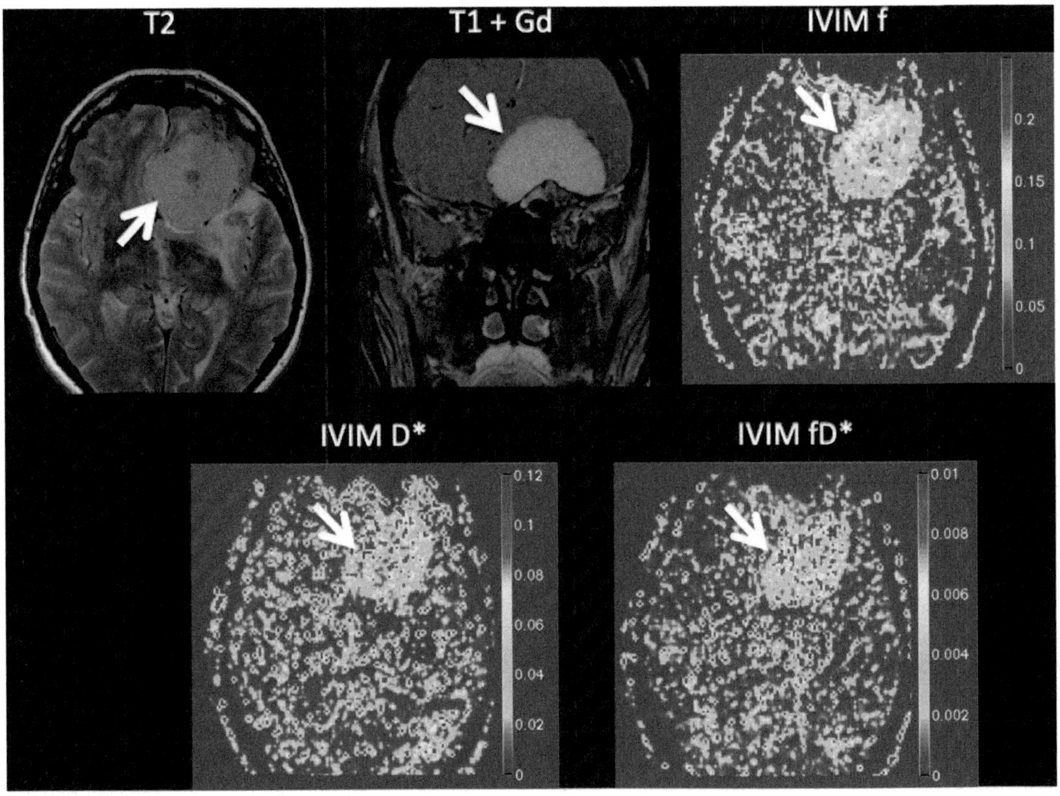

Fig. 7. Meningioma (*arrows*) are extra-axial tumors with increased perfusion, as can be clearly seen on all IVIM perfusion contrasts (the perfusion fraction f, the pseudodiffusion coefficient D*, and the blood flow–related fD*).

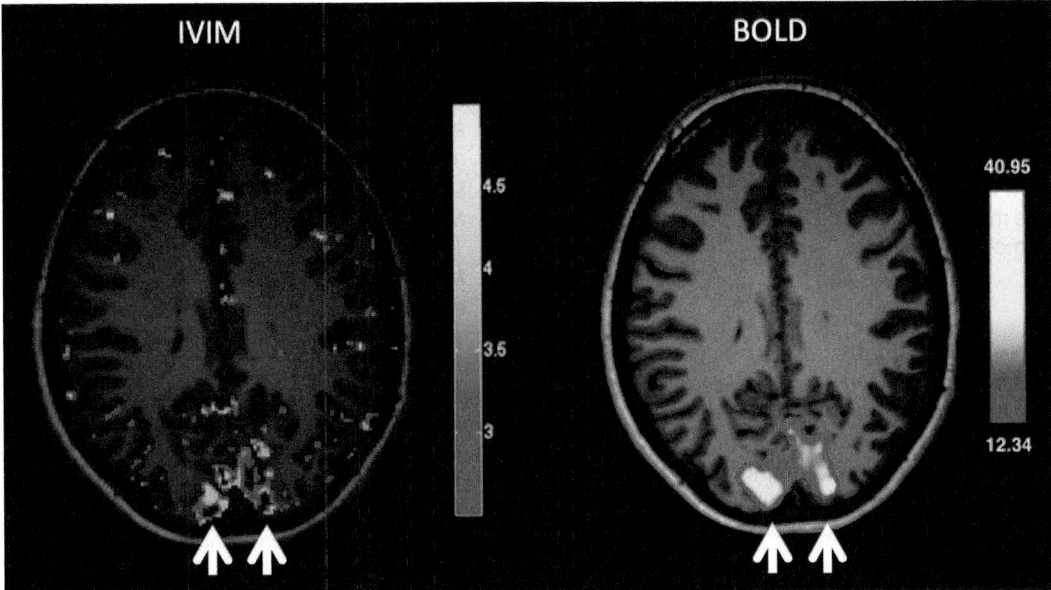

Fig. 8. Functional imaging showing an activation in the primary visual cortex (*arrows*) after visual stimulus (blinking checkerboard) on both the blood flow–related IVIM parameter (fD*) and on the blood oxygenation level–dependent (BOLD) map. The IVIM fD* maps were obtained with a high in-plane resolution (1.2 × 1.2 mm). Scale of the color bars: 10^{-3} mm^2s^{-1} (IVIM) and t-value (BOLD). (Modified with permission from.[52])

independent of any artifacts that could have occurred proximally to the plane of measurement. This contrasts to all other perfusion methods, which depend on the inflow. For example, a failed contrast injection could mimic an absence of brain perfusion on DSC MR imaging or CT perfusion, as well as important calcifications or carotid stenosis on arterial spin labeling (ASL). ASL can be also impaired in the presence of metallic artifacts, for example, from carotid stenting or dental treatments. Lack of cerebral perfusion as assessed by IVIM for brain death have been reported, to our knowledge, only in a case report of 2 patients,[44] and in rats.[45] Results in accordance with those findings, using a low b-value ADC measure rather than the IVIM biexponential model, were reported in a larger patient cohort (n = 64).[46]

Neurovascular and Neurodegenerative Diseases

A reduction in IVIM perfusion fraction f and blood flow–related parameter fD* was found to correlate with delayed cerebral ischemia and proximal artery vasospasm development after cerebral aneurysmal rupture.[47] Alteration of IVIM parameters has recently been found in Alzheimer disease,[48] systemic lupus erythematosus,[49] and moyamoya disease.[50]

Functional MR Imaging

An interesting indirect application of brain perfusion imaging is the application to functional MR imaging, where brain neural activity maps are derived from perfusion-related maps, as focal brain neural activity increases local perfusion through neurovascular coupling.[51] Functional MR imaging has been demonstrated to be feasible using the biexponential IVIM model in the visual cortex[52] (**Fig. 8**); however, perfusion effects observed at low b-values in the context of functional imaging have mostly been studied using an ADC model, for example, in the motor cortex.[53]

SUMMARY

In this review, the authors summarized the idea behind IVIM perfusion imaging method and its clinical application to diagnostic neuroradiology, including stroke, central nervous system tumor diagnosis, grading and prognostication, cerebral death evaluation, neurovascular and neurodegenerative diseases, and functional imaging.

DISCLOSURE

The author is supported by the Swiss National Science Foundation (Grant No PZ00P3_173952 and CRSK-2_190697).

REFERENCES

1. Chehabeddine L, Al Saleh T, Baalbaki M, et al. Cumulative administrations of gadolinium-based contrast agents: risks of accumulation and toxicity of linear vs macrocyclic agents. Crit Rev Toxicol 2019;49(3):262–79.
2. Le Bihan D, Breton E, Lallemand D, et al. MR imaging of intravoxel incoherent motions: application to diffusion and perfusion in neurologic disorders. Radiology 1986;161(2):401–7.
3. Stejskal EO, Tanner JE. Spin diffusion measurements: spin echoes in the presence of a time-dependent field gradient. J Chem Phys 1965; 42(1):288–92.
4. Federau C, Maeder P, O'Brien K, et al. Quantitative measurement of brain perfusion with intravoxel incoherent motion MR imaging. Radiology 2012;265(3): 874–81.
5. Conklin J, Heyn C, Roux M, et al. A simplified model for intravoxel incoherent motion perfusion imaging of the brain. AJNR Am J Neuroradiol 2016;37(12): 2251–7.
6. Hino T, Togao O, Hiwatashi A, et al. Clinical efficacy of simplified intravoxel incoherent motion imaging using three b-values for differentiating high- and low-grade gliomas. PLoS One 2018;13(12):e0209796.
7. Wang X, Cao M, Chen H, et al. Simplified perfusion fraction from diffusion-weighted imaging in preoperative prediction of IDH1 mutation in WHO grade II–III gliomas: comparison with dynamic contrast-enhanced and intravoxel incoherent motion MRI. Radiol Oncol 2020;1. https://doi.org/10.2478/raon-2020-0037.
8. Cao M, Suo S, Han X, et al. Application of a simplified method for estimating perfusion derived from diffusion-weighted MR imaging in glioma grading. Front Aging Neurosci 2018;9. https://doi.org/10.3389/fnagi.2017.00432.
9. Levenberg K. A method for the solution of certain non-linear problems in least squares. Q Appl Math 1944;2(2):164–8.
10. Marquardt DW. An algorithm for least-squares estimation of nonlinear parameters. Journal of the Society for Industrial and Applied Mathematics 1963; 11(2):431–41.
11. Orton MR, Collins DJ, Koh DM, et al. Improved intravoxel incoherent motion analysis of diffusion weighted imaging by data driven Bayesian modeling. Magn Reson Med 2014;71(1):411–20.
12. Lin C, Shih YY, Huang SL, et al. Total variation-based method for generation of intravoxel incoherent motion parametric images in MRI: TV-based method for generating IVIM parametric images in MRI. Magn Reson Med 2017;78(4):1383–91.
13. Freiman M, Perez-Rossello JM, Callahan MJ, et al. Reliable estimation of incoherent motion parametric

maps from diffusion-weighted MRI using fusion bootstrap moves. Med Image Anal 2013;17(3): 325–36.
14. van Rijssel MJ, Froeling M, van Lier Astrid LHMW, et al. Untangling the diffusion signal using the phasor transform. NMR Biomed 2020;33(12):e4372.
15. Federau C. Intravoxel incoherent motion MRI as a means to measure in vivo perfusion: a review of the evidence. NMR Biomed 2017;30(11). https://doi.org/10.1002/nbm.3780.
16. Neil JJ, Bosch CS, Ackerman JJ. An evaluation of the sensitivity of the intravoxel incoherent motion (IVIM) method of blood flow measurement to changes in cerebral blood flow. Magn Reson Med 1994;32(1):60–5.
17. Federau C, Hagmann P, Maeder P, et al. Dependence of brain intravoxel incoherent motion perfusion parameters on the cardiac cycle. PLoS One 2013;8(8):e72856.
18. Heit JJ, Zaharchuk G, Wintermark M. Advanced neuroimaging of acute ischemic stroke. Neuroimaging Clin N Am 2018;28(4):585–97.
19. Federau C, Sumer S, Becce F, et al. Intravoxel incoherent motion perfusion imaging in acute stroke: initial clinical experience. Neuroradiology 2014; 56(8):629–35.
20. Yao Y, Zhang S, Tang X, et al. Intravoxel incoherent motion diffusion-weighted imaging in stroke patients: initial clinical experience. Clin Radiol 2016; 71(9):938.e11-16.
21. Suo S, Cao M, Zhu W, et al. Stroke assessment with intravoxel incoherent motion diffusion-weighted MRI. NMR Biomed 2016;29(3):320–8.
22. Federau C, Wintermark M, Christensen S, et al. Collateral blood flow measurement with intravoxel incoherent motion perfusion imaging in hyperacute brain stroke. Neurology 2019;92(21):e2462–71.
23. Federau C, Meuli R, O'Brien K, et al. Perfusion measurement in brain gliomas with intravoxel incoherent motion MRI. AJNR Am J Neuroradiol 2014;35(2): 256–62.
24. Bisdas S, Koh TS, Roder C, et al. Intravoxel incoherent motion diffusion-weighted MR imaging of gliomas: feasibility of the method and initial results. Neuroradiology 2013;55(10):1189–96.
25. Togao O, Hiwatashi A, Yamashita K, et al. Differentiation of high-grade and low-grade diffuse gliomas by intravoxel incoherent motion MR imaging. Neuro Oncol 2016;18(1):132–41.
26. Keil VC, Mädler B, Gielen GH, et al. Intravoxel incoherent motion MRI in the brain: impact of the fitting model on perfusion fraction and lesion differentiability. J Magn Reson Imaging 2017;46(4): 1187–99.
27. Zou T, Yu H, Jiang C, et al. Differentiating the histologic grades of gliomas preoperatively using amide proton transfer-weighted (APTW) and intravoxel incoherent motion MRI. NMR Biomed 2018;31(1): e3850.
28. Shen N, Zhao L, Jiang J, et al. Intravoxel incoherent motion diffusion-weighted imaging analysis of diffusion and microperfusion in grading gliomas and comparison with arterial spin labeling for evaluation of tumor perfusion. J Magn Reson Imaging 2016; 44(3):620–32.
29. Wang X, Chen X-Z, Shi L, et al. Glioma grading and IDH1 mutational status: assessment by intravoxel incoherent motion MRI. Clin Radiol 2019;74(8):651.e7–14.
30. Catanese A, Malacario F, Cirillo L, et al. Application of intravoxel incoherent motion (IVIM) magnetic resonance imaging in the evaluation of primitive brain tumours. Neuroradiol J 2018;31(1):4–9.
31. Federau C, O'Brien K. Increased brain perfusion contrast with T_2-prepared intravoxel incoherent motion (T2prep IVIM) MRI. NMR Biomed 2015;28(1): 9–16.
32. Suh CH, Kim HS, Lee SS, et al. Atypical imaging features of primary central nervous system lymphoma that mimics glioblastoma: utility of intravoxel incoherent motion MR imaging. Radiology 2014;272(2): 504–13.
33. Yamashita K, Hiwatashi A, Togao O, et al. Diagnostic utility of intravoxel incoherent motion mr imaging in differentiating primary central nervous system lymphoma from glioblastoma multiforme. J Magn Reson Imaging 2016;44(5):1256–61.
34. Federau C, Cerny M, Roux M, et al. IVIM perfusion fraction is prognostic for survival in brain glioma. Clin Neuroradiol 2017;27(4):485–92.
35. Puig J, Sánchez-González J, Blasco G, et al. Intravoxel incoherent motion metrics as potential biomarkers for survival in glioblastoma. PLoS One 2016;11(7):e0158887.
36. Zhu L, Wu J, Zhang H, et al. The value of intravoxel incoherent motion imaging in predicting the survival of patients with astrocytoma. Acta Radiol 2020. https://doi.org/10.1177/0284185120926907. 284185120926907.
37. Zhang J, Xue W, Xu K, et al. Dual inhibition of PFKFB3 and VEGF normalizes tumor vasculature, reduces lactate production, and improves chemotherapy in glioblastoma: insights from protein expression profiling and MRI. Theranostics 2020; 10(16):7245–59.
38. Togao O, Hiwatashi A, Yamashita K, et al. Measurement of the perfusion fraction in brain tumors with intravoxel incoherent motion MR imaging: validation with histopathological vascular density in meningiomas. Br J Radiol 2018;20170912. https://doi.org/10.1259/bjr.20170912.
39. Bohara M, Nakajo M, Kamimura K, et al. Histological grade of meningioma: prediction by intravoxel incoherent motion histogram parameters. Acad Radiol 2020;27(3):342–53.

40. Zampini MA, Buizza G, Paganelli C, et al. Perfusion and diffusion in meningioma tumors: a preliminary multiparametric analysis with dynamic susceptibility contrast and IntraVoxel incoherent motion MRI. Magn Reson Imaging 2020;67:69–78.
41. Kamimura K, Nakajo M, Yoneyama T, et al. Assessment of microvessel perfusion of pituitary adenomas: a feasibility study using turbo spin-echo-based intravoxel incoherent motion imaging. Eur Radiol 2020;30(4):1908–17.
42. Wijdicks EFM. The diagnosis of brain death. N Engl J Med 2001;344(16):1215–21.
43. Shankar JJS, Vandorpe R. CT perfusion for confirmation of brain death. AJNR Am J Neuroradiol 2013;34(6):1175–9.
44. Federau C, Nguyen A, Christensen S, et al. Cerebral perfusion measurement in brain death with intravoxel incoherent motion imaging. Neurovasc Imaging 2016;2(1):9.
45. Neil JJ, Ackerman JJH. Detection of pseudodiffusion in rat brain following blood substitution with perfluorocarbon. J Magn Reson 1992;97(1):194–201.
46. Peckham ME, Anderson JS, Rassner UA, et al. Low b-value diffusion weighted imaging is promising in the diagnosis of brain death and hypoxic-ischemic injury secondary to cardiopulmonary arrest. Crit Care 2018;22(1). https://doi.org/10.1186/s13054-018-2087-9.
47. Heit JJ, Wintermark M, Martin BW, et al. Reduced intravoxel incoherent motion microvascular perfusion predicts delayed cerebral ischemia and vasospasm after aneurysm rupture. Stroke 2018;49(3):741–5.
48. Bergamino M, Nespodzany A, Baxter LC, et al. Preliminary assessment of intravoxel incoherent motion diffusion-weighted MRI (IVIM-DWI) metrics in Alzheimer's disease. J Magn Reson Imaging 2020. https://doi.org/10.1002/jmri.27272.
49. DiFrancesco MW, Lee G, Altaye M, et al. Cerebral microvascular and microstructural integrity is regionally altered in patients with systemic lupus erythematosus. Arthritis Res Ther 2020;22(1). https://doi.org/10.1186/s13075-020-02227-7.
50. Hara S, Hori M, Ueda R, et al. Intravoxel incoherent motion perfusion in patients with Moyamoya disease: comparison with ^{15}O-gas positron emission tomography. Acta Radiol Open 2019;8(5). 205846011984658.
51. Roy CS, Sherrington CS. On the regulation of the blood-supply of the brain. J Physiol 1890;11(1–2):85–158.17.
52. Federau C, O'Brien K, Birbaumer A, et al. Functional mapping of the human visual cortex with intravoxel incoherent motion MRI. PLoS One 2015;10(2):e0117706.
53. De Luca A, Schlaffke L, Siero JCW, et al. On the sensitivity of the diffusion MRI signal to brain activity in response to a motor cortex paradigm. Hum Brain Mapp 2019;40(17):5069–82.

Neurofluid as Assessed by Diffusion-Weighted Imaging

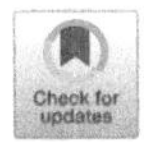

Toshiaki Taoka, MD, PhD*

KEYWORDS

• Interstitial fluid dynamics • Magnetic resonance image • Diffusion image • Glymphatic system

KEY POINTS

- The glymphatic system facilitates clearance of neurofluids and waste removal via glia-supported perivascular channels.
- There have been many attempts made to visualize the glymphatic function by MR imaging, including the diffusion techniques.
- "Central nervous system interstitial fluidopathy" is a new concept proposed to encompass diseases, the pathogenesis of which is predominantly associated with abnormalities in neurofluids dynamics.

INTRODUCTION

Glymphatic System Hypothesis

The glymphatic system hypothesis is associated with the circulation of cerebrospinal fluid (CSF) in the skull and interstitial fluid (ISF) in the brain. This term was coined based on the combination of the words glia and lymphatic system. The concept has garnered attention in several fields since its proposition by Iliff and colleagues[1] in 2012, which were followed by several other reports. This hypothesis does not represent discovery of a previously unknown anatomic structure. Instead, it appears to be based on observation of an already known structure from the perspective of waste product clearance from the brain. The hypothesis is outlined as follows. The perivascular space functions as a conduit that drains CSF into the brain parenchyma. The driving force of this system is arterial pulsation. CSF guided to the perivascular space around the arteries enters the interstitium of brain tissue via water channels controlled by aquaporin 4 (AQP4), which are distributed in the foot processes of astrocytes that constitute the outer wall of the perivascular space. CSF that enters the interstitium washes waste proteins in tissues. Following clearance of the intercellular spaces in this manner, the CSF flows into the perivascular space around the veins and is drained from the brain (**Fig. 1**A).

The glymphatic system theory has attracted attention because of its association with sleep, among other reasons. Drainage by the glymphatic system is suppressed during awakening and markedly increases during sleep. This increased drainage during sleep is because the volume of the glial cells decreases during sleep, and the interstitial space expands more than during awakening, facilitating mass transport of tissues.[2] Studies have shown that a similar effect can be obtained by anesthesia. A study reported that the volume ratio of interstitial space of tissues is 13% to 15% when a person is awake, as opposed to 22% to 24% when sleeping.[3] Furthermore, a

Department of Innovative Biomedical Visualization (iBMV), Department of Radiology, Nagoya University Graduate School of Medicine, Nagoya, Aichi 464-8601, Japan
* Corresponding author. Department of Innovative Biomedical Visualization (iBMV), Nagoya University Graduate School of Medicine, 65 Tsurumai-cho, Showa-ku, Nagoya, Aichi 466-8550, Japan.
E-mail address: ttaoka@med.nagoya-u.ac.jp

Magn Reson Imaging Clin N Am 29 (2021) 243–251
https://doi.org/10.1016/j.mric.2021.01.002

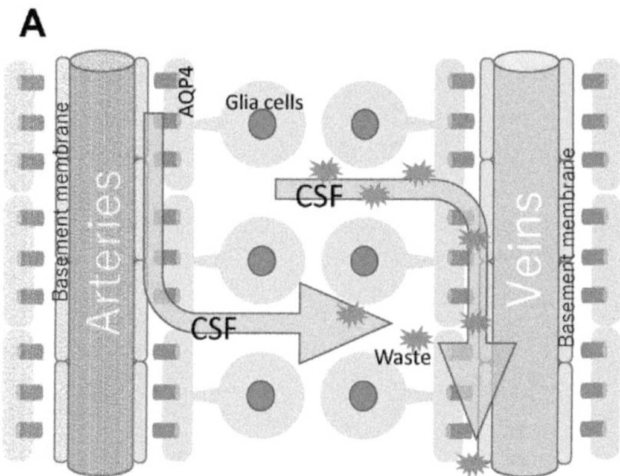

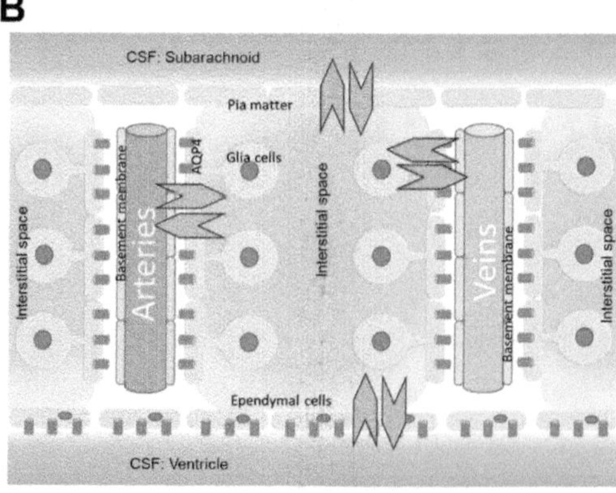

Fig. 1. Outline of the glymphatic system and concept of neurofluids in the brain. (*A*) Perivascular clearance comprises perivascular drainage and glymphatic pathways. CSF flows into the brain parenchyma via the periarterial space and enters the interstitial space of the brain tissue via AQP4-controlled water channels, which are distributed in the end feet of astrocytes that constitute the outer wall of the perivascular space. CSF entering the interstitial space removes waste proteins in the tissue. Following this, CSF flows into the perivenous space and is discharged outside the brain. (*B*) The concept of neurofluids. Interstitial space or CSF space of the brain tissue is considered a common space, which not only acts as a supportive structure but also functions as a space for mass transportation, immune function, or intercellular signal transmission. This space is filled with "neurofluids," a term that is used to indicate all fluids that fill the CNS, including CSF, ISF, and blood. Exchanges occur among the compartments of neurofluids. (*Adapted from* Taoka et al. Glymphatic imaging using MR. J Magn Reson Imaging 2020;51:11-24; with permission.)

continuous scanning 3-dimensional electron microscope study reported that the axon-spine interface was reduced during sleep, and the interstitial space was relatively enlarged at most synapses in the motor and sensory cortices of mice.[4]

Neurofluids Concept

The term "Neurofluids" first appeared in 2018 in the International Society for Magnetic Resonance in Medicine, in which there was a session on the glymphatic system. The term was first used by Professor E.F. Toro, an Italian applied mathematician (University of Trento), as the project title of a series of studies simulating the entire fluid dynamics of the central nervous system (CNS) using a mathematical model. The model was used to apply for a grant supported by the European Research Council. "Neurofluids" is the collective term for the fluids in which the CNS is immersed, which includes blood, CSF, and ISF. The term "neurofluids" helps to understand the dynamics of the fluids (see **Fig. 1**B). In this review, the authors aimed to introduce the glymphatic system hypothesis and its association with neurofluid dynamics, as well as with sleep and diseases.

NEUROFLUID DYNAMICS

Classical Understanding of Cerebrospinal Fluid Dynamics

The concept established by Cushing[5] and Weed[6,7] in the early twentieth century regarding the production, circulation, and absorption of CSF was supported by several studies. Accordingly, CSF was thought to be produced by the choroid plexus in the ventricle and to flow out of the ventricular system from the foramens of Luschka and Magendie. CSF was then thought to flow up into the subarachnoid space on the surface of the brain and be absorbed by the arachnoid granules distributed in the parasagittal area. However, this concept has been questioned since the end of the twentieth century, and various studies have disproved it.

Modern Understanding of Neurofluid Dynamics: Production of Cerebrospinal Fluid/Interstitial Fluid

The currently accepted idea is that production of CSF is mainly induced by hydrostatic pressure exerted by capillaries in the brain. It is known that 70% to 90% of water molecules in the arteries are transferred into the brain parenchyma in a single passage.[8,9] Oreskovic and Klarica[10] stated that both production and absorption of CSF occur in capillaries (Oreskovic and Klarica hypothesis). According to their hypothesis, the difference in hydrostatic pressure causes movement of water from the capillaries to tissues, producing ISF. Conversely, there is a bidirectional movement of water molecules, wherein ISF is absorbed by capillaries because of the difference in osmotic pressure. Part of the ISF passes through the surface of the brain and the perivascular space to fill the ventricles and subarachnoid space as CSF. In contrast, there is a bidirectional movement of water, wherein a part of the CSF is indirectly discharged into the capillaries. Cerebral ISF, together with CSF, is considered a source of CSF to the ventricles.[10,11] In addition to the production of ISF/CSF from capillaries of the brain parenchyma, migration of water also occurs from the ependymal tissue of the ventricle, pia matter of the brain surface, and perivascular space.[12]

Modern Understanding of Neurofluid Dynamics: Absorption of Cerebrospinal Fluid/ Interstitial Fluid

Multiple pathways have been identified pertaining to the absorption of CSF, in addition to the classical pathway via the arachnoid granules. Those absorption routes include the brain parenchyma, spinal arachnoid granules, dural lymphatic system, nasal cavity, and other lymphatic systems. It is considered that multiple pathways function in parallel in a complementary or compensatory manner. The drainage of CSF is broadly divided into the venous and lymphatic systems. In the venous system, as the passage of water is bidirectional in the wall of the ventricle and pia matter, which results in a rapid transfer of ISF and CSF, it is thought that an indirect drainage route exists through the ISF and the capillary wall.[11] In addition, CSF drains into the venous system via the classical arachnoid granule pathway. The arachnoid granules are covered with an endothelial structure and project into the sinus and are thought to drain CSF into the venous system. Arachnoid granules are present in the intracranial sinuses as well as in the spinal epidural venous plexus, which is also associated with drainage of CSF.[13]

IMAGING EVALUATION OF NEUROFLUID DYNAMICS IN HUMANS USING TRACERS

Intrathecal Gadolinium-Based Contrast Agent

Evaluations using intrathecally injected gadolinium-based contrast agent (GBCA) as tracers have been reported in humans. For example, a study reported accidental intrathecal injection of relatively high doses of GBCA in a clinical setting.[14] Other studies have reported systematic injection of small doses of GBCA into the intrathecal space for diagnostic purposes.[15,16] All of these reports have shown that contrast penetrates from the surface to the cortex and further into deep tissues of the brain. These findings confirm that CSF flows from the surface of the brain into the parenchyma, as stated by the glymphatic system hypothesis, and suggest that GBCA could be used to evaluate the activity of glymphatic system. A study reported intrathecal injection of GBCA to evaluate decreased activity of the glymphatic system in normal pressure hydrocephalus.[17] However, intrathecal injection of GBCA is not yet clinically approved, making its application practically impossible. Evaluation using radioisotope cisternography may be a possible solution to observe the tracers injected intrathecally over time. However, presently, there are no systematic reports on the glymphatic system using the radioisotope cisternography technique.

Intravenous Gadolinium-Based Contrast Agent

Intravenous injection of contrast has also been reported in the evaluation of the glymphatic system. A study assessed the permeation of GBCA into normal brain tissue using permeability imaging. This tracer study reported that the transfer coefficient of the blood-brain barrier was elevated in patients with Alzheimer disease.[18] Furthermore, transfer of intravenously injected gadolinium into the CSF has also been confirmed. It has been reported that contrast agents even leak into the CSF in healthy subjects.[19] Transfer of the contrast agent into the CSF and the perivascular space at the base of the brain could be observed at approximately 4 hours after intravenous injection of gadolinium on heavily T2-weighted fluid-attenuated inversion recovery images.[20,21] Another interesting aspect that has been reported is about the intravenously administrated GBCA demonstrating leakage from the cortical veins on delayed imaging, and the leakiness of the cortical veins significantly correlated with age.[21]

EVALUATION OF NEUROFLUID DYNAMICS ON DIFFUSION IMAGES

Diffusion Tensor Image Analysis Along the Perivascular Space

Attempts have been made to evaluate the activity of the glymphatic system using diffusion images. In the abovementioned tracer studies, the behaviors of the tracers after injection are assessed using "integral evaluation." Contrary to this, assessment by diffusion images will enable direct capture of the behavior of water molecules at the time of imaging. The latter would enable evaluation of the activity of the glymphatic system at any given point in time. The method is based on the hypothesis that diffusivity limited to the direction of the perivascular space correlates with the activity of the glymphatic system. An evaluation technique called diffusion tensor image analysis along the perivascular space (DTI-ALPS) has been proposed. In this DTI-ALPS technique, the behavior of water molecules in the deep white matter is evaluated using DTIs.[22] Upon the evaluation of the diffusivity in the brain, the effects of diffusion along the large white matter fibers bundles will dominate; therefore, evaluation of diffusion along the perivascular space is difficult. However, if the large white matter fibers and perivascular space intersect at a right angle, the effects of the former should be separable. In the human brain, the medullary arteries and veins intersect with the ventricular wall at a right angle, at the outer side of the body of the lateral ventricle. In the DTI-ALPS technique, the diffusivity along the perivascular space in the white matter, on the outer side of the body of the lateral ventricle, is evaluated as a ratio of the diffusivity along the perivascular space to that perpendicular to the running direction of the main white matter fibers (ALPS index).

Evaluations performed in healthy volunteers, patients with mild cognitive decline, and patients with Alzheimer disease showed that the ALPS index is inversely correlated with the Mini-Mental State Examination score (MMSE) and with age (**Fig. 2**). As several animal experiments have demonstrated impaired ISF dynamics in Alzheimer disease models,[1,23,24] the aforementioned result suggests that the ALPS index might be an indicator of the function of the glymphatic system.

Advanced Diffusion Methods

Several studies, including animal experiments and human studies, have evaluated the glymphatic system by diffusion imaging. TGN-020 is a compound that blocks AQP4 channels in vivo.[25] An animal study has used this TGN-020 for diffusion imaging,[26] and it determined the shifted apparent diffusion coefficient (sADC) and S-index, which are diffusion markers of tissue microstructure. The sADC and S-index are derived from diffusion MR signals acquired at 2 key b values (low and high), indicating the degree of diffusion hindrance to discriminate malignant from benign tissue.[27] Following inhibition of the AQP4 channel with a TGN-020 solution, a decrease in the S-index and increase in sADC were readily observed in the cortex, more in the hippocampus, but not in the striatum, reflecting local differences in astrocyte and vascular density. The decrease and increase in the S-index and sADC, respectively, jointly indicated a decrease in the degree of hindrance to water diffusion in astrocyte-rich areas (cortex and hippocampus) under acute AQP4 channel inhibition induced by TGN-020.[26]

A human study used multishell diffusion tensor imaging (b values = 0, 50, 300, and 1000 s/mm^2) to measure slow and fast components of the ADC of water in the brain. The findings of the study revealed an increase in slow ADC as well as a decrease in fast ADC in relation to sleep, which reflected the distinct biological significance of fast- and slow-ADC values and sleep-induced changes on the volume of CSF.[28] One study used the intravoxel incoherent motion (IVIM) method to investigate the intermediate diffusion component by the nonnegative least-squares method to evaluate functions of the glymphatic system. The values of both the parenchymal diffusivity and the microvascular perfusion could be detected, and the perivascular fluid motion in relation to the glymphatic system could be evaluated by the IVIM method.[29]

Cerebrospinal Fluid Dynamics on Diffusion MR Imaging

Diffusion-weighted imaging (DWI) enables visualization of the water molecules' motion as a decrease in signal because of the phase shift induced by motion. When the phase shift becomes larger than $\pm\pi$ or when various velocities exist in a single voxel, signal decrease on the DWI becomes prominent depending on the b values (motion-related signal dephasing; see **Fig. 1**). CSF has been reported to cause a prominent decrease in the signal because of its substantial and/or nonuniform motion.[30] A study reported that a diffusion-weighted image of b = 500 s/mm^2 reflected changes in the dynamics of CSF.[31] The study has shown that CSF within the lateral ventricles at b = 500 s/mm^2 on DWI showed higher signal in the ventricle dilatation group compared with the control group. However, a single b value, such as b = 500 s/mm^2, cannot depict the detailed distribution of the CSF dynamics. DWI based on different b values would enable visualization of the degree of CSF motion. As explained earlier, DWI with lower b value will demonstrate signal dephasing only in areas with substantial CSF motion. In contrast, DWI with higher b value will show signal dephasing of the CSF in a wide area with minimal to substantial CSF motions. Diffusion ANalysis of fluid DYnamics with Incremental Strength of Motion proving gradient (DANDYISM) images indicated that the motion of the CSF was prominent in areas such as the ventral portion of the posterior fossa, suprasellar cistern, and Sylvian fissure. However, the motion was limited in the lateral ventricles and parietal subarachnoid space, thereby creating uncertainty regarding the classical model of CSF dynamics. A study also indicated that the motion of the CSF correlated with age in the third ventricle and interhemispheric fissure[32] (**Fig. 3**).

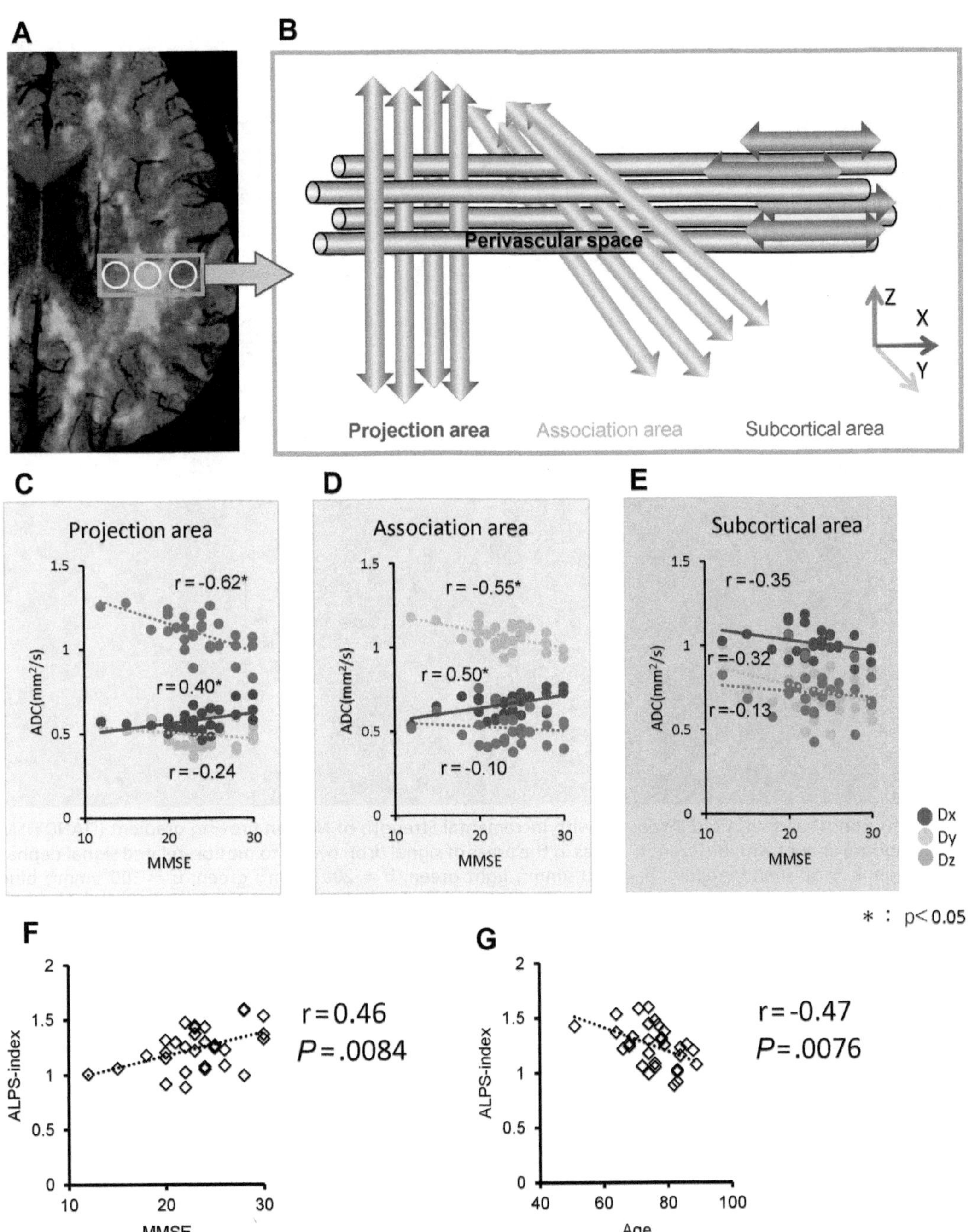

Fig. 2. Concept for the DTI-ALPS method and its result for Alzheimer disease cases. (*A*) Superimposed color display of DTI on SWI indicating the distribution of projection fibers (*z-axis: blue*), association fibers (*y-axis: green*), and the subcortical fibers (*x-axis: red*). Three regions of interest (ROIs) are placed in the area with projection fibers (projection area), association fibers (association area), and subcortical fibers (subcortical area) to measure diffusivities of the three directions (*X, Y, Z*). (*B*) Schematic indicating the relationship between the direction of the perivascular space (gray cylinders) and directions of the fibers. Note that the direction of the perivascular space is perpendicular to both the projection and association fibers. (*C-E*) Correlation between directional diffusivity and Mini-Mental State Examination (MMSE) scores. Correlation between MMSE and diffusivities of the three directions of the three areas (projection: *C*, association: *D*, subcortical: *E*). Diffusivity of the x-axis is plotted as red, y-axis as green, and z-axis as blue. In the projection area (*C*), a significant positive correlation was found between the diffusivity along the perivascular space (*x-axis*) and the MMSE scores. Similarly, in the association

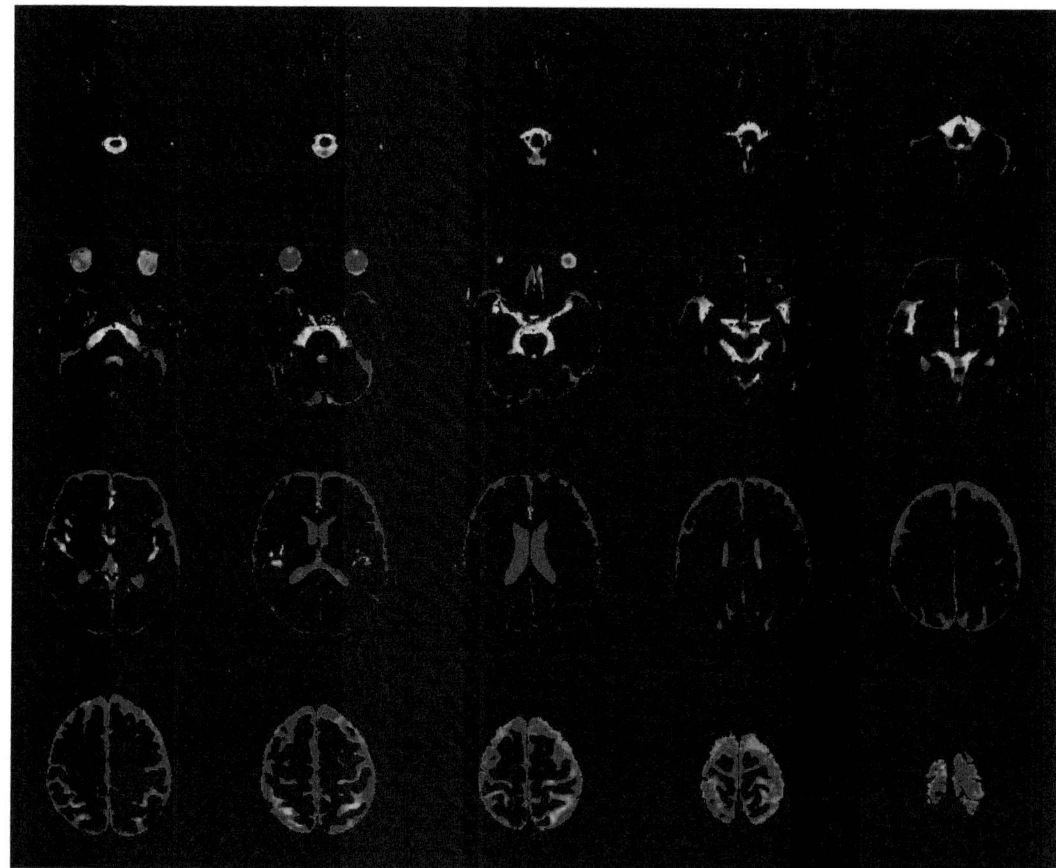

Fig. 3. Diffusion ANalysis of fluid DYnamics with Incremental Strength of Motion proving gradient (DANDYISM) color composite images with different b values in the areas of signal drop owing to motion-related signal dephasing: Orange: b = 50 s/mm^2; yellow: b = 100 s/mm^2; light green: b = 200 s/mm^2; green: b = 300 s/mm^2; blue: b = 500 s/mm^2; indigo: b = 700 s/mm^2; purple: b = 1000 s/mm^2. Note that the signal drops occurred in instances of lower b value in the ventral portion of the posterior fossa, suprasellar cistern, and Sylvian fissure, indicating substantial motion of the CSF. In contrast, a signal drop in the lateral ventricle and the subarachnoid space of the parietal region occurred only with a higher b value, indicating limited motion of the CSF.

DISORDERS IN THE DYNAMICS OF NEUROFLUIDS: CENTRAL NERVOUS SYSTEM INTERSTITIAL FLUIDOPATHY

The glymphatic system hypothesis has provided new insights into the physiology and pathophysiology of the CNS, including the concept of neurofluids. An increasing number of studies are reporting on the dynamics of ISF and CSF within the brain. Many diseases are known to develop because of abnormality of the glymphatic system. As previously explained, several studies have reported impaired dynamics of the ISF in Alzheimer disease.[1,23,24] Moreover, glymphatic influx of the

area (*D*), a significant positive correlation was found between the diffusivity along the perivascular space (*x-axis*) and the MMSE scores. (*F*) Correlation between ALPS index and MMSE. The ALPSindex is calculated in order to evaluate the activity of the glymphatic system. In this index, it was hypothesized that the ratio of x-axis diffusivity in the projection fibers and association fibers area (Dxproj and Dxassoc) to the diffusivity which is perpendicular to them (Dyproj and Dzassoc) would express the influence of the water diffusion along the perivascular space which will reflect activity of the glymphatic system. Thus, ALPS index are shown, which was assessed based on the following ratio: ALPS index = mean (Dxproj, Dxassoc)/mean (Dyproj, Dzassoc). There was a significant positive correlation (r = 0.46, p = 0.0084) between the ALPS index and the MMSE scores. (*G*) Correlation between ALPS index and the age. There was a significant positive correlation (r = -0.47, p = 0.00764) between the ALPS index and the age. (*Adapted from* Taoka et al. Evaluation of glymphatic system activity with the diffusion MR technique: diffusion tensor image analysis along the perivascular space (DTI-ALPS) in Alzheimer's disease cases. Jpn J Radiol 2017;35:172-178, with permission.)

CSF tracer was reduced in a Parkinson disease mouse model, causing severe accumulation of α-synuclein, glial activation, inflammation, dopaminergic neuronal loss, and motor deficits.[33] An experimental model of moderate to severe head trauma demonstrated that migration of the tracer injected into the perivascular cortex of mice after injury was significantly reduced compared with the region ipsilateral to the trauma, suggesting reduced activity of the glymphatic system.[34] Another study reported severe impairment of the glymphatic system after SAH and in the acute phase of ischemic stroke.[35]

Arteriolosclerosis is the most common small vessel alteration in aged brains. An animal experiment, wherein MR imaging was performed following intrathecal administration of GBCA on spontaneously hypertensive rats, reported that ventricular reflux of the agent was observed only in the hypertensive rats, indicating abnormal ISF dynamics.[36]

Glaucoma has also been hypothesized to occur because of alterations in fluid dynamics in the intraocular and intracranial spaces. These alterations might result in impaired entry of the CSF into the subarachnoid and perivascular spaces of the optic nerve, thereby inhibiting glymphatic clearance of waste products from the retrobulbar or retrolaminar portion of the optic nerve.[37]

Box 1
Disease or disorders categorized as "central nervous system interstitial fluidopathy"

- Alzheimer disease[1,23,24]
- Parkinson disease[33]
- Traumatic brain injury[34]
- Stroke
  - Subarachnoid hemorrhage[35]
  - Ischemic stroke[35]
- Small vessel diseases of CNS
  - Arteriolosclerosis[36]
  - Cerebral amyloid angiopathy[44]
  - Cerebral autosomal dominant arteriopathy with subcortical infarcts and leukoencephalopathy (CADASIL)[45]
  - COL4A1 mutation related disorders[46]
- Glaucoma[37]
- Meniere disease[47]
- Idiopathic normal pressure hydrocephalus[17]
- Mucopolysaccharidoses[48]

Meniere disease is a complex, heterogeneous disorder associated with many underlying factors, including endolymphatic hydrops. The disorder occurs because of excessive accumulation of endolymph in the inner ear, which damages the ganglion cells. Endolymphatic hydrops shares the characteristics of dysfunction of ISF dynamics in the inner ear.[38,39] Several reports have indicated altered dynamics of the ISF of the CNS in idiopathic normal pressure hydrocephalus.[17] One study used the DTI-ALPS method and evaluated the aforementioned diffusivity limited to the direction of the perivascular space.[40]

Box 1 presents the list of the disorders that are reported to demonstrate altered glymphatic function or neurofluid dynamics. The listed disorders, including Alzheimer disease, traumatic brain injury, stroke, and other disorders, share the characteristics of glymphatic system dysfunction or other mechanisms related to dynamics of the ISF. In this context, CNS interstitial fluidopathy has been proposed as a new concept encompassing diseases with pathologic conditions that are predominantly associated with abnormal dynamics of the ISF or CSF.[41]

Currently, the glymphatic system hypothesis is not yet well established, and there are several reports to point out the problems of the hypothesis.[42,43] However, no study has been able to oppose the fact that CSF and ISF play important roles in the maintenance of brain function and homeostasis. Therefore, visualizing the dynamics of neurofluids using various methods, including diffusion MR technique, will provide significant information on the maintenance of healthy brain function in humans.

FINANCIAL DISCLOSURE

The Department of Innovative Biomedical Visualization (iBMV), Nagoya University Graduate School of Medicine is financially supported by Canon Medical Systems Corporation.

REFERENCES

1. Iliff JJ, Wang M, Liao Y, et al. A paravascular pathway facilitates CSF flow through the brain parenchyma and the clearance of interstitial solutes, including amyloid beta. Sci Transl Med 2012; 4(147):147ra11.
2. Xie L, Kang H, Xu Q, et al. Sleep drives metabolite clearance from the adult brain. Science 2013; 342(6156):373–7.
3. DiNuzzo M, Nedergaard M. Brain energetics during the sleep-wake cycle. Curr Opin Neurobiol 2017;47: 65–72.

4. de Vivo L, Bellesi M, Marshall W, et al. Ultrastructural evidence for synaptic scaling across the wake/sleep cycle. Science 2017;355(6324):507–10.
5. Cushing H. The third circulation and its channels (Cameron lecture). Lancet 1925;206(5330):851–7.
6. Weed LH. Studies on cerebro-spinal fluid. No. III: the pathways of escape from the subarachnoid spaces with particular reference to the arachnoid villi. The J Med Res 1914;31(1):51–91.
7. Dandy WE. Where is cerebrospinal fluid absorbed? J Amer Med Assoc 1929;92:2012–4.
8. Eichling JO, Raichle ME, Grubb RL Jr, et al. Evidence of the limitations of water as a freely diffusible tracer in brain of the rhesus monkey. Circ Res 1974;35(3):358–64.
9. Hladky SB, Barrand MA. Elimination of substances from the brain parenchyma: efflux via perivascular pathways and via the blood-brain barrier. Fluids Barriers CNS 2018;15(1):30.
10. Oreskovic D, Klarica M. The formation of cerebrospinal fluid: nearly a hundred years of interpretations and misinterpretations. Brain Res Rev 2010;64(2):241–62.
11. Carare RO, Hawkes CA, Weller RO. Afferent and efferent immunological pathways of the brain. Anatomy, function and failure. Brain Behav Immun 2014;36:9–14.
12. Abbott NJ. Evidence for bulk flow of brain interstitial fluid: significance for physiology and pathology. Neurochem Int 2004;45(4):545–52.
13. Sakka L, Coll G, Chazal J. Anatomy and physiology of cerebrospinal fluid. Eur Ann Otorhinolaryngol Head Neck Dis 2011;128(6):309–16.
14. Samardzic D, Thamburaj K. Magnetic resonance characteristics and susceptibility weighted imaging of the brain in gadolinium encephalopathy. J Neuroimage 2015;25(1):136–9.
15. Eide PK. MRI with intrathecal MRI gadolinium contrast medium administration: a possible method to assess glymphatic function in human brain. Acta Radiol Open 2015;4(11):1–5.
16. Oner AY, Barutcu B, Aykol S, et al. Intrathecal contrast-enhanced magnetic resonance imaging-related brain signal changes: residual gadolinium deposition? Invest Radiol 2017;52(4):195–7.
17. Ringstad G, Vatnehol SAS, Eide PK. Glymphatic MRI in idiopathic normal pressure hydrocephalus. Brain 2017;140:2691–705.
18. van de Haar HJ, Burgmans S, Jansen JF, et al. Blood-brain barrier leakage in patients with early Alzheimer disease. Radiology 2016;281(2):527–35.
19. Naganawa S, Suzuki K, Yamazaki M, et al. Serial scans in healthy volunteers following intravenous administration of gadoteridol: time course of contrast enhancement in various cranial fluid spaces. Magn Reson Med Sci 2014;13(1):7–13.
20. Naganawa S, Nakane T, Kawai H, et al. Gd-based contrast enhancement of the perivascular spaces in the basal ganglia. Magn Reson Med Sci 2017;16(1):61–5.
21. Naganawa S, Nakane T, Kawai H, et al. Age dependence of gadolinium leakage from the cortical veins into the cerebrospinal fluid assessed with whole brain 3D-real inversion recovery MR Imaging. Magn Reson Med Sci 2019;18(2):163–9.
22. Taoka T, Masutani Y, Kawai H, et al. Evaluation of glymphatic system activity with the diffusion MR technique: diffusion tensor image analysis along the perivascular space (DTI-ALPS) in Alzheimer's disease cases. Jpn J Radiol 2017;35(4):172–8.
23. Wang L, Zhang Y, Zhao Y, et al. Deep cervical lymph node ligation aggravates AD-like pathology of APP/PS1 mice. Brain Pathol 2019;29(2):176–92.
24. Da Mesquita S, Louveau A, Vaccari A, et al. Functional aspects of meningeal lymphatics in ageing and Alzheimer's disease. Nature 2018;560(7717):185–91.
25. Igarashi H, Huber VJ, Tsujita M, et al. Pretreatment with a novel aquaporin 4 inhibitor, TGN-020, significantly reduces ischemic cerebral edema. Neurol Sci 2011;32(1):113–6.
26. Debacker C, Djemai B, Ciobanu L, et al. Diffusion MRI reveals in vivo and non-invasively changes in astrocyte function induced by an aquaporin-4 inhibitor. PLoS One 2020;15(5):e0229702.
27. Iima M, Le Bihan D. Clinical intravoxel incoherent motion and diffusion MR imaging: past, present, and future. Radiology 2016;278(1):13–32.
28. Demiral SB, Tomasi D, Sarlls J, et al. Apparent diffusion coefficient changes in human brain during sleep - does it inform on the existence of a glymphatic system? Neuroimage 2019;185:263–73.
29. Wong SM, Backes WH, Drenthen GS, et al. Spectral diffusion analysis of intravoxel incoherent motion MRI in cerebral small vessel disease. J Magn Reson Imaging 2020;51:1170–80.
30. Le Bihan D, Breton E, Lallemand D, et al. MR imaging of intravoxel incoherent motions: application to diffusion and perfusion in neurologic disorders. Radiology 1986;161(2):401–7.
31. Taoka T, Naganawa S, Kawai H, et al. Can low b value diffusion weighted imaging evaluate the character of cerebrospinal fluid dynamics? Jpn J Radiol 2019;37(2):135–44.
32. Taoka T, Kawai H, Nakane T, et al. Diffusion analysis of fluid dynamics with incremental strength of motion proving gradient (DANDYISM) to evaluate cerebrospinal fluid dynamics. Jpn J Radiol, in press. doi:10.1007/s11604-020-01075-4.
33. Zou W, Pu T, Feng W, et al. Blocking meningeal lymphatic drainage aggravates Parkinson's disease-like pathology in mice overexpressing

mutated alpha-synuclein. Transl Neurodegener 2019;8:7.
34. Iliff JJ, Chen MJ, Plog BA, et al. Impairment of glymphatic pathway function promotes tau pathology after traumatic brain injury. J Neurosci 2014;34(49):16180–93.
35. Gaberel T, Gakuba C, Goulay R, et al. Impaired glymphatic perfusion after strokes revealed by contrast-enhanced MRI: a new target for fibrinolysis? Stroke 2014;45(10):3092–6.
36. Mortensen KN, Sanggaard S, Mestre H, et al. Impaired glymphatic transport in spontaneously hypertensive rats. J Neurosci 2019;39(32):6365–77.
37. Wostyn P. Glaucoma as a dangerous interplay between ocular fluid and cerebrospinal fluid. Med Hypotheses 2019;127:97–9.
38. Naganawa S, Suzuki K, Nakamichi R, et al. Semi-quantification of endolymphatic size on MR imaging after intravenous injection of single-dose gadodiamide: comparison between two types of processing strategies. Magn Reson Med Sci 2013;12(4):261–9.
39. Nakashima T, Sone M, Teranishi M, et al. A perspective from magnetic resonance imaging findings of the inner ear: relationships among cerebrospinal, ocular and inner ear fluids. Auris Nasus Larynx 2012;39(4):345–55.
40. Yokota H, Vijayasarathi A, Cekic M, et al. Diagnostic performance of glymphatic system evaluation using diffusion tensor imaging in idiopathic normal pressure hydrocephalus and mimickers. Curr Gerontol Geriatr Res 2019;2019:5675014.
41. Taoka T, Naganawa S. Imaging for central nervous system (CNS) interstitial fluidopathy: disorders with impaired interstitial fluid dynamics. Jpn J Radiol 2021;39:1–14.
42. Albargothy NJ, Johnston DA, MacGregor-Sharp M, et al. Convective influx/glymphatic system: tracers injected into the CSF enter and leave the brain along separate periarterial basement membrane pathways. Acta Neuropathol 2018;136(1):139–52.
43. Asgari M, de Zelicourt D, Kurtcuoglu V. Glymphatic solute transport does not require bulk flow. Sci Rep 2016;6:38635.
44. Peng W, Achariyar TM, Li B, et al. Suppression of glymphatic fluid transport in a mouse model of Alzheimer's disease. Neurobiol Dis 2016;93:215–25.
45. Yamamoto Y, Craggs L, Baumann M, et al. Review: molecular genetics and pathology of hereditary small vessel diseases of the brain. Neuropathol Appl Neurobiol 2011;37(1):94–113.
46. Morris AW, Sharp MM, Albargothy NJ, et al. Vascular basement membranes as pathways for the passage of fluid into and out of the brain. Acta Neuropathol 2016;131(5):725–36.
47. Nakashima T, Pyykko I, Arroll MA, et al. Meniere's disease. Nat Rev Dis Primers 2016;2:16028.
48. Abbott NJ, Pizzo ME, Preston JE, et al. The role of brain barriers in fluid movement in the CNS: is there a 'glymphatic' system? Acta Neuropathol 2018;135(3):387–407.

Temperature Measurement by Diffusion-Weighted Imaging

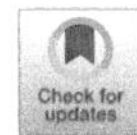

Gianvincenzo Sparacia, MD[a,*], Koji Sakai, PhD[b]

KEYWORDS

- Diffusion-weighted imaging (DWI) temperature • DWI thermometry • MR imaging
- Ventricular temperatures

KEY POINTS

- Diffusion-weighted imaging (DWI) thermometry refers to the capability of measuring the brain core temperature from postprocessing of standard DWI magnetic resonance images.
- DWI thermometry is based on a phenomenon in which higher thermal diffusion of proton leads to reduced echo signal.
- DWI thermometry is a potential method to elucidate the pathophysiology of several brain diseases and neurologic syndromes.

INTRODUCTION

The brain is an intensively heat-producing organ; it produces 16% of the total heat generated in the whole body (13W–20W), even in a resting state, despite comprising approximately only 2% of the bodyweight.[1] Heat generation in the brain results from the neuronal activity, and this heat is removed mainly by the blood flow. Blood has temperature similar to that of the body core, so brain temperature usually is approximately 1°C higher than the body core temperature.[2]

Brain core temperature is determined by the balance between heat generation and heat removal, involving 3 essential elements: brain metabolism, cerebral blood flow (CBF), and body core temperature.[3] Under normal conditions, the brain metabolizes glucose, which are oxidized via the Krebs cycle to carbon dioxide and water. Adenosine triphosphate is generated through this chain of chemical reactions. Cells in the brain use this as an energy resource and, consequently, generate heat. Heat production in the brain thus is related closely to the cerebral metabolic rates of glucose (CMRGlu) and oxygen (CMRO2), whereas CBF is essential to cool down the brain.[2] Hayward and Baker[4] showed, in an animal study, that the temperature of deep brain regions increases during the initial 10 minutes after circulatory arrest because of continued metabolic heat production without heat removal by CBF. Recent studies have shown that both CMRGlu and CMRO2 decline with age,[5] whereas CBF shows no such trend and is much less age dependent.[6]

Methods of brain core temperature measurement based on magnetic resonance imaging (MRI)[7] and magnetic resonance spectroscopy (MRS)[8–10] have been attempted and are shown to be potentially useful. Numbers of magnetic resonance (MR) parameters show sensitivity to temperature: the proton density, the T1 and T2 relaxation times, the diffusion coefficient, magnetization transfer, and the proton resonance frequency. In addition to these intrinsic parameters, temperature-sensitive contrast agents have been developed.

Depending on the technique, the temperature measurement is absolute (eg, in spectroscopy) or

[a] Department of Diagnostic and Therapeutic Services, IRCCS-ISMETT, Via Tricomi, 5, Palermo 90127, Italy; [b] Clinical AI Research Laboratory, Department of Radiology, Kyoto Prefectural University of Medicine, 465 Kajii-cho, Kawaramachi-Hirokoji, Kamigyo-ku, Kyoto 602-8566, Japan
* Corresponding author.
E-mail address: gsparacia@ismett.edu

Magn Reson Imaging Clin N Am 29 (2021) 253–261
https://doi.org/10.1016/j.mric.2021.02.005
1064-9689/21/

gives a relative temperature change by comparing the acquired data to reference data, acquired under identical experimental conditions at a known temperature. The sensitivity of these methods, however, is limited and strongly subject dependent. Therefore, the methods suitable for actual clinical use are limited. Among these methods, studies are being conducted on methods using diffusion-weighted imaging (DWI), which is more easily acquired because it is used routinely as part of the standard brain imaging examination.

DWI-based brain temperature measurement (ie, diffusion thermometry) is based on a phenomenon in which higher thermal diffusion of proton leads to reduced echo signal. The higher the temperature is, the more the signal intensity is decreased due to more actively moving water molecules,[11–13] based on the Stokes-Einstein equation,[14] which describes the relationship between diffusion and temperature. This fundamental relationship is important to understand because diffusion has a direct proportion to temperature and inverse proportion to viscosity.

In recent years, DWI thermometry has been demonstrated as capable of indicating intraventricular cerebrospinal fluid (CSF) temperature, and such information may greatly contribute to assessment of brain diseases and aging, because it was demonstrated that ventricular temperature declines with the normal aging process.[5]

To better understand the basic physical principles and the principal applications of DWI thermometry, a brief overview is presented in this article.

DIFFUSION AND TEMPERATURE

In 1889, a Swedish chemist, S. A. Arrhenius, advocated a formula[15] expressing the relationship between the chemical reaction rate constant, k, and the absolute temperature, T, expressed as follows:

$$k = A \exp(-E/RT) \tag{1}$$

where A represents the frequency at which atoms and molecules collide in a way that leads to a reaction, E is the activation energy for the reaction, R is the ideal gas constant (8.314 joules per kelvin per mole), and T is the absolute temperature. The equation is commonly given in the form of an exponential function $k = A\exp(-E/RT)$. This formula is widely applicable to the uniform gas phase and liquid phase reactions; general chemical reactions, such as nonuniform contact reactions and solid reactions; and dynamic phenomena, such as viscosity and diffusion, except for fast reactions, such as ionic reactions.

To apply Equation (1) to the relation between the diffusion of water molecules and temperature, k can be replaced with diffusion coefficient, D:

$$D = A \exp(-E/RT) \tag{2}$$

Using the logarithm of both sides of Equation (2), it is possible to represent the temperature (T) as follows:

$$T = (E/R)/\ln(A/D) \tag{3}$$

In Equation (3), E/R and A were experimentally determined by Mills[16]: $E/R = 2256.74$ and $A = 4.39221$.

From these, Equation (4) showing the relationship between temperature and diffusion is obtained[11]:

$$T = \frac{2256.74}{\ln\left(\frac{4.39221}{D}\right)} - 273.15 \tag{4}$$

DIFFUSION-WEIGHTED IMAGING THERMOMETRY

Diffusion thermometry is a relatively straightforward method that already has been utilized clinically.[5,17] Kozak and colleagues[11] confirmed this relationship on a water phantom using a 3.0T clinical MR scanner. They proposed that temperature could be estimated by calculating the average number of voxels within a predetermined threshold (ie, 30°C–55°C). They also tried to avoid the influence of cardiac pulsation by selecting only certain diffusion gradient directions. Despite their successful results, a more objective method of assessing temperature, without any arbitrary threshold, is preferable.

Sakai and colleagues[2] established a data analysis method for DWI thermometry of CSF. The workflow of the DWI thermometry proposed is summarized in **Fig. 1** and is explained in the following paragraphs.

Diffusion-weighted Imaging Acquisition

The first step of DWI thermometry is to acquire DWIs. Typical DWI imaging parameters are as follows: using a 1.5T or 3T MR unit, single-shot, echo-planar imaging sequence with sensitivity encoding (parallel imaging factor of 2.5).[18] Typical imaging matrix used is 96 × 96 with a field-of-view of 240 mm × 240 mm (nominal resolution, 2.5 mm), zero-filled to 256 pixels × 256 pixels. Transverse sections of 2.5-mm thickness are acquired parallel to the anterior commissure–posterior commissure line. A total of 50 to 55 sections covering the entire brain and brainstem without gaps typically are acquired. Diffusion-weighting encoding along 3 to 30 independent orientations typically is used, with a b-value of 700 s/mm^2 to 1000 s/mm^2.[19] Scan time per data set is approximately 5 minutes. To enhance the signal-to-noise ratio, imaging is repeated 2 to 3 times.

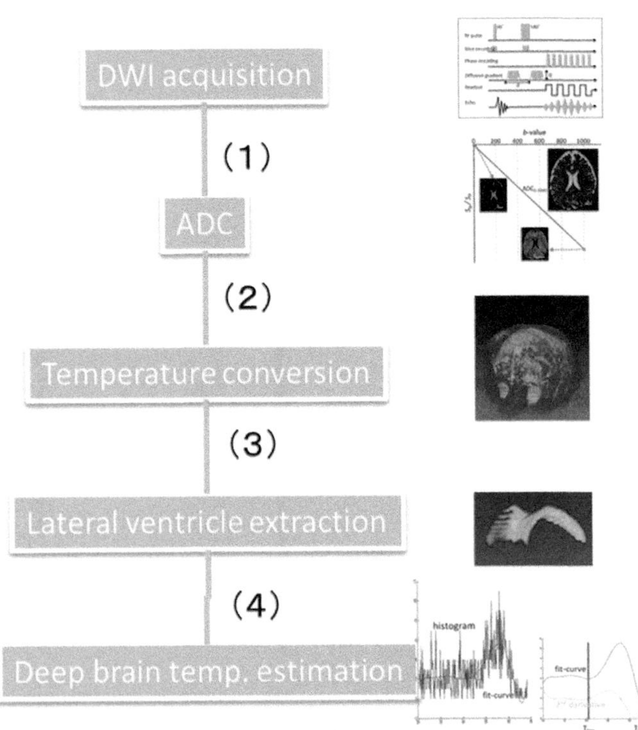

Fig. 1. DWI thermometry proposed workflow. (1) DWI acquisition. (2) Diffusion constant calculation. (3) Temperature from diffusion constant. (4) Deep brain temperature estimation. ADC, apparent diffusion coefficient.

Diffusion Constant Calculation

From the 2 signals with different b-values obtained from DWI, the diffusion coefficient is calculated by the following formula:

$$D = \frac{\ln(S_0/S)}{b} \quad \textbf{(5)}$$

where D is the diffusion constant (mm^2/s), b is the applied diffusion weighting (s/mm^2), and S_0 and S are the voxel signal intensities of the reference and DWIs, respectively.

Temperature Conversion from Diffusion Constant

The D value is converted to the corresponding temperature using Equation (4).

Lateral Ventricle Extraction

Lateral ventricles for each subject are extracted manually from the b0 images with intensity thresholding using image processing software (Image J, National Institute of Mental Health, Bethesda, Maryland). The extracted lateral ventricles were termed, *lateral ventricle mask*.

DEEP BRAIN TEMPERATURE ESTIMATION

DWI thermometry cannot be calculated by Equation (4) alone. The converted diffusion coefficients in the brain contain pixels with high and low temperatures that do not fit within the appropriate brain temperature. Kozak and colleagues[11] determined the effective temperature range by simple thresholding (30°C–44°C). The motion of water molecules in the lateral ventricles are affected not only by self-diffusion but also by flow from the choroid plexus and interventricular foramen. Therefore, it is necessary to select a suitable threshold that enables extraction of the motion of water molecules caused by self-diffusion.

Sakai and colleagues[2] employed polynomial fitting to the temperature distribution of the lateral ventricles and selected the majority of the distribution.

Accordingly, they determined an effective apparent ventricle temperature as follows:

1. Histograms (bin = 256) were generated for values in the extracted region.
2. A polynomial curve was fitted to the histogram.
3. The lowest and highest peaks of the first derivative of the fit curve were assigned to the range of effective apparent ventricular temperatures (**Fig. 2**).

DIFFUSION COEFFICIENT DISTRIBUTION IN THE LATERAL VENTRICLE

The diffusion coefficient of water molecules in the lateral ventricles is not constant. For that reason, it

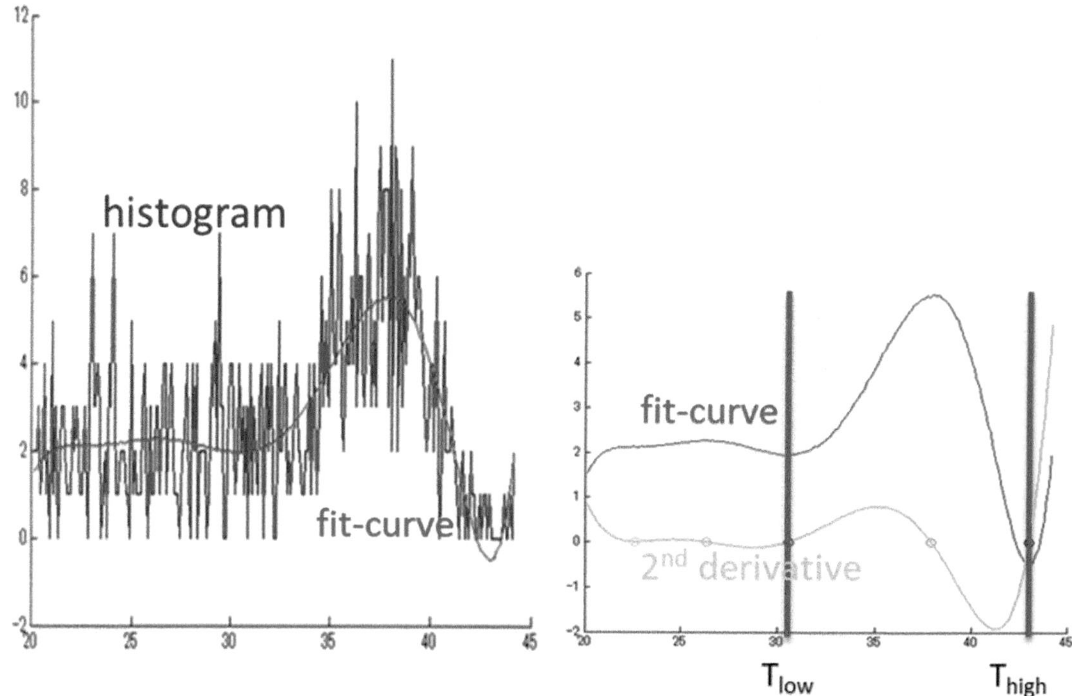

Fig. 2. Polynomial fitting to the temperature distribution of the lateral ventricle. (*Left*) Histogram (bin = 256) was generated for values in the extracted region. (*Right*) A polynomial curve was fitted to the histogram: the lowest and highest peaks of the first derivative of the fit curve were assigned to the range of effective apparent ventricle temperatures. (Tlow) = temperature lower than the lower threshold; (Tmax) = Temperature higher than higher temperature threshold.

is necessary to select appropriately and without bias. When the value was smaller than the threshold value, a small diffusion area was observed around the margin of the lateral ventricle. If an appropriate threshold value is selected, the diffusion region of water molecules near the body temperature is used for the average temperature calculation. When it is larger than the threshold value, a highly diffused region was observed near the foramen of Monro (**Fig. 3**).

DIFFUSION-WEIGHTED IMAGING THERMOMETRY AT OTHER CISTERNS

From a pilot study by Sakai and colleagues (unpublished data, 2016), fast and complex flows can impact DWI temperature measurements. Of these areas, the lateral ventricles were suitable for DWI temperature measurements.

COMPARISONS WITH DIFFUSION-WEIGHTED IMAGING THERMOMETRY AND MAGNETIC RESONANCE SPECTROSCOPY THERMOMETRY

Because the method based on T1 relaxation is capable of capturing only temperature changes, it is necessary to induce temperature changes, such as cooling and heating, to estimate the temperature. On the other hand, for MRS and DWI, a formula for converting a measured value into a temperature is possible. Therefore, the temperature can be estimated from a normal measurement. Although these methods have different calculation principles, it was considered that a certain correlation was observed when the target was the deep brain.

Sumida and colleagues[20] estimated brain temperature at lateral ventricle (T_v) and brain parenchyma (T_p) from data gathered simultaneously by MR DWI and MRS, respectively, in 35 healthy volunteers (17 men and 18 women; ages 25–78 years). Their results showed brain parenchymal temperature is a little bit higher than that of CSF at the deep brain.

$$T_v = 0.534 \times T_p + 17.379$$

(R = 0.611; $P<.001$; Pearson product–moment correlation coefficient controlling for ventricular volume).

DIFFUSION-WEIGHTED IMAGING THERMOMETRY IN CLINICAL PRACTICE

Diffusion-weighted thermometry has been applied clinically to brain disorders, such as moyamoya

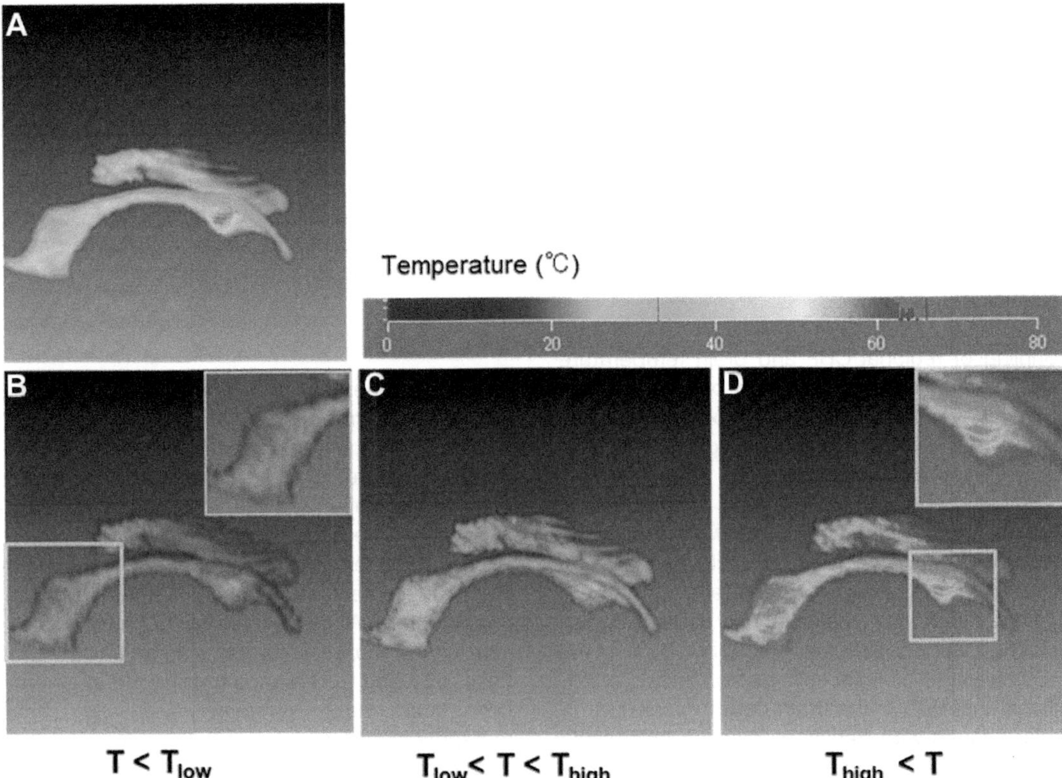

Fig. 3. Temperature mapping in the lateral ventricle. These figures show the distributions of temperature within the ventricle for different thresholds. (*A*) All voxels within the lateral ventricle. (*B*) Voxels with a temperature lower than the lower threshold (T_{low}). Such low-temperature voxels are distributed mainly at the edges of the lateral ventricle. (*C*) The distribution of voxels used for analysis. (*D*) Voxels with a higher temperature threshold (T_{high}). This figure clearly shows that voxels with higher temperatures are distributed mainly near the foramen of Monro and around the choroid plexus.

disease,[21] multiple sclerosis (MS),[22] mild traumatic brain injury,[23] schizophrenia,[24] epilepsy,[25] and parkinsonian syndromes.[26]

In patients with moyamoya disease, a progressive steno-occlusive disease of bilateral distal internal carotid arteries that predisposes the patients to vascular events, the brain's thermal balance is altered with evidence of elevated ventricular temperature, which in turn represents a mismatch between cerebral metabolism and cerebral perfusion due to decreased blood flow resulting from the bilateral internal carotid artery stenoses.[21] Although the brain represents only 2% of the human body weight, it receives 10% of the cardiac output, mainly by the internal carotid arteries, and accounts for 20% of the total oxygen consumption. Thus, the brain is one of the most energy-demanding organs, and this large quantity of energy used for metabolism subsequently is transformed into heat, which is removed chiefly by blood flow through the cranial vessels. The balance between heat production and removal maintains the brain at a constant temperature.[1,3] This thermal balance may become disturbed in patients with steno-occlusive disease, such as moyamoya disease patients, because there is less blood flow to the brain and, as a result, less heat removed.

In patients with MS, Sai and colleagues[22] demonstrated that brain temperature is significantly lower than in normal healthy controls without correlation between either disease duration or Expanded Disability Status Scale,[27] possibly reflecting decreased brain metabolism. Decreased brain metabolism in MS patients has been demonstrated by fluorodeoxyglucose-PET, which has shown that MS patients not only have a lower mean brain metabolism compared with healthy controls but also localized sites within the brain in which metabolism is decreased.[22]

A global decrease in cerebral metabolism occurs in severe head trauma, which causes direct destruction of the brain parenchyma, metabolic dysfunction, and a decrease in blood flow.[23] In patients with severe head trauma, a Glasgow Coma Scale score of less than 8 is known to be associated with increased brain temperature, because CBF is decreased, limiting the heat removal function. Tazoe and colleagues[23] assessed the brain core temperature of patients with mild traumatic brain injury by means of DWI thermometry of the CSF in the lateral ventricles, demonstrating a reduction in brain core temperature, possibly due to a global decrease in cerebral metabolism.

Ota and colleagues[24] demonstrated altered coupling of regional CBF and brain temperature in schizophrenia compared with bipolar disorder and healthy subjects. This could be explained by the fact that brain temperature is highly dependent on cerebral metabolism and CBF.

Similarly, Sone and colleagues[25] demonstrated regional uncoupling of blood flow and cerebral metabolism in temporal lobe epilepsy patients, indicating that ipsilateral area (inferior frontal gyrus) in temporal lobe epilepsy has different metabolic regulation systems in the brain.

Sumida and colleagues[26] demonstrated a significant increase in the brain core temperature of male patients with Parkinson disease or multiple system atrophy compared with that of healthy male controls using DWI thermometry. The altered brain core temperature in men with Parkinson disease or multiple system atrophy indicates the possible involvement of mitochondrial and autonomic dysfunction.

Increasing brain core temperature in idiopathic normal pressure hydrocephalus due to lack of CSF circulation with insufficient heat removal was suggested by Kuriyama and colleagues.[28] DWI thermometry also was applied in physiologic conditions demonstrating an increased brain core temperature in the luteal phase of the menstrual cycle in healthy women.[29]

Recently, Sparacia and colleagues[3] assessed DWI thermometry in Alzheimer disease patients reporting a counterbalancing between a global decline in brain metabolism and factors that positively or negatively influence temperature calculation, such as the positive effect of the pulsatile movement of the CSF and the negative effect of the coefficient of viscosity, which results in no significant decrease in lateral ventricle temperature in Alzheimer disease patients compared with healthy volunteers.

Another retrospective study was aimed at assessing brain-core temperature in end-stage liver disease patients undergoing orthotopic liver transplantation. In this study, Sparacia and colleagues[30] reported the feasibility in the routine clinical setting of the measurement of brain core temperature using the routine DWI sequence acquired as part of the standard brain MR examination and postprocessing the DWI images later to obtain DWI thermometry measurement. They reported successful measurement in all the patients using retrospective DWI data with a stable brain-core temperature in patients as a potential supplementary brain biomarker to confirm that CBF and cerebral metabolism are stable in patients undergoing orthotopic liver transplantation.

FUTURE DIRECTIONS

Although further research is needed on the clinical use of DWI thermometry, DWIs are easier to obtain than MRS images, and the measurement of temperature can be achieved along with daily clinical brain MR examinations in a short time, even retrospectively. The observation that the temperature of deep brain regions increases after circulatory arrest in an animal model[4] may be a potential field of research for DWI thermometry in brain infarction.

Brain thermoregulation remains an unclear process reflecting the balance between heat generation and heat removal, involving brain metabolism, cerebrovascular perfusion, and body core temperature. The disturbance of this delicate balance of heat-producing and heat-dissipating mechanisms, which ensures thermal homeostasis, may lead to a catastrophic brain injury. Temperature dysregulation is particularly deleterious as a potentiator of CNS injury following various background insults, such as cerebrovascular ischemia.[31] Postischemic cerebral MR thermography assessed in a nonhuman primate infarction model demonstrated the existence of a disturbance and decoupling of physiologic brain-systemic temperature gradients.[31]

In an experimental animal infarction model,[32] MRS thermometry demonstrated different temperature gradients during the arterial occlusion stage. The brain temperature of different ischemic tissue was higher than the contralateral hemisphere, including infarct core, ischemic penumbra, and oligemic region.

In the future, in vivo human brain DWI thermometry may be used as an adjunctive neuroimaging biomarker in brain infarction.

DIFFUSION-WEIGHTED IMAGING THERMOMETRY LIMITATION

A limitation of this technique is that various pathologic features of the CSF suggest the calculated temperature cannot be expected to be as accurate as in laboratory experiments using pure water. The pulsatile movement of the CSF increases the

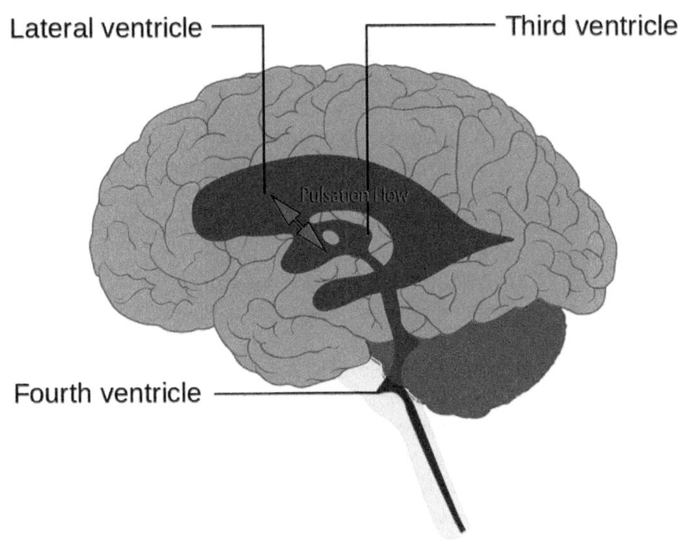

Fig. 4. Pulsatile flow. DWI at the lateral ventricle in the brain might be influenced by the pulsation flow of CSF.

diffusion coefficient. In certain locations, such as the foramen of Monro, overestimation of the temperature could be problematic (Fig. 4). DWI thermometry acquired with synchronization to electrocardiograms or CSF flow could be helpful to take into account the effects of the pulsatile movement of the CSF for DWI thermometry measurement[3,30] (Fig. 5).

Moreover, the substrates contained in the CSF, including glucose, protein, electrolytes, and blood cells, can lead to underestimation of the brain temperature. Thus, the altered composition of CSF with aging could lead to an apparent thermic change in ventricular CSF.[3] Future research involving the DWI method to obtain more accurate CSF temperature estimates may improve this technique.

Another limitation to this measurement technique is that the measurement can be performed only in the ventricles where there is nonrestricted water (ie, CSF); thus, this method is not applicable for brain parenchyma because of restricted diffusion.

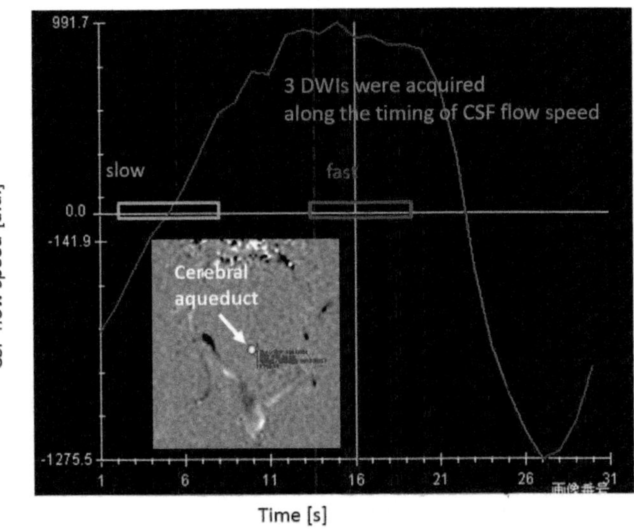

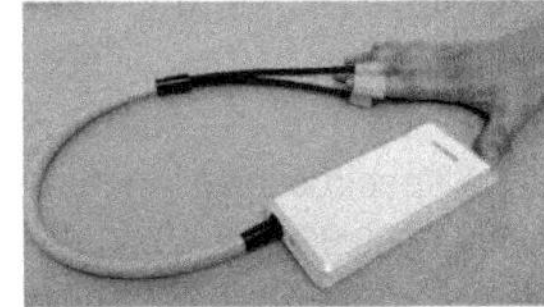

Fig. 5. DWI thermometry acquired with synchronization to electrocardiograms or CSF flow at the level of the cerebral aqueduct. a.u., arbitrary unit.

Finally, the artifacts induced by field inhomogeneities potentially could alter the measured temperature, and this would be problematic in patients with monitoring devices or dental prostheses.

DISCLOSURE

The authors have nothing to disclose.

REFERENCE

1. Guyton AC, Hall JE. Textbook of medical physiology. Philadelphia: Elsevier Inc.; 2006.
2. Sakai K, Yamada K, Sugimoto N. Calculation methods for ventricular DWI thermometry: phantom and control studies. NMR Biomed 2012;25(2):340–6.
3. Sparacia G, Sakai K, Yamada K, et al. Assessment of brain core temperature using MR DWI-thermometry in Alzheimer disease patients compared to healthy subjects. Jpn J Radiol 2017; 35:168–71.
4. Hayward JN, Baker MA. Role of cerebral arterial blood in the regulation of brain temperature in the monkey. Am J Physiol 1968;215:389–403.
5. Sakai K, Yamada K, Mori S, et al. Age dependent brain temperature decline as assessed by DWI thermometry. NMR Biomed 2011. https://doi.org/10.1002/nbm.1656.
6. Yamaguchi T, Kanno I, Uemura K, et al. Reduction in regional cerebral metabolic rate of oxygen during human aging. Stroke 1986;17:1220–8.
7. Rieke V, Pauly KB. MR thermometry. J Magn Reson Imaging 2008;27:376–90.
8. Kuroda K, Takei N, Mulkern RV, et al. Feasibility of internally referenced brain temperature imaging with a metabolite signal. Magn Reson Med Sci 2003;2:17–22.
9. Corbett RJ, Purdy PD, Laptook AR, et al. Noninvasive measurement of brain temperature after stroke. AJNR Am J Neuroradiol 1999;20:1851–7.
10. Karaszewski B, Wardlaw JM, Marshall I, et al. Measurement of brain temperature with magnetic resonance spectroscopy in acute ischemic stroke. Ann Neurol 2006;60:438–46.
11. Kozak LR, Bango M, Szabo M, et al. Using diffusion MRI for measuring the temperature of cerebrospinal fluid within the lateral ventricle. Acta Paediatr 2010; 99:237–43.
12. Sakai K, Yamada K, Sugimoto N. Calculation methods for ventricular diffusion-weighted imaging thermometry: phantom and volunteer studies. NMR Biomed 2012;25:340–6.
13. Sakai K, Yamada K, Sugimoto N. Automated temperature calculation method for DWI-thermometry: the usefulness of LV probability map on healthy subjects. Conf Proc IEEE Eng Med Biol Soc 2013; 2013:499–502.
14. Einstein A. Über die von der molekularkinetischen Theorie der Wärme geforderte Bewegung von in ruhenden Flüssigkeiten suspendierten Teilchen. Annalen der Physik 1905;322:549–60.
15. Arrhenius S. Über die Reaktionsgeschwindigkeit bei der Inversion von Rohrzucker durch Säuren. Zeitschrift für Physikalische Chemie, Walter de Gruyter GmbH eds 1889. https://doi.org/10.1515/zpch-1889-0416.
16. Mills R. Self-diffusion in normal and heavy-water in range 1–45 degrees. J Phys Chem 1973;77: 685–8.
17. Yamada K, Sakai K, Akazawa K, et al. Brain temperature of moyamoya patients is higher than normal controls; a study by noninvasive assessment of ventricular temperature using DWI. NeuroReport 2010; 21:851–5.
18. Pruessmann KP, Weiger M, Scheidegger MB, et al. SENSE: sensitivity encoding for fast MRI. Magn Reson Med 1999;42:952–62.
19. Jones DK, Horsfield MA, Simmons A. Optimal strategies for measuring diffusion in anisotropic systems by magnetic resonance imaging. Magn Reson Med 1999;42:515–25.
20. Sumida K, Sato N, Ota M, et al. Intraventricular temperature measured by diffusion-weighted imaging compared with brain parenchymal temperature measured by MRS *in vivo*. NMR Biomed 2016; 29(7). https://doi.org/10.1002/nbm.3542.
21. Yamada K, Sakai K, Akazawa K, et al. Moyamoya patients exhibit higher brain temperatures than normal controls. Neuroreport 2010;21:851–5.
22. Sai A, Shimono T, Sakai K, et al. Diffusion-weighted imaging thermometry in multiple sclerosis. J Magn Reson Imaging 2014;40:649–54.
23. Tazoe J, Yamada K, Sakai K, et al. Brain core temperature of patients with mild traumatic brain injury as assessed by DWI-thermometry. Neuroradiology 2014;56:809–15.
24. Ota M, Sato N, Sakai K, et al. Altered coupling of regional cerebral blood flow and brain temperature in schizophrenia compared with bipolar disorder and healthy subjects. J Cereb Blood Flow Metab 2014;34:1868–72.
25. Sone D, Ota M, Yokoyama K, et al. Noninvasive evaluation of the correlation between regional cerebral blood flow and intraventricular brain temperature in temporal lobe epilepsy. Magn Reson Imaging 2016;34(4):451–4.
26. Sumida K, Sato N, Ota M, et al. Intraventricular cerebrospinal fluid temperature analysis using MR diffusion-weighted imaging thermometry in Parkinson's disease patients, multiple system atrophy patients, and healthy subjects. Brain Behav 2015; 5(6):e00340.
27. Kurtzke JF. A new scale for evaluating disability in multiple sclerosis. Neurology 1955;5:580–3.

28. Kuriyama N, Yamada K, Sakai K, et al. Ventricular temperatures in idiopathic normal pressure hydrocephalus (iNPH) measured with DWI-based MR Thermometry. Magn Reson Med Sci 2015;14:305–12.
29. Tsukamoto T, Shimono T, Sai A, et al. Assessment of brain temperatures during different phases of the menstrual cycle using diffusion-weighted imaging thermometry. Jpn J Radiol 2016;34:277–83.
30. Sparacia G, Cannella R, Lo Re V, et al. Brain-core temperature of patients before and after orthotopic liver transplantation assessed by DWI thermometry. Jpn J Radiol 2018;36(5):324–30.
31. Dehkharghani S, Fleischer CC, Qiu D, et al. Cerebral temperature dysregulation: mr thermographic monitoring in a nonhuman primate study of acute ischemic stroke. AJNR Am J Neuroradiol 2017;38:712–20.
32. Sun Z, Chen Y, Zhang J, et al. [Evolution of brain temperature in ischemic tissues by H magnetic resonance spectroscopy]. Zhonghua Yi Xue Za Zhi 2014;94:2297–9.

Overview of Diffusion Tensor, Diffusion Kurtosis, and Q-space Imaging and Software Tools

Khader M. Hasan, PhD[a,*], Kei Yamada, MD, PhD[b]

KEYWORDS

• Diffusion tensor imaging • Diffusion spectrum imaging • Diffusion kurtosis • DTI • DSI • DKI

KEY POINTS

1. Diffusion-weighted MR imaging (dMRI) provides neuroimage markers of tissue architecture in health and disease.
2. dMRI can be used to map multiple fibers and multicompartments (ie, neurofluids and capillary blood).
3. There are a host of methods that require multishells with different diffusion strength sensitizations and orientations.
4. Consolidated dMRI data may be acquired in a clinically feasible time.
5. There are freely available software packages that may be used to model and fit the dMRI data.

INTRODUCTION

The Stejskal-Tanner experiment allows the phase encoding of spin displacements by applying a strong pulse gradient of duration,δ, and magnitude ,G_d, on each side of the 180° radiofrequency pulse of a conventional spin-echo sequence (**Fig. 1**A).[1,2] The MR signal is proportional to the average dephasing of a spin ensemble for a specified diffusion duration, Δ, which is the time elapsed between the beginning of the first and second diffusion gradients. The gradient wave vector is defined as, $q = \gamma\delta G\, g$, where γ is the gyromagnetic ratio and g is the diffusion gradient vector. S(q, Δ) is diffusion-weighted signal.

$$S(q,\Delta) = S(0)\langle \exp(i\phi(r))\rangle \tag{1}$$

$$E(q,\Delta) = \frac{S(q,\Delta)}{S(0)} = \int P(r,\Delta)\exp(iq\cdot r)dr \tag{2}$$

$$P(r) = \int E(q,\Delta)\exp(-iq\cdot r)dq \tag{3}$$

The P(r) is the water displacement probability density function or diffusion propagator, and most dMRI methods are designed to estimate or model this marker to assign to microstructural or physiologic attributes of the tissue by proper selection of the diffusion time and gradient pulse orientation (see **Fig. 1**B). This is a general q-space formalism that allows diffusion spectrum imaging (DSI)[2] analysis of the acquired data along with other high angular diffusion resolution diffusion models.[3,4] For example, the single diffusion tensor[5] and diffusion kurtosis[6,7] are the second

[a] Department of Diagnostic and Interventional Radiology, The University of Texas Health Science Center, McGovern Medical School, Houston, Texas, USA; [b] Department of Radiology, Kyoto Prefectural University of Medicine, 465 Kajii-cho, Kamigyo-ku, Kyoto 6028566, Japan
* Corresponding author. Department of Diagnostic and Interventional Imaging, The University of Texas Health Science Center, McGovern Medical School at Houston, 6431 Fannin Street, MSB 2.100, Houston, Texas 77030.
E-mail address: Khader.M.Hasan@uth.tmc.edu

Magn Reson Imaging Clin N Am 29 (2021) 263–268
https://doi.org/10.1016/j.mric.2021.02.003

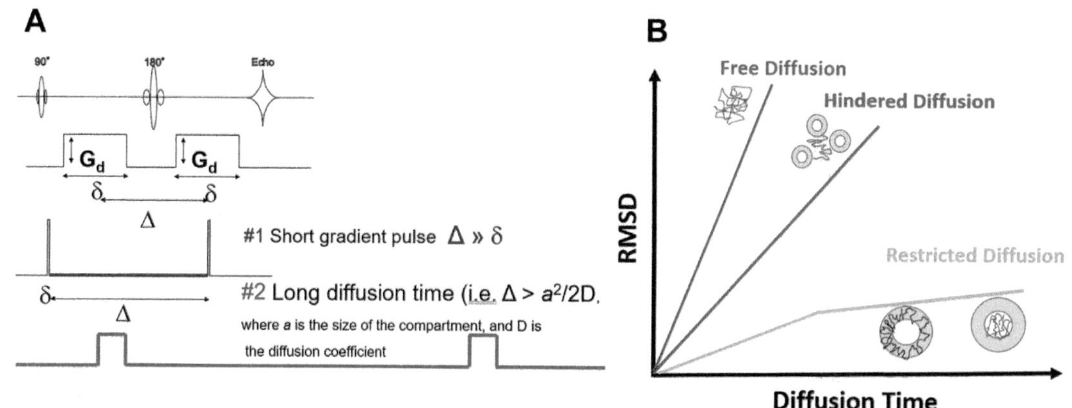

Fig. 1. *(A)* Simplified version of the sequence used to acquire diffusion-sensitized data and *(B)* illustration of the variation of diffusion root-mean squared distance (RMSD) with diffusion time as a probe of tissue microstructure.

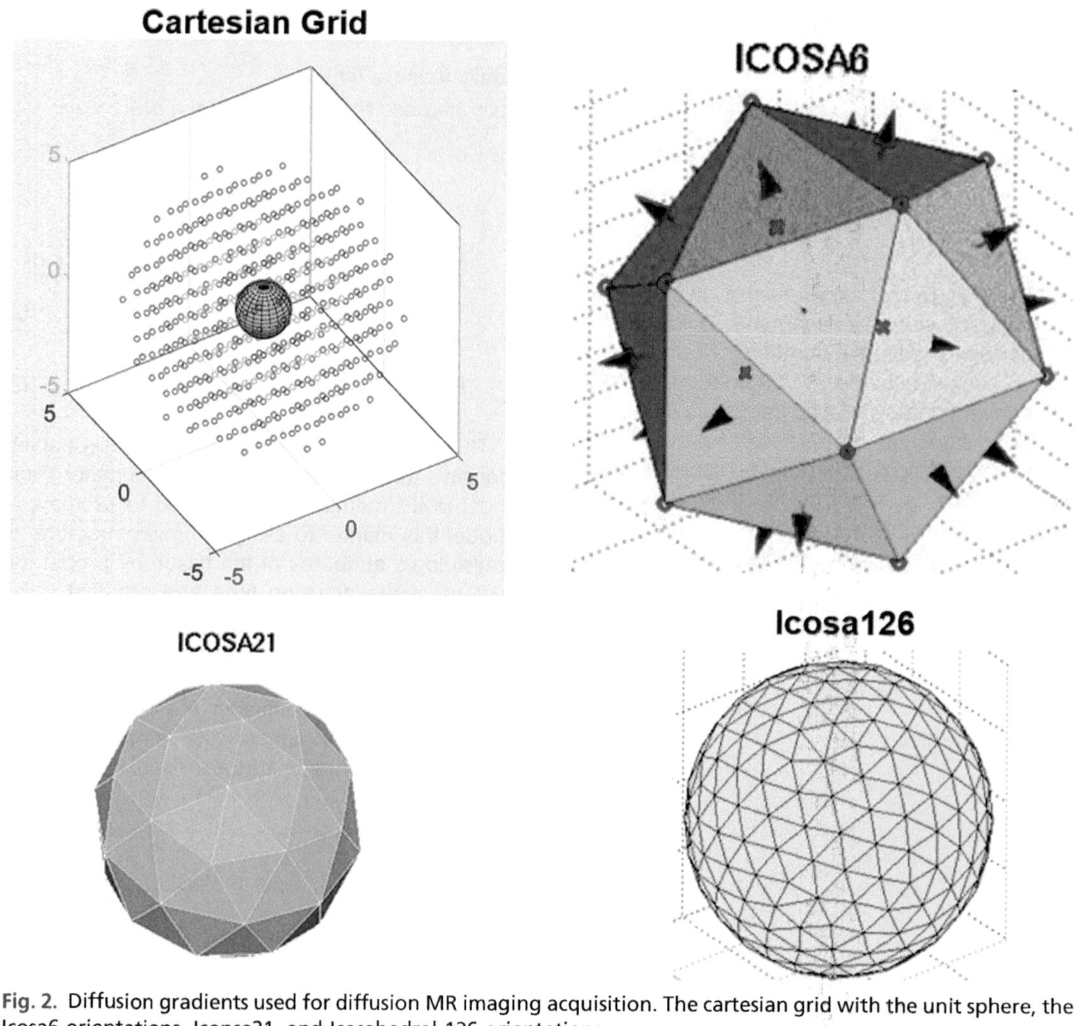

Fig. 2. Diffusion gradients used for diffusion MR imaging acquisition. The cartesian grid with the unit sphere, the Icosa6 orientations, Icopsa21, and Icosahedral 126 orientations.

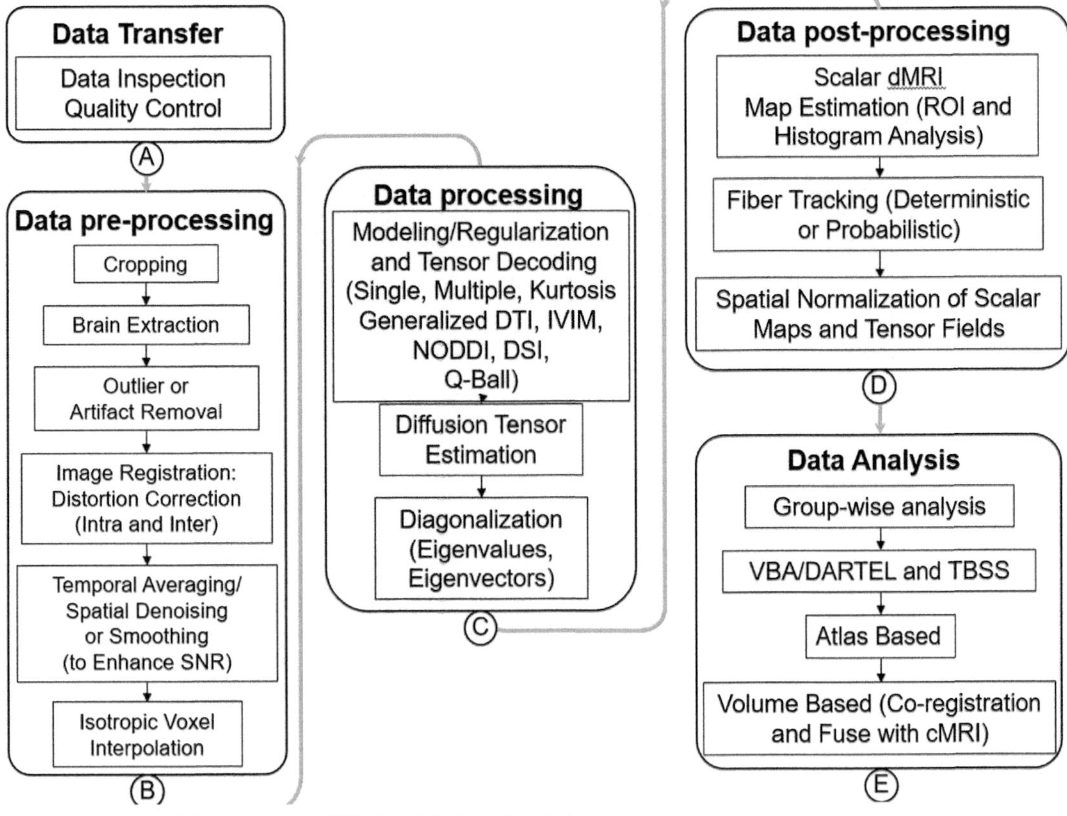

Fig. 3. Stages used in processing diffusion MR imaging data.

Table 1
A list of popular free software tools to analyze diffusion MR imaging data

Diffusion Tensor Imaging Software	Purpose	Web Location
CAMINO	Diffusion MR imaging tool kit	http://web4.cs.ucl.ac.uk/research/medic/camino/pmwiki/pmwiki.php?n=Main.HomePage
DIPY	Diffusion imaging in Python	https://dipy.org/
DTI Studio MRICloud	Deterministic fiber tracking Atlas-based DTI processing	https://www.mristudio.org/wiki/installation https://mricloud.org/
DSI Studio	Handles QBI, DSI, DTI, RSI	http://graphics.stanford.edu/projects/dti/software/ http://dsi-studio.labsolver.org/Manual/Reconstruction
DKE	Diffusion kurtosis	https://www.nitrc.org/projects/dke/
DTI-Query	DTI	http://graphics.stanford.edu/projects/dti/
ExploreDTI	DTI tracking DTI and DKI	http://www.exploredti.com/
FDT TBSS Probtrack	FSL diffusion tools Voxel-based Problem tracking	http://www.fmrib.ox.ac.uk/fslcourse/lectures/practicals/fdt/index.htm#tbss http://www.fmrib.ox.ac.uk/fsl/tbss/index.html http://www.fmrib.ox.ac.uk/fslcourse/lectures/fdt.pdf
INRIA	DTI	http://www-sop.inria.fr/asclepios/software/MedINRIA/
SLICER-DTMRI	DTI	http://www.na-mic.org/Wiki/index.php/Slicer:DTMRI
SPM	Spatial normalization	http://www.fil.ion.ucl.ac.uk/spm/ http://www.fil.ion.ucl.ac.uk/spm/ext/#toolboxes
TrackVis	Q-ball, DTI, DSI	http://www.trackvis.org/
NODDI	Neurite mapping	https://www.nitrc.org/projects/noddi_toolbox/

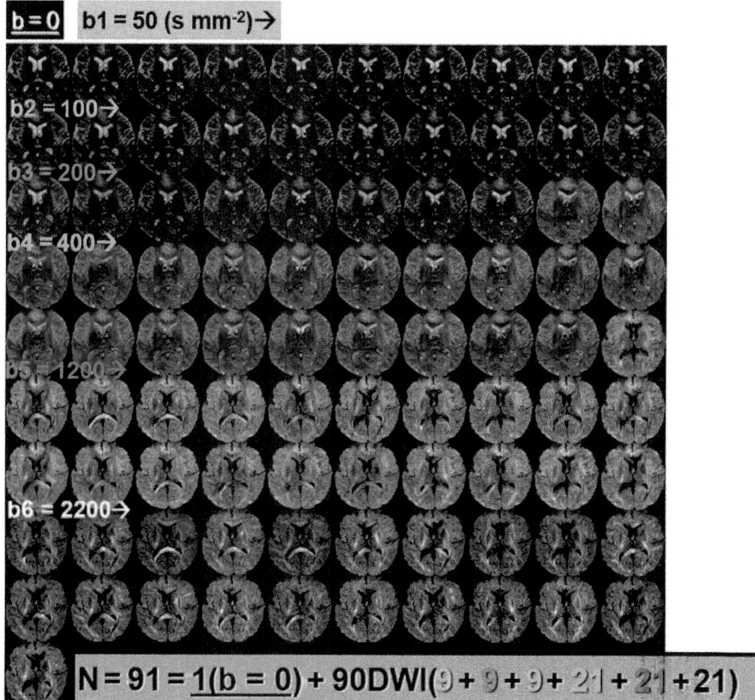

Fig. 4. Example of a multishell diffusion MR imaging acquisition to map neurofluids, tissue microstructural attributes using the DTI and DKI models.

and fourth moments of this propagator. Methods of analyzing the data include Fourier transform and linear or nonlinear fitting models. Diffusion MRI data acquisition is multidimensional because the diffusion encoding vector may be altered, along with the diffusion sensitization $b_{factor} \sim G^2{}_d (\gamma\delta)^2(\Delta\text{-}\delta/3)$. Cartesian data grids for q-space imaging–DSI and uniformly distributed diffusion encoding orientations have been used for diffusion tensor imaging (DTI) (N>6) and diffusion kurtosis imaging (DKI) (N>15) (Fig. 2).

TISSUE MULTICOMPARTMENTS

Mathematically, the k-th signal, S_k obtained from a volume element upon applying a diffusion-weighting or b-factor, b_k along the unit vector, g_k, can be modeled[2] using the gaussian mixture model as the superposition of different slowly exchanging positive-definite and symmetric tensors, D_n, each with a population fraction, f_n.

$$S_k = S_0 \sum_{n=1}^{N} f_n \exp\left(- b_k \hat{g}_k D_n \hat{g}_k \right) + \eta_k \qquad \textbf{(4)}$$

The signal acquired may originate from random thermal diffusion, which can be free gaussian, hindered or restricted nongaussian, and nonthermal diffusion originating from randomly distributed capillaries or the so-called intravoxel incoherent motion (IVIM).[8] The IVIM pseudodiffusion amounts to mapping the blood volume in the voxel and requires low b-factors (ie, b<300 s/mm^{-2}). Gaussian diffusion modeling usually is adopted in single DTI, which requires a minimum of 6 directions uniformly distributed over the unit hemisphere, with b-factor approximately 1000 s/mm^2. The gaussian model also may include free water in the extracellular space. Restricted diffusion has been shown to be modeled best with high b-factors (ie, b>2000) using high-order tensors,[2] diffusion kurtosis imaging (DKI), and neurite orientation dispersion and density imaging (NODDI).[9,10,11,12] In general, a host of b-factors and diffusion gradient pulses are acquired, and the nonlinear model, described later, is used to fit the acquired data.

$$\begin{aligned} S = S(0) * \left(f_{IVIM} * \exp(-bD_f)\right. \\ + fw * \exp(-ADC_{fw}) + (1 - f_{IVIM} - fw) \\ \left. * \exp\left(- b * ADC + (b * ADC)^2 * K / 6\right)\right) \end{aligned} \qquad \textbf{(5)}$$

A simplified version of this model to account for diffusion, spin-spin (T2-decay) and spin-lattice (T1-effects) has been described recently.[13]

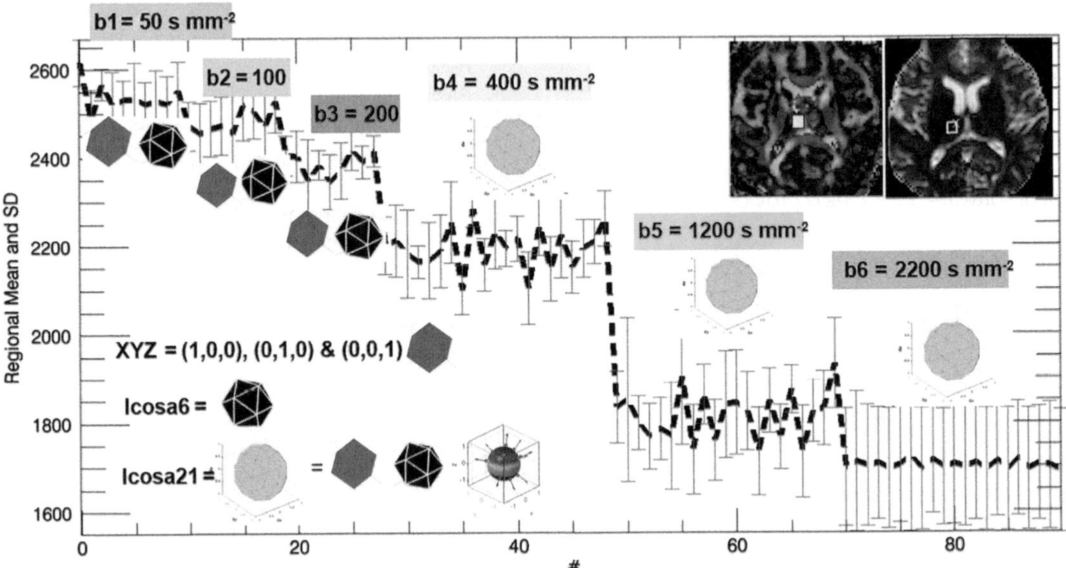

Fig. 5. Illustration of signal attenuation of a voxel at the right thalamus of the data acquired using the scheme described previously.[5]

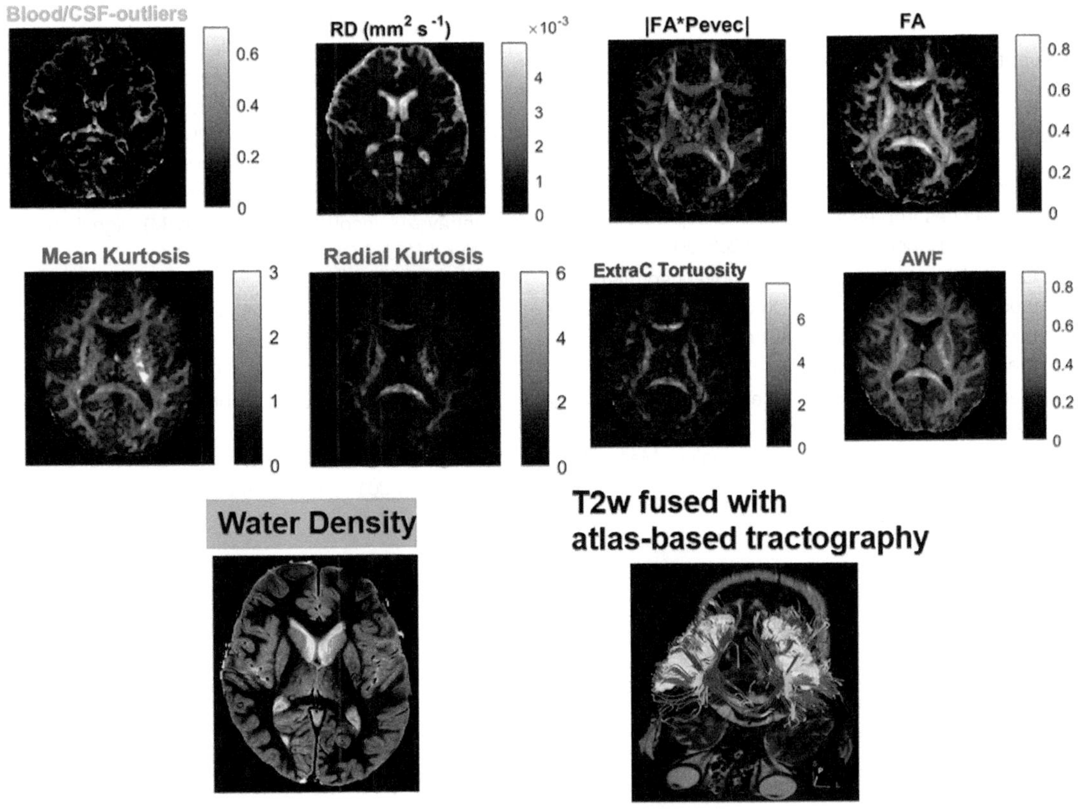

Fig. 6. Example of MR imaging maps generated using the IVIM, DTI, and DKI models.

DIFFUSION MR IMAGING ANALYSIS AND SOFTWARE PACKAGES

Multidimensional diffusion MR imaging data undergo extensive processing that includes geometric distortion correction, spatial smoothing, and fusion with high-resolution anatomic data (**Fig. 3**). A brief list of software packages is provided in **Table 1**.[14,15]

EXAMPLE OF DIFFUSION MR IMAGING DATA TO CONSOLIDATE DIFFUSION TENSOR IMAGING, DIFFUSION KURTOSIS IMAGING, AND INTRAVOXEL INCOHERENT MOTION

Fig. 4 shows an example from 1 section of a 3-dimensional dMRI data set acquired using multi-shells (b = 0, b = 50, b = 100, and b = 200 at 9 diffusion gradient orientations; and b = 400, b = 1200, and b = 2200 at 21 orientations—a total of 91 acquisitions). **Fig. 5** shows the signal attenuation at the right thalamus as for all diffusion shells acquired. **Fig. 6** shows the ability to provide IVIM fraction using low b values, DTI maps using b = 400 and b = 1200, and DKI axonal water fraction using b = 0 s/mm^2, b = 400 s/mm^2, b = 1200 s/mm^2, and b = 2200 s/mm^2, along with other models.

DISCLOSURES

The authors have nothing to disclose.

REFERENCES

1. Stejskal E, Tanner J. Spin diffusion measurements—spin echoes in presence of a time-dependent field gradient. J Chem Phys 1965;42:288–300.
2. Ghosh A, Ianus A, Alexander D. Advanced diffusion models. In: Cercignanic M, Dowell NG, Tofts PS, editors. Quantitative MRI of the brain. New York: CRC press; 2018. p. 139–60.
3. Wedeen VBJ, Hagmann P, Tseng WYI, et al. Mapping complex tissue architecture with diffusion spectrum magnetic resonance imaging. Magn Reson Med 2005;54:1377–86.
4. Frank LR. Characterization of anisotropy in high angular resolution diffusion-weighted MRI. Magn Reson Med 2002;47:1083–99.
5. Basser PJ, Pierpaoli C. Microstructural and physiological features of tissues elucidated by quantitative-diffusion-tensor MRI. J Magn Reson B 1996;111(3):209–19.
6. Jensen JH, Helpern JA, Ramani A, et al. Diffusional kurtosis imaging: the quantification of non-Gaussian water diffusion by means of magnetic resonance imaging. Magn Reson Med 2005;53:1432–40.
7. Novikov DS, Fieremans E, Jespersen SN, et al. Quantifying brain microstructure with diffusion MRI: Theory and parameter estimation. NMR Biomed 2019;32(4):e3998.
8. Iima M, Le Bihan D. Clinical intravoxel incoherent motion and diffusion MR imaging: past, present, and future. Radiology 2016;278:13–32.
9. Zhuo J, Xu S, Proctor JL, et al. Diffusion kurtosis as an in vivo imaging marker for reactive astrogliosis in traumatic brain injury. Neuroimage 2012;59:467–77.
10. Afzali M, Pieciak T, Newman S, et al. The sensitivity of diffusion MRI to microstructural properties and experimental factors. J Neurosci Methods 2021. https://doi.org/10.1016/j.jneumeth.2020.108951.
11. Assaf Y, Johansen-Berg H, Thibaut de Schotten M. The role of diffusion MRI in neuroscience. NMR Biomed 2019;32(4):e3762.
12. Fieremans E, Jensen JH, Helpern JA. White matter characterization with diffusional kurtosis imaging. Neuroimage 2011;58(1):177–88.
13. Rydhög A, Pasternak O, Ståhlberg F, et al. Estimation of diffusion, perfusion and fractional volumes using a multi-compartment relaxation-compensated intravoxel incoherent motion (IVIM) signal model. Eur J Radiol Open 2019;6:198–205.
14. Hangy Jiang, Peter CMvan Zijl, et al. DtiStudio: resource program for diffusion tensor computation and fiber bundle tracking. Comput Methods Programs Biomed 2006;81(2):106–16.
15. Hasan KM, Walimuni IS, Abid H, et al. A review of diffusion tensor magnetic resonance imaging computational methods and software tools. Comput Biol Med 2011;41(12):1062–72.

9780323759960